NUTRITIONAL ADAPTATION
OF THE GASTROINTESTINAL
TRACT OF THE NEWBORN

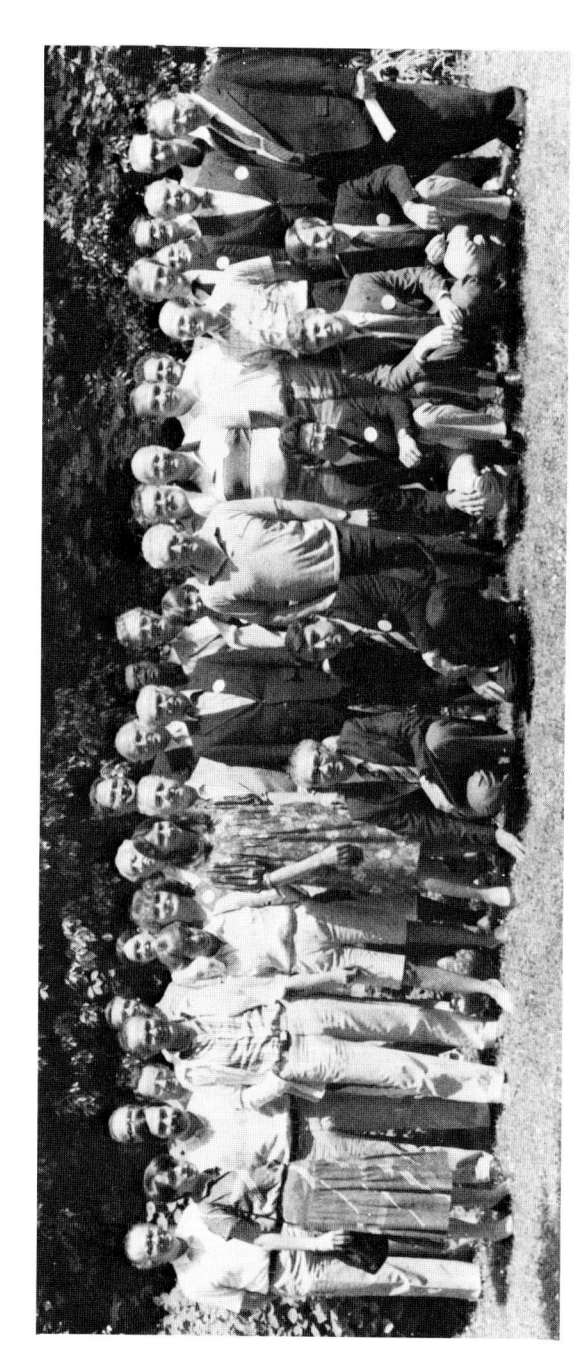

Nutritional Adaptation of the Gastrointestinal Tract of the Newborn, Third Nestlé Nutrition Workshop, Talloires, France, June 3-6, 1982

Kneeling: G. Semenza, P. Guesry, L. Marin, G. Putet, J. Rigo. *Standing* (from left to right): R. Eeckels, C. Maurage, F. Arnaud-Battandier, S. Auricchio, B. Ribadeau Dumas, J. Rey, J. P. Relier, F. Rey, E. Gamarra, A. Ferguson, A. Minkowski, P. Colony, E. Demaeyer, R. Theuer, N. Räihä, N. Kretchmer, O. Ransome-Kuti, R. Zetterström, A. Malbeau-Jacquot, L. Strang, R. Jacquot, P. Sunshine, R. Greenberg, P. Rambaud, J. P. Chouraqui, S. Hagelberg, J. Riby, J. Metcoff, B. Halikowski, H. Schwachman.

Nutritional Adaptation of the Gastrointestinal Tract of the Newborn

Editors

Norman Kretchmer, M.D.
Department of Nutritional Sciences
University of California at Berkeley
Berkeley, California, and
Department of Obstetrics and Pediatrics
University of California at San Francisco
San Francisco, California

Alexandre Minkowski, M.D.
Centre de Recherche de Biologie
du Développement Foetal
et Neonatal
Hôpital Port Royal
Paris, France

Nestlé Nutrition
Workshop Series
Volume 3

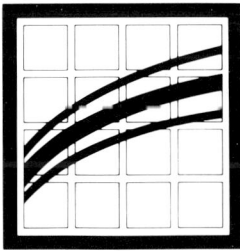

NESTLÉ NUTRITION, VEVEY

RAVEN PRESS ■ NEW YORK

Raven Press, 1140 Avenue of the Americas, New York, New York 10036

© 1983 by Nestlé Nutrition, S.A., and Raven Press Books, Ltd. All rights reserved. This book is protected by copyright. No part of it may be reproduced, stored in a retrieval system, or transmitted, in any form or by any means, electronic, mechanical, photocopying, recording, or otherwise, without the prior written permission of Nestlé Nutrition and Raven Press.

Made in the United States of America

The material contained in this volume was submitted as previously unpublished material, except in the instances in which credit has been given to the source from which some of the illustrative material was derived.

Great care has been taken to maintain the accuracy of the information contained in the volume. However, Nestlé Nutrition or Raven Press cannot be held responsible for errors or for any consequences arising from the use of the information contained herein.

Library of Congress Cataloging in Publication Data
Main entry under title:

Infant adaptation of the gastrointestinal tract and nutrition.

(Nestlé Nutrition workshop series; v. 3)
"Based on a conference sponsored by Nestlé Nutrition S.A. . . . the International Organization for the Study of Human Development . . . and Aide à la Recherche Médicale pour l'Enfance."—Acknowledgments.
Includes index.
1. Gastrointestinal system—Congresses. 2. Infants—Physiology—Congresses. 3. Infants—Nutrition—Congresses. I. Kretchmer, Norman, 1923– . II. Minkowski, Alexandre. III. Aide à la Recherche Médicale pour l'Enfance. IV. International Organization for the Study of Human Development. V. Nestlé Nutrition S.A.
RJ125.I53   1983   618.92'39   83-48665
ISBN 0-89004-905-X (Raven Press)

Preface

The gastrointestinal tract is an incredibly important organ, one of the primary organs in contact with the environment. Technically, any nutritional event that takes place requires the participation of the gastrointestinal tract. This volume, the third in the Nestlé Nutrition series, updates the most recent advances in developmental gastroenterology and relates these advances to human nutrition.

In order to lay a solid foundation for understanding the relationship between structure and function of the gastrointestinal tract, the volume opens with a section on fundamental biology. Structural studies are the first steps in the understanding of differences in cellular activity. Intestinal cells are in a continuous developmental cycle. In general, intestinal epithelial cells function in digestion and absorption, but there are also cells with specific functions that involve synthesis and elaboration of specific peptide hormones while others are concerned with synthesis of mucopolysaccharides.

The site of absorption and digestion of peptides and disaccharides is the brush border. Peptide absorption is a main contributor to the nutritional economy of the organism. In general, peptides are absorbed more rapidly by the cells of a young animal and transit the cell more quickly than in the cells of an older animal. Differences between young and old are also apparent with carbohydrates. Lactose is an example of a disaccharide that is digested more effectively by the young animal. Sucrase does not appear as an active enzyme nor is sucrose digested by the epithelia of the rat until two weeks after birth, after which the enzyme adapts to the concentration of sucrose in the diet.

Adaptation is a characteristic of all organisms and is specifically encountered in the gastrointestinal tract. Possibly, the fact that the gastrointestinal tract has direct contact with the environment emphasizes its structural and functional capability for adaptation to dietary change. This important aspect of intestinal physiology is clearly demonstrated by all the enzymes of the pancreas and many of the enzymes of the intestinal epithelium.

The second section, "Clinical Aspects of Gastrointestinal Function," is composed of two important chapters. The first discusses noninvasive techniques for the evaluation of intestinal function. The second covers the puzzling and elusive necrotizing enterocolitis.

The last section of the book is concerned with infant nutrition. The first complete food to gain entrance to the gastrointestinal tract postnatally is milk, and its constituents are exceedingly important to the well-being of the recipient. These substances are a result of the millenia of evolutionary adaptation of the mammary gland. This biological fact alone should indicate that the milk produced by the human has been carefully biologically molded for the human.

This fact should not obviate against usefulness of specially created preparations of milk for those babies or mothers who need them.

Nutrition of the fetus and infant is critical since malnourishment early in life can have an effect over an entire lifetime. The fetus is completely dependent on the maternal diet and maternal physiologic viscissitudes. The small-for-gestational-age baby and the large-for-gestational-age baby are remarkable examples of the results of poor maternal nutrition. The former is an indication of undernutrition and the latter typifies overnutrition. There are also many environmental factors that could participate in the pathogenesis of these particular situations. Large-for-gestational-age and small-for-gestational-age infants are subjected to a variety of immediate and long-term risks. In the very-low-birth-weight infant there is a definite immaturity of the gastrointestinal tract. Often, in order to provide adequate nutrition for these infants, there is a need for complete or partial parenteral nutrition to provide for normal growth while waiting for the gastrointestinal tract to attain an adequate stage of development. Initially, the large-for-gestational-age infant also has a great deal of difficulty adjusting to the extrauterine environment. The problem of macrosomia derives in part from the inability for regulation of carbohydrate metabolism as a result of hyperinsulinism during pregnancy.

The conference was organized to exchange ideas, increase communication between disciplines, and to stimulate new thoughts and research activities. The material that follows gives evidence of the fulfillment of these goals. This volume will be of interest to pediatricians, internists and general practitioners, as well as specialists in epidemiology, nutrition, microbiology, immunology, and infectious diseases.

Norman Kretchmer, M.D.
Alexandre Minkowski, M.D.

Foreword

The Nestlé Nutrition Workshops are now well established. This volume is the third in the series, and four more workshops have been held in the period since the Talloires meeting.

The first two volumes in the series are *Maternal Nutrition in Pregnancy—Eating for Two?*, edited by J. Dobbing (Academic Press, 1981) and *Acute Diarrhea: Its Nutritional Consequences in Children,* edited by J. A. Bellanti (Raven Press, 1983). Upcoming volumes are: *Iron Deficiency in Infancy and Childhood,* edited by A. Stekel; *Human Milk Processing and the Nutrition of the Very-Low-Birth-Weight Infant,* edited by J. D. Baum and A. F. Williams; and *Chronic Diarrhea in Children,* edited by E. Lebenthal; *Nutritional Needs and Assessment of Normal Growth,* edited by F. Falkner and M. Gracey.

By bringing together leading specialists in the field and widely diffusing the findings of each workshop we aim to contribute to an improved understanding of the important problems in pediatric nutrition.

P. R. Guesry, M.D.
Vice-President
Nestlé Nutrition S.A.

Acknowledgments

This volume is the third in a series based on workshops sponsored by Nestlé Nutrition, which is now an important contributor in the field of infant and young child nutrition. The meeting also represented a solid effort to establish cooperation among researchers throughout the world, as exemplified by the co-sponsorship by ARME (Aide à la Recherche Médicale pour l'Enfance) and the International Organization for the Study of Human Development.

Research in nutrition is a priority with the present state of our world. We intend to pursue that effort in the future with the help of Nestlé Nutrition.

Alexandre Minkowski, M.D.

Contents

Fundamental Biology

Successive Phases of Human Fetal Intestinal Development ... 3
Pamela C. Colony

Anchoring and Biosynthesis of Small-Intestinal Sucrase–
Isomaltase 29
Giorgio Semenza

Effect of Variation of Dietary Intake of Starch and Sucrose on
the Activity of Sucrase and Lactase in Jejunum of Adult
Rats 43
*Otakar Koldovský, Sergio Bustamante, Toshinao Goda, and
Kazuhiko Yamada*

Fetal Forms of Enzymes of Intestinal Brush Border 53
S. Auricchio

Influence of Lymphocytes and of Cell-Mediated Immunity on
the Epithelial Cell Kinetics in the Intestine 59
Anne Ferguson, Allan McI. Mowat, and Stephan Strobel

Protein Digestion and Absorption 73
D. M. Matthews

Clinical Aspects of Gastrointestinal Function

Noninvasive Techniques for the Evaluation of Gastrointestinal
Function 95
Jay A. Perman

Necrotizing Enterocolitis 107
John Barnard, Harry Greene, and Robert Cotton

Infant Nutrition

Some Pathophysiologic Changes in Experimental Intrauterine
Malnutrition 131
A. Minkowski and C. Chanez

Fetal Growth Retardation Caused by Maternal Dietary Amino
 Acid Imbalance 151
Jack Metcoff, T. Cole, P. Lunn, and S. Salem

The Use of Intravenous Fat Emulsions in Preterm Infants 163
Philip Sunshine and John A. Kerner, Jr.

Nutrient Deposit in Low-Birth-Weight Infants 177
G. Putet and J. Senterre

Nutrition of the Low-Birth-Weight Infant 185
Niels C. R. Räihä

Parenteral Nutrition in the Very-Low-Birth-Weight Infant 191
J. Rigo and J. Senterre

Modifications of Human Milk Composition During the Early
 Stages of Lactation 209
B. Ribadeau Dumas

Introduction of Weaning Foods into the Infant's Diet 215
Olikoye Ransome-Kuti

Subject Index 223

Contributors

*S. Auricchio
Clinica Pediatrica II
Facoltà di Medicina e Chirurgia di
  Napoli
Università Napoli
Naples, Italy

John Barnard
Department of Pediatrics
Division of Pediatric Gastroenterology/
  Nutrition
Nutrition Center
Vanderbilt School of Medicine
Nashville, Tennessee 37232

Sergio Bustamante
Departments of Pediatrics and
  Physiology
University of Arizona Health Sciences
  Center
Tucson, Arizona 85724

C. Chanez
Centre de Recherches Biologiques du
  Développement Foetal et Neonatal
INSERM U29
Université René Descartes
Hôpital Port-Royal
F-75014 Paris, France

T. Cole
MRC–Dunn Nutritional Laboratories
Cambridge, United Kingdom

*Pamela C. Colony
Department of Anatomy
Pennsylvania State University
Milton S. Hershey Medical School
Hershey, Pennsylvania 17033

---

* Conference participants.

Robert Cotton
Department of Pediatrics
Division of Pediatric Gastroenterology/
  Nutrition
Nutrition Center
Vanderbilt School of Medicine
Nashville, Tennessee 37232

*Anne Ferguson
Gastrointestinal Unit
Western General Hospital and
  University of Edinburgh
Crewe Road
Edinburgh EH4, United Kingdom

Toshinao Goda
Departments of Pediatrics and
  Physiology
University of Arizona Health Sciences
  Center
Tucson, Arizona 85724

*Harry Greene
Department of Pediatrics
Division of Pediatric Gastroenterology/
  Nutrition
Nutrition Center
Vanderbilt School of Medicine
Nashville, Tennessee 37232

John A. Kerner, Jr.
Department of Pediatrics
Division of Neonatology and
  Gastroenterology
Stanford University School of Medicine
Stanford, California 94305

*Otakar Koldovský
Departments of Pediatrics and
  Physiology
University of Arizona Health Sciences
  Center
Tucson, Arizona 85724

P. Lunn
MRC–Dunn Nutritional Laboratories
Cambridge, United Kingdom

* **D. M. Matthews**
Department of Experimental Chemical
  Pathology
Vincent Square Laboratories of
  Westminster Hospital
124 Vauxhall Bridge Road
London SW1V 2RH, United Kingdom

* **Jack Metcoff**
University of Oklahoma Health
  Sciences Center
Oklahoma City, Oklahoma 73190

A. Minkowski
Centre de Recherches Biologiques du
  Développement Foetal et Neonatal
INSERM U29
Université René Descartes
Hôpital Port-Royal
F-75014 Paris, France

* **Allan McI. Mowat**
Department of Bacteriology and
  Immunology
Western Infirmary
Glasgow, United Kingdom

* **Jay A. Perman**
Department of Pediatrics
University of California at San
  Francisco
San Francisco, California 94143

* **G. Putet**
INSERM U34 and Departement
  Neonatal (Professeur B. Salle)
Hôpital Edouard-Herriot
69374 Lyon Cedex 08, France

* **Niels C. R. Räihä**
Department of Pediatrics
University of Lund
214 01 Malmö, Sweden

* **Olikoye Ransome-Kuti**
Department of Paediatrics and Primary
  Care
Institute of Health and Primary Care
College of Medicine
University of Lagos
P.M.B. 12003 Lagos, Nigeria

* **B. Ribadeau Dumas**
Institut National de la Recherche
  Agronomique, C.N.R.Z.
78350 Jouy-en-Josas, France

* **J. Rigo**
Departement de Pédiatrie
Université de Liège et
  Hôpital de Bavière
B-4020 Liège, Belgium

S. Salem
MRC–Dunn Nutritional Laboratories
Cambridge, United Kingdom

* **Giorgio Semenza**
Laboratorium für Biochemie der ETH
ETH-Zentrum
CH-8092 Zürich, Switzerland

J. Senterre
Departement de Pédiatrie
Université de Liège et
  Hôpital de Bavière
B-4020 Liège, Belgium

Stephan Strobel
Gastrointestinal Unit
Western General Hospital and
  University of Edinburgh
Crewe Road
Edinburgh EH4, United Kingdom

*Philip Sunshine
Department of Pediatrics
Division of Neonatology and Gastroenterology
Stanford University School of Medicine
Stanford, California 94305

Kazuhiko Yamada
Departments of Pediatrics and Physiology
University of Arizona Health Sciences Center
Tucson, Arizona 85724

Invited Attendees

Franck Arnaud-Battandier/*Paris, France*
Jean-Jacques Baudon/*Paris, France*
J. P. Chouraqui/*La Tronche, France*
Edouard Demaeyer/*Louvain, Belgium*
Roger Eeckels/*Leuven, Belgium*
Edurne Gamarra/*Paris, France*
Robert Greenberg/*Albuquerque, New Mexico*
Stefan Hagelberg/*Stockholm, Sweden*
Bogustaw Halikowski/*Szczecin, Poland*
Robert Jacquot/*Reims, France*
Norman Kretchmer/*Berkeley, California*

Anne Malbeau-Jacquot/*Reims, France*
Luis Marin/*Stockholm, Sweden*
Chantal Maurage/*Tours, France*
Pierre Rambaud/*La Tronche, France*
Jean-Jacques Relier/*Paris, France*
Jean Rey/*Paris, France*
Jacques Riby/*Berkeley, California*
Bernard Salle/*Lyon, France*
Harry Schwachman/*Boston, Massachusetts*
Leonard Strang/*London, United Kingdom*
Rolf Zetterström/*Stockholm, Sweden*

Nestlé Participants

Y. Barbicux
Senior Vice President
Nestlé Products Technical Assistance Company Ltd.
1814 La Tour-de-Peilz, Switzerland

Pierre R. Guesry
Vice President
Nestlé Nutrition, S. A.
1800 Vevey, Switzerland

J. J. Pahud
Nestlé Research Department
1814 La Tour-de-Peilz, Switzerland

Beat Schürch
Director
Nestlé Foundation
Lausanne, Switzerland

Richard Theuer
Vice President
Beech-Nut Nutrition Corporation
Fort Washington, Pennsylvania 19034

FUNDAMENTAL BIOLOGY

Nutritional Adaptation of the Gastrointestinal Tract of the Newborn, edited by N. Kretchmer and A. Minkowski. Nestlé, Vevey/Raven Press, New York © 1983.

Successive Phases of Human Fetal Intestinal Development

*Pamela C. Colony

Department of Anatomy, The Milton S. Hershey Medical Center, The Pennsylvania State University, Hershey, Pennsylvania 17033

Adequate nutrition, a critical factor to the health and well being of the newborn infant, is dependent on the digestive and absorptive capacities of the intestinal epithelial cells at birth. These cells must also function as a "barrier" to the nonspecific uptake and transport of lumenal macromolecules. These digestive, absorptive, and barrier functions are all directly related to the structural maturity of the intestinal mucosa. This structural maturity, in turn, is a function of many factors including: (a) the cell types present; (b) the distribution, composition, and organization of the intracellular organelles within the different cell types; and (c) the presence and continuity of an epithelial barrier with tight junctional complexes between adjacent lumenal cells. The aim of this chapter is to review these three aspects of morphological maturation in the developing human intestine. Knowledge of this maturation process will provide insights into the functional potential of the intestinal tract at different gestational ages.

Data on the structural maturation of the human fetal intestine are limited. Detailed histological studies have defined the major architectural changes occurring during gestation, particularly during the early period of morphogenesis (7,12,31,53,54). Additional scattered reports provide detailed histochemical (8,22,38) and ultrastructural (2,33,62) information at different gestational ages. Only recently have systematic analyses of the sequential ultrastructural changes occurring within the human fetal intestinal mucosa been conducted (42–44). The following discussion reviews these earlier findings in conjunction with more recent biochemical, histochemical, and ultrastructural data. This discussion encompasses several successive stages of intestinal maturation. In particular, based on the analysis of intestinal tissue from 44 fetuses between 8 and 22 weeks of gestation, it is possible to delineate at least three phases of development: (a) an early period of epithelial proliferation and morphogenesis; (b) an intermediate period of cellular differentiation characterized by the appearance of a wide variety of distinctive cell types, some of which are unique

---

* Formerly Pamela C. Moxey.

to the fetal intestine; and (c) a later period of cellular "maturation" which results in the formation of an epithelial mucosa capable of handling the nutritional demands of the neonate.

FIRST PHASE OF DEVELOPMENT: PROLIFERATION AND MORPHOGENESIS

Formation of the Intestinal Tract

As in other animal species the human fetal intestinal tract is derived from the endodermal germ cell layer. During the first 3 to 4 weeks of development a simple tube lined by undifferentiated cells is formed. This primitive tube can be divided into three parts, each with a separate blood supply: (a) the foregut and its derivatives (pharynx, respiratory tract, esophagus, stomach, proximal duodenum, liver, gallbladder, and pancreas) are all supplied by the coeliac axis; (b) the midgut, which includes the entire small intestine from the distal duodenum through the proximal two-thirds of the transverse colon, is supplied by the superior mesenteric artery; and (c) the hindgut, which extends to the upper part of the anal canal, is supplied by the inferior mesenteric artery. This tripartite blood supply is retained in the adult.

At the end of the third week, a physical connection between the amniotic cavity and the intestinal lumen is established. The buccopharyngeal membrane, an ectodermal–endodermal membrane located at the cephalic end of the foregut, ruptures, and a connection between the amniotic cavity and the primitive intestine is established. During the seventh week of gestation the cloacal membrane, located at the posterior end of the hindgut, ruptures, and the continuity between the amniotic cavity, the intestinal tract, and the urogenital tract is completed. This continuity is essential for the circulation of the amniotic fluid through the intestinal tract later in fetal life.

After its initial formation, the primitive intestinal tube increases dramatically in length and diameter resulting in a temporary "physiological umbilical herniation" between 6 and 12 weeks' gestation. This period of rapid growth introduces and encompasses the first developmental stage of proliferation and morphogenesis. Between 8 and 10 weeks' gestation, columnar cells 2 to 4 cell layers thick line the entire length of the small intestine (Figs. 1A and 2B). These cells are undifferentiated with few intracellular organelles, a high nuclear to cytoplasmic ratio, short irregular microvilli bordering the lumen, and small glycogen deposits. A high proliferative capacity is suggested by the frequent presence of mitotic figures at all levels of the stratified epithelium (Fig. 2B). Cellular kinetic data on labeling indices are not available for human fetal intestinal tissue, but in animal models such as the fetal rat, labeling indices (percent labeled cells of total epithelial cell population) ranging from 27% to 35% are noted during comparable periods of epithelial growth and morphogenesis in both the small (29) and large (19) intestine. A high proliferative

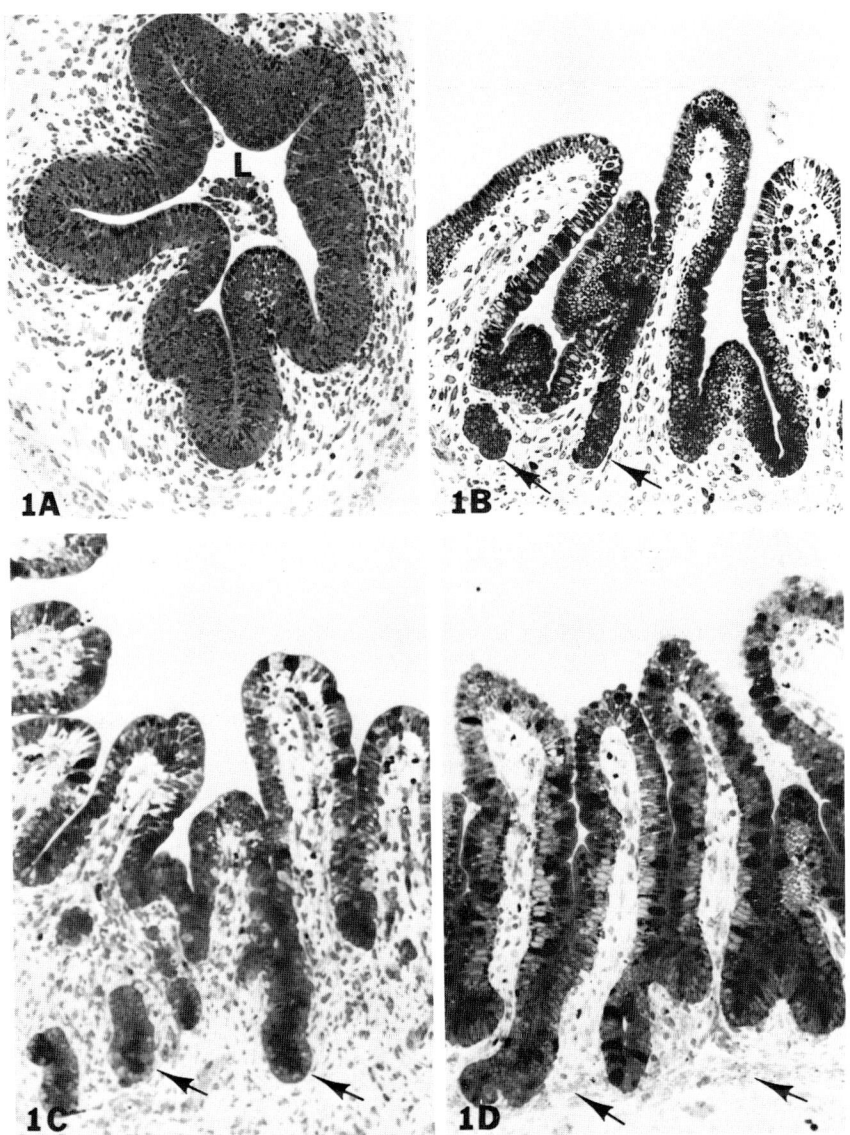

FIG. 1.A: In this 1-μ epoxy section the proximal intestinal lumen (L) of a 9–10-week fetus is surrounded by a stratified epithelium, 2–4 cell layers thick. The undifferentiated epithelial cells are characterized by darkly staining glycogen deposits. Richardson's stain. ×180. **B:** This 1-μ epoxy section of an 11–12-week fetus demonstrates early crypt formation with cords of epithelial cells penetrating the underlying mesenchyme (*arrows*). PAS stain. ×170. **C:** This 1-μ epoxy section from the proximal small intestine of a 14–15-week fetus illustrates the continuity of early crypts with Brunner's gland acini (*arrows*). Richardson's stain. ×160. **D:** This 1-μ epoxy section from a 22-week fetus has well-defined villi and crypts with a presumptive muscularis mucosa. The cells of this muscularis (*arrows*) are oriented perpendicular to the base of the crypts. Richardson's stain. ×180. (From Moxey and Trier, ref. 43, with permission of the Wistar Institute Press.)

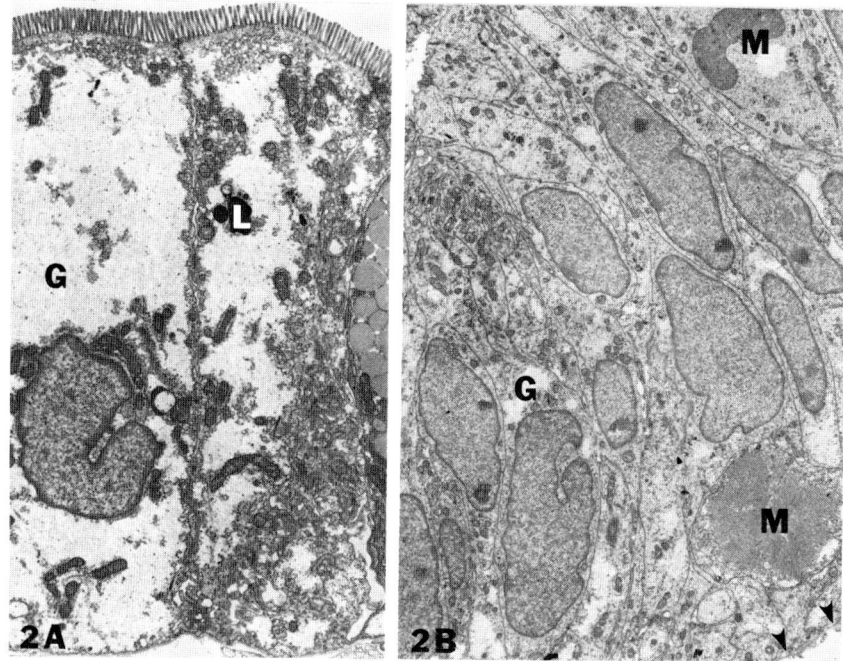

FIG. 2.A: The proximal small intestine of this 9–10-week fetus is lined by a simple columnar epithelium. The cells are characterized by short regular microvilli, occasional electron-dense lysosomal elements (L) and glycogen (G) deposits. ×6,700. **B:** The distal small intestine from the same fetus as in **A** is still highly stratified. The lumen in the *upper left* is bordered by cells with short irregular microvilli. Mitoses (M) are common in the superficial epithelium as well as near the basal lamina (*arrowheads*). G, glycogen. ×2,000. (From Moxey and Trier, ref. 43, with permission of the Wistar Institute Press.)

capacity in the primitive human fetal intestine is also indicated by the size and location of the proliferative zone. Whereas mitosis is restricted to the crypts in adult epithelium, mitotic figures are noted at all levels of the stratified epithelium prior to villus formation as well as on the sides of the villi between 10 and 16 weeks of gestation. It appears, therefore, that the intestinal epithelial cells of the first trimester human fetus resemble the immature crypt cells of the adult intestine to a limited extent both morphologically and in their proliferative capacity.

Morphogenesis of Villi and Crypts

The end of the first stage of intestinal development is marked by the morphogenesis of villi and crypts. Villus formation commences in the stratified epithelium of the proximal intestine at 9 weeks' gestation, proceeds distally, and by 11 weeks the entire intestine is lined by short villi with a simple columnar epithelium (Figs. 1B–D and 2A). Crypt development also proceeds along a craniocaudal axis. The first knoblike crypts, which appear to be the result of simple epithelial downgrowth into the mesenchyme between the newly formed villi (31,43,53), appear proximally at 10 to 11 weeks (Fig. 1B) and are present in the ileum and colon by 11 to 12 weeks. Although villi and crypts develop in a sequential temporal and spatial pattern along the length of the intestine, the actual conversion of the epithelium from stratified to simple columnar varies regionally. In the proximal intestine vacuoles develop within the stratified epithelium (Fig. 3A) between 6 and 9 weeks' gestation (31,43). These vacuoles resemble the "secondary lumina" present deep in the stratified epithelium of 17- to 18-day fetal rat proximal intestine (41) and of 18- to 20-day fetal rat colon (14,15). In the rat these secondary lumina have a crucial role in the formation of villi. Initially, as determined by the luminal injection of macromolecular markers, they are not in continuity with the primary lumen. The cells surrounding these lumina, however, resemble the cells bordering the main lumen in two important respects. First, the apical membrane in both rat and human small intestine is highly specialized with a well-developed microvillous border and an occasional luminal cilia (Fig. 3B). In the fetal rat colon this brush border of cells surrounding the secondary lumina even exhibits alkaline phosphatase activity similar to that seen on the apical membrane of cells bordering the main lumen (14,15). Secondly, in both the fetal rat small intestine (40) and colon (15) the cells lining the secondary lumina are joined by continuous tight junctional strands. The presence of these junctions maintains a physical barrier between the lumen and the bloodstream even as the secondary lumina enlarge and eventually fuse with the main lumen.

The precise steps in the transformation of the stratified epithelium of the fetal rat proximal intestine have been described previously (41). Briefly, a sequence of events including expansion of the secondary lumina, sloughing of degenerating superficial cells, and invagination of the underlying mesenchyme all contribute to the formation of short villi lined by a simple columnar epithelium. Due to limited samples, it is uncertain if a similar process occurs in the proximal intestine of the human, though the appearance of occasional lumina deep in the stratified epithelium (Fig. 3A), and the apparent degeneration and sloughing of superficial cells, suggests a similar process. Even less is known about the remodeling mechanism in the distal intestine or colon in either humans or animal models. Based on published reports (27,32) and cumulative data in the author's lab from both human and rat fetal colon, it seems that a combination of secondary lumina and deep cleft-like invaginations of the primary lumen contribute to the epithelial conversion in the colon (14,15). In contrast, no vacuoles or deep extensions appear in the distal intestine of human or rat. The mechanism of epithelial conversion in this region is, as yet, undetermined. It is also unknown if, as in the rat, the epithelial barrier is maintained during villus formation in any region of the human fetal small or large intestine.

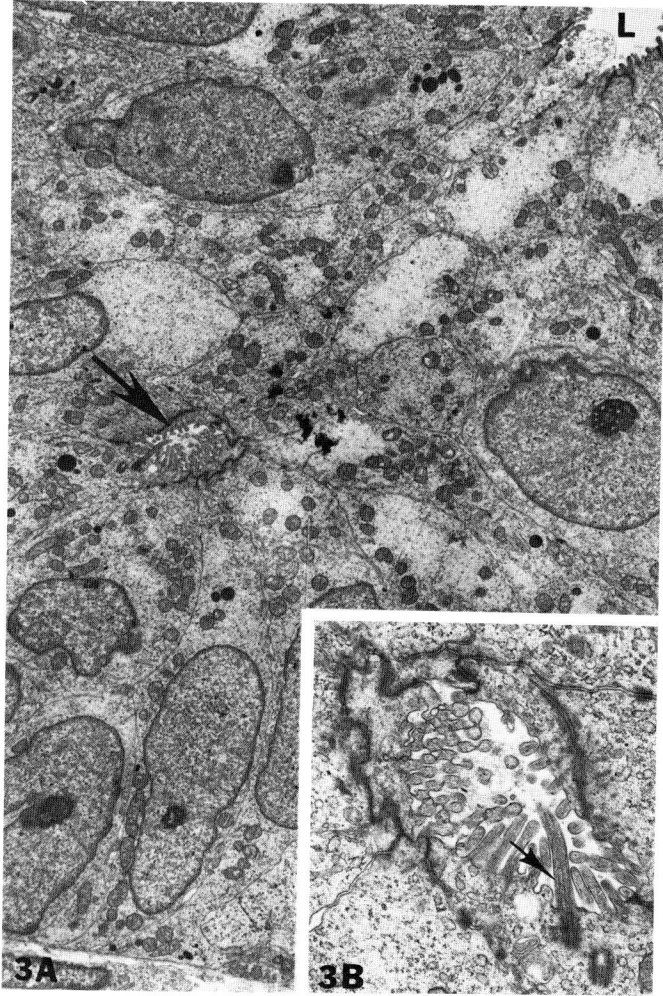

FIG. 3.A: A presumptive secondary lumina (*arrow*) is present deep in the stratified epithelium of the proximal small intestine of this 9–10-week fetus. L, main lumen. ×2,700. **B:** Higher magnification of the secondary lumina illustrated in **A**. Note the well-developed microvilli and the single cilium (*arrow*) projecting into the lumen. ×10,800. (From Moxey and Trier, ref. 43, with permission of the Wistar Institute Press.)

Cellular Differentiation

The second stage of human intestinal development, defined in this chapter as the period of cellular differentiation, overlaps with the preceding period of morphogenesis to a limited extent. Two distinct cell types differentiate within the stratified epithelium of 9- to 10-week fetuses. These are the goblet cells and two different enteroendocrine cells (42). Both immature (oligomucous) and mature appearing goblet cells can be defined early in development. As in the adult mucosa, the former are characterized by the presence of short strands of dilated rough endoplasmic reticulum (RER) and small secretory granules which often have a dense core surrounded by a less dense halo, while the latter have a well-developed theca filled with large secretory granules, a well-developed Golgi complex, and abundant RER. Some of these fetal goblet cells are unusual in that the secretory granules are infranuclear rather than supranuclear (Fig. 4). The significance of this orientation towards the basal lamina rather than the lumen is unclear, though it has been previously noted (37).

The second class of differentiated cells present in the stratified epithelium are endocrine. By 9 weeks two unique enteroendocrine cells which are not present in the adult mucosa can be identified (42). These cells, which appear to be limited to the proximal mucosa, have been arbitrarily termed "primitive" and "precursor" cells. The primitive cells are characterized by a pale cytoplasm, a large nucleus, abundant free ribosomes, little formed ER, numerous small

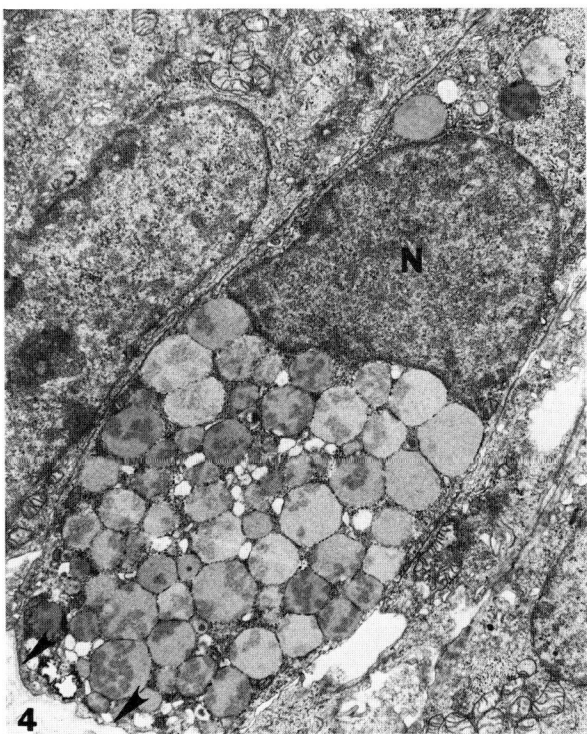

FIG. 4. A well-developed goblet cell from the proximal intestine of an 18-week fetus. Note the unusual orientation of the secretory granules towards the basal lamina (*arrowheads*). N, nucleus, ×7,000.

mitochondria, and secretory granules (SG) with a mean diameter of 200 to 330 nm. These granules often have electron opaque cores surrounded by electron lucent regions and an outer complete or incomplete membrane. Other granules vary in electron density and may lack or have only a very thin electron lucent halo. Similar to the primitive cells, precursor cells have a pale cytoplasm, abundant free ribosomes, few well-developed organelles, and a characteristic population of SGs. These granules, which have an average diameter ranging from 530 to 1450 nm, are pale to moderately electron dense with a closely apposed membrane. Some of these precursor cells have a second population of SGs resembling those found in the primitive cells, suggesting a potential developmental relationship between these two cell types (Fig. 5A). Though the precise relationship and the role(s) of these cells are unknown, it appears that both of them may represent developmental precursors of adult endocrine cells. This is supported by their early appearance, their apparent decrease with increasing age, their absence in adult intestine, the presence of morphologically similar cells in lower vertebrates (21,46) and in some pancreatic tumors (10),

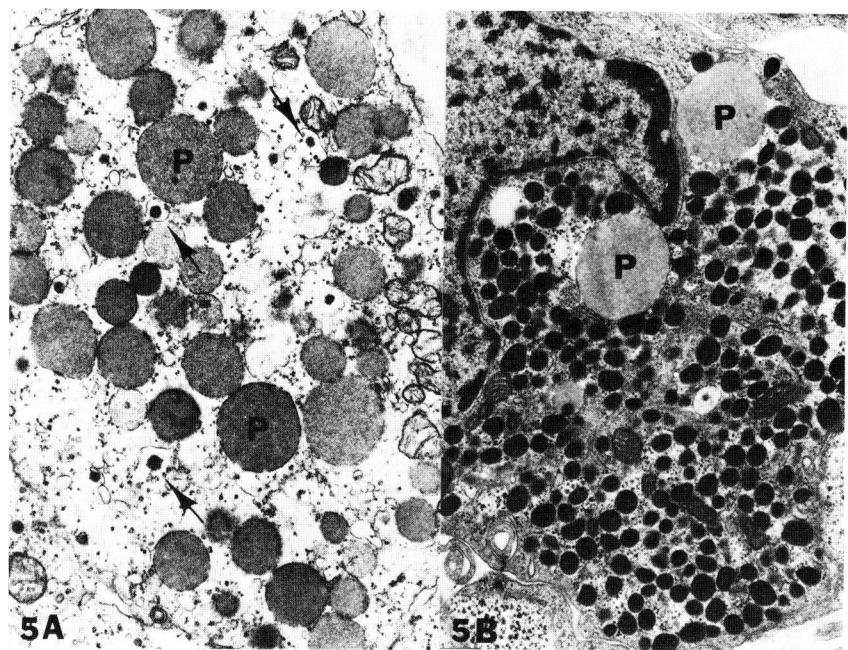

FIG. 5. A: A "precursor" endocrine cell from the proximal small intestine of a 9–10-week fetus. The characteristic large homogeneous granules (P) are prevalent. Interspersed among this population are smaller electron-dense granules surrounded by an incomplete membrane (*arrows*) that resembles those found in "primitive" endocrine cells. ×13,500. **B:** A "transitional" I cell from the proximal small intestine of a 16-week fetus with two distinct populations of granules. The large homogeneous granules characteristic of "precursor" cells (P) are surrounded by smaller electron-dense granules averaging 250 nm and resembling the granules of adult I (cholecystokinin) cells. ×13,500.

and the appearance of "transitional" cells intermediate in type between the precursor and adult-type endocrine cells.

SECOND PHASE OF DEVELOPMENT: CELLULAR DIFFERENTIATION

Endocrine Cells

At least four types of "transitional" endocrine cells have been identified in the human fetal small (42) and large (13; P. C. Colony, *unpublished observations*) intestine. All of these cells have two separate populations of SGs (Fig. 5B). One, common to all transitional cells, is indistinguishable from the large homogeneous granules of the "precursor" cells. The second population is characteristic of adult-type endocrine cells and is the basis for classifying these cells as "transitional" EC, S, I (Fig. 5B), or G cells. These cells are commonly observed at the time of their initial appearance at 10 to 12 weeks' gestation, but are rarely observed after 16 to 18 weeks. In contrast, seven additional endocrine cell types which appear at the same time, but which have only a single population of SGs resembling those of adult type endocrine cells (EC, S, I, G, D, L, and D_1), can be readily identified at all ages. These findings support the suggestion that the "transitional" cells, like the "primitive" and "precursor" cells, represent immature precursors of adult endocrine cells which are only present transiently during intestinal maturation.

The sudden appearance of various endocrine cell types in the fetal intestine immediately following villus and crypt formation at 10 to 12 weeks exemplifies the second phase of development, the period of cellular differentiation. During this period, which roughly corresponds to the second trimester, new highly specialized cell types such as Paneth cells, M cells, and Tuft cells first appear. Other cell types such as the endocrine cells diversify, and still others such as the prevalent columnar "absorptive" cells undergo successive developmental changes that vary regionally and with increasing age. The final result of this period of cellular differentiation is the establishment of an epithelium that is morphologically similar to the adult.

Crypt Cells

Undifferentiated Crypt Cells and Paneth Cells

The appearance of undifferentiated crypt cells (UCC) is coincident with crypt formation in both the proximal and distal intestine. As in the adult intestine the fetal UCCs are morphologically immature cells with large elongate basal nuclei with prominent nucleoli, abundant free ribosomes, a moderately well-developed Golgi, and little formed ER. The cells can be distinguished from their adult counterparts, however, by the regular occurrence of glycogen deposits, the relative absence of lysosomes, and the reduced size and number of apical dense SGs (Fig. 6). A second cell type restricted to the crypts, the Paneth cell, also appears early in the second trimester. These cells exhibit long strands of RER, a well-developed Golgi complex, and highly heterogeneous SGs of variable size and number (Fig. 7). In contrast to the homogeneous internal structure of the SGs in adult Paneth cells, some granules in the fetal cells have crystalline-like inclusions similar to those described in young rats (6), while others have dense cores with pale halos or pale cores with denser halos similar to those seen in adult mice (61). The significance of this heterogeneity or the functional capacity of these cells is unknown.

Brunner's Gland Cells

In the proximal intestine of a single 14- to 15-week fetus, the crypt bases are continuous with glandular extensions leading to acini deep in the lamina propria that resemble Brunner's glands (Fig. 1C). These extensions penetrate the mesenchyme to a depth comparable to the submucosa, though no mus-

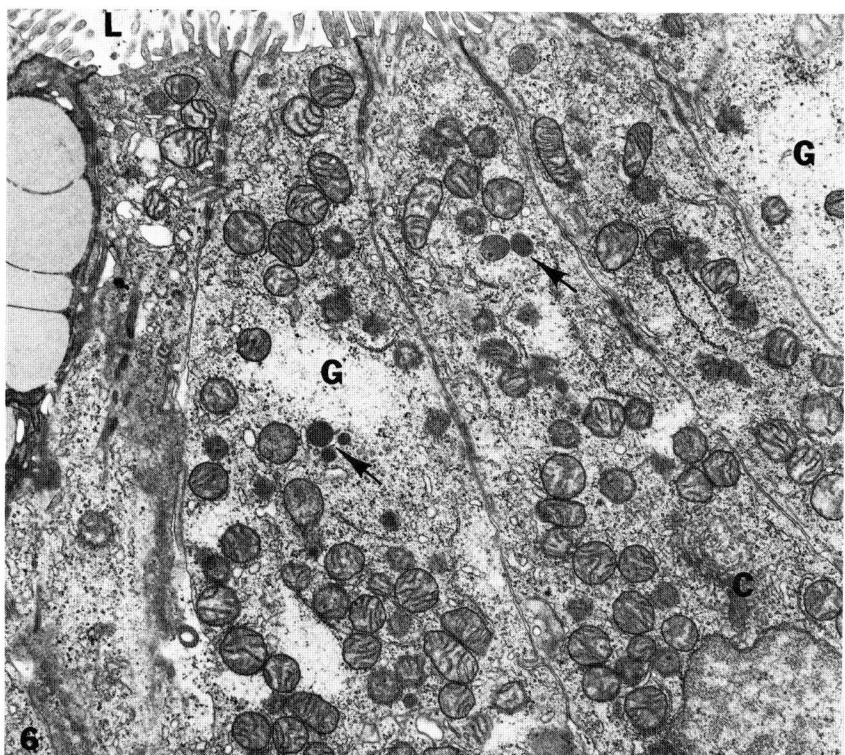

FIG. 6. Irregular microvilli line the lumen (L) of the apical cytoplasm of undifferentiated crypt cells from the proximal intestine of a 16-week fetus. The cytoplasm is characterized by small round mitochondria, a moderately well-developed Golgi complex (C), glycogen deposits (G), and occasional small electron-dense secretory granules (*arrows*). ×6,500.

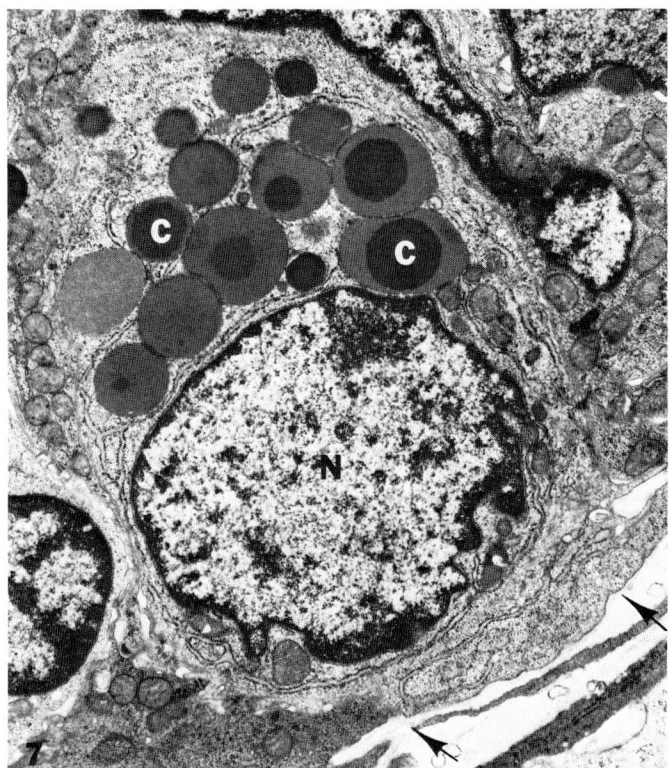

FIG. 7. A well-developed Paneth cell is present on the basal lamina (*arrows*) at the base of a crypt in the proximal intestine of a 20–22-week fetus. Long strands of RER are present throughout the cytoplasm, while the large secretory granules with electron-dense cores (C) are restricted to the apical cytoplasm. N, nucleus. ×8,700. (From Moxey and Trier, ref. 43, with permission of the Wistar Institute Press.)

cularis mucosa demarcating this zone appears until the 20 to 22nd week (Fig. 1D). The simple columnar cells comprising these glandular acini resemble adult secretory cells with their basal nuclei and apical secretory granules. The fetal cells do not, however, have organized parallel arrays of basal RER. Rather, short dilated strands of RER are interspersed throughout the cytoplasm (Fig. 8). Also, as in all fetal intestinal cells, free ribosomes and numerous small mitochondria are common. Finally, although the SGs of these cells are smaller and less numerous than in the adult, their size and number suggest that they may have differentiated earlier in gestation.

Specialized Villous Cells

Tuft Cells

The villi in the fetal intestine are lined primarily by columnar epithelial cells. Interspersed among these cells are several other cell types including the

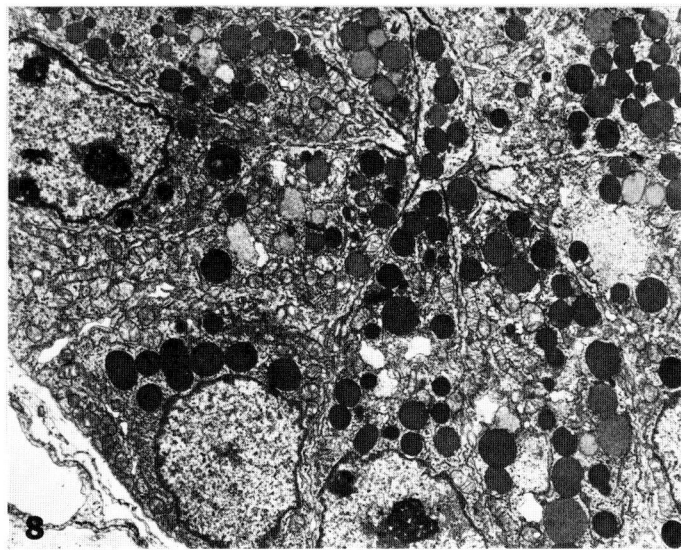

FIG. 8. Cells within the Brunner's gland acini deep in the mesenchyme of the proximal intestine of a 14–15-week fetus. Secretory granules of variable size and density are prevalent in all cells. ×4,700.

endocrine cells (see above), Tuft (caveolated) cells, and putative M cells. Tuft cells are first noted at 16 weeks' gestation. Though infrequent, these cells could be identified by the presence of bundles of dense filaments extending from the microvillous cores deep into the supranuclear region, a filamentous cytoplasm particularly around the nucleus, occasional lysosomal or multivesicular structures, and dense apical granules (Fig. 9). The presence of apical vesicles and caveoli, a distinguishing feature in adult Tuft cells (45), is rarely observed in the fetal cells. The role of these cells in either the adult or the fetal intestine remains to be determined.

M Cells

Another highly specialized cell type identified within the fetal intestine during the period of cellular differentiation is the putative M cell. M cells were first described by scanning and transmission electron microscopy as a unique group of cells restricted to the dome epithelium overlying the lymphoid follicles of Peyer's patches in adult intestine (50,51). The cytoplasm of these cells is attenuated forming a thin "membrane" between the intestinal lumen and the underlying lymphoid cells. The apical plasma membrane typically consists of irregular "microfolds" in place of a regular microvillous border, and abundant vesicles are present within the apical cytoplasm. These vesicles appear to have a role in the uptake and transcellular transport of lumenal macromolecules including microorganisms (9,49,63,67). This transport system provides a spe-

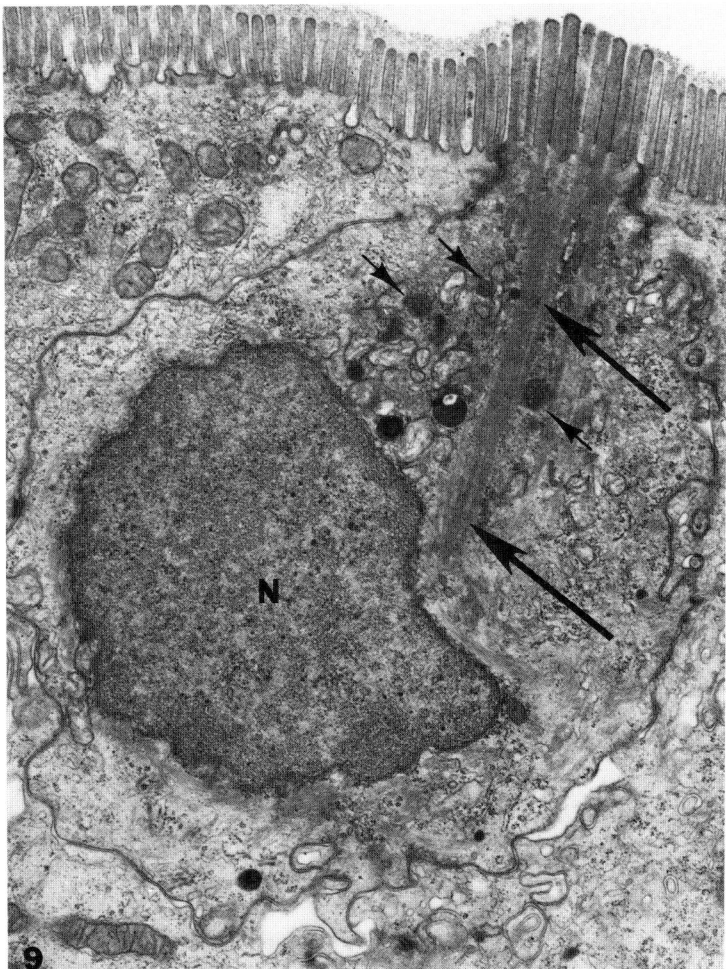

FIG. 9. A caveolated or Tuft cell located on the villus of a 20-week fetus. The microfilaments of the microvillous cores extend deep into the supranuclear region (*long arrows*). The cytoplasm is characterized by abundant filaments, particularly around the nucleus (N), and apical multivesicular bodies (*short arrows*). ×13,800.

cific route for the transport of lumenal antigens, microorganisms, and other macromolecules to the lymphoid system. It is speculated, in fact, that M cells continually sample the lumenal contents.

At 17 weeks' gestation cells resembling the adult M cells are first noted in the distal intestinal epithelium overlying an aggregation of lymphocytes (43). As in the adult, some of the cells in this dome epithelium are attenuated with irregular microfolds and apical vesicles (Fig. 10), while others remain columnar and have a typical microvillus border. The appearance of this specialized dome

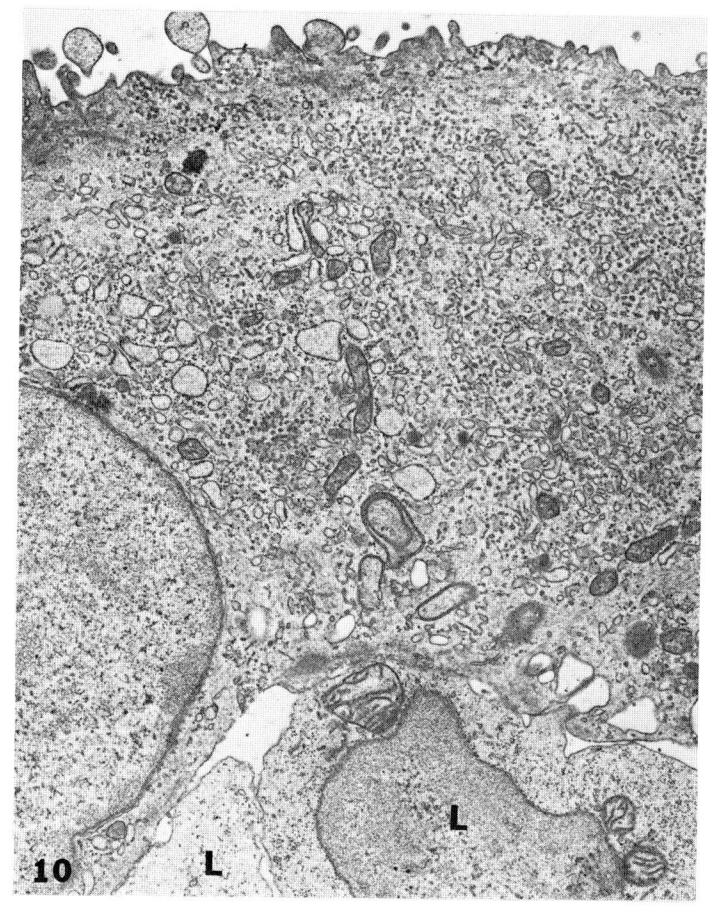

FIG. 10. A presumptive M cell is in direct contact with the underlying lymphocytes (L) in the distal intestine of this 17–18-week fetus. Characteristic microfolds are present along the luminal plasma membrane, and membrane-bound vesicles are abundant in the cytoplasm. ×7,900. (From Moxey and Trier, ref. 43, with permission of the Wistar Institute Press.)

epithelium seems to be temporally associated with the initial formation of Peyer's patches. Thus, although individual lymphocytes appear in the lamina propria late in the first trimester, aggregates are not seen until 16 to 20 weeks. This observation is consistent with earlier studies in human fetal intestine where accumulations of lymphocytes were first noted between 15 (20) and 20 (16,53) weeks' gestation.

As noted in several animal models (for review see Bockman and Cooper, ref. 9), the temporal association between the appearance of lymphoid aggregates and the differentiation of the dome epithelium suggests a developmental relationship between these two cellular compartments. A potential interaction between the dome epithelium and the lamina propria lymphocytes is supported by the finding that there is direct contact between these two cell types in the fetal intestine (Figs. 10 and 11). The intestinal epithelium is bordered by a continuous basal lamina at all ages of fetal development except in the regions of the developing M cells. In these regions the basal lamina departs from its course along the basal aspect of the intestinal epithelial cells and surrounds the epithelial–lymphocyte cells as a single complex (Fig. 11), returning to the basal aspect of the epithelium immediately after this area of lymphocyte accumulation. Due to limited samples the prevalence of this phenomenon cannot be determined. It appears to be restricted, however, to areas of significant lymphocyte infiltration since individual lymphocytes adjacent to the epithelium remain separated by a continuous basal lamina. In contrast, individual lymphocytes, which are present between adjacent epithelial cells as early as 11 weeks of gestation (48), are in direct contact with the epithelial cells. These cells, which correspond to the adult intraepithelial lymphocytes (IEL), are also

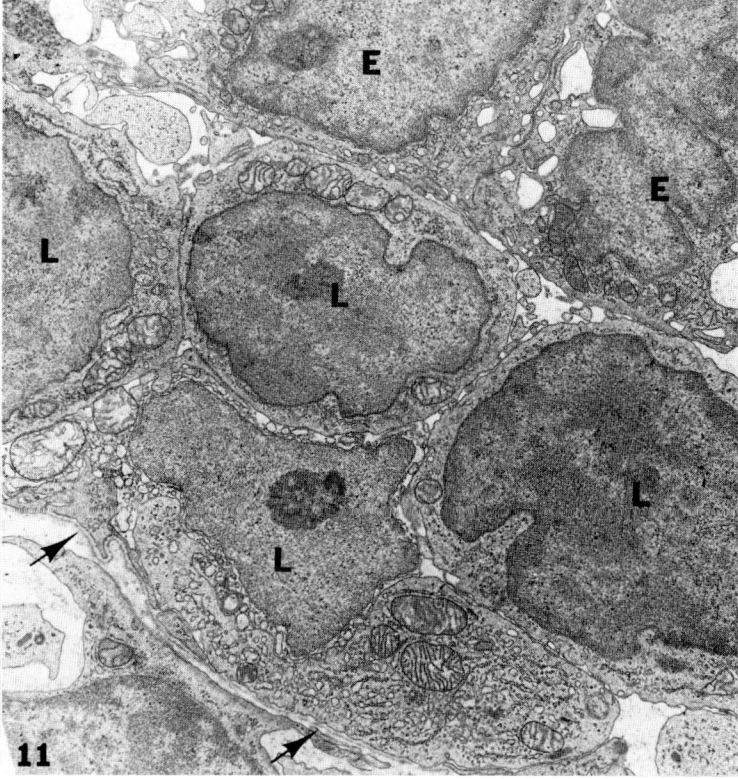

FIG. 11. In this 17-week fetus an aggregate of lymphocytes (L) is in direct contact with the overlying epithelial cells (E). The basal lamina surrounds this entire epithelial–lymphocytic complex as a single entity (*arrows*). ×6,800. (From Moxey and Trier, ref. 43, with permission of the Wistar Institute Press.)

enclosed by the epithelial basal lamina. It is not known if, as in the adult, the IELs in fetal intestine are primarily T lymphocytes and the Peyer's patch lymphocytes primarily B cells. Nor is the significance of the potential direct contact between developing epithelium and immature lymphocytes known.

In the adult, macromolecular transport across the epithelium is largely restricted to the M cells in the dome epithelium, though some transport also occurs through the villous absorptive cells (64). Paracellular transport of macromolecules is prevented by the presence of continuous tight junctions between adjacent epithelial cells (60). The pathway for transport across the fetal intestine is less clearly defined. Since junctional complexes are present between adjacent epithelial cells, at least between 9 and 22 weeks of gestation, it seems unlikely that significant paracellular transport occurs, though freeze fracture studies are needed to define the complexity and continuity of these junctions. In contrast, the cellular pathway across the absorptive cells may be relatively important in the fetal life. Thus, during the second trimester morphological specializations differentiate within the columnar cells of the human fetal intestine which are known in other animal species to function in the transport of macromolecules. To understand the potential significance of these morphological specializations it is necessary to consider the sequential differentiation of the final cell type appearing in the human fetal intestine during the period of cellular differentiation, the villous absorptive cell.

Villous Absorptive Cells

The simple columnar epithelial cells lining the newly formed villi of 10- to 12-week fetuses are characterized by short regular microvilli, large supra- and infranuclear glycogen deposits, a moderately well-developed Golgi complex, and the presence of electron-dense lysosomal elements and vesicles in the apical cytoplasm (Fig. 2A). Several of these characteristics have functional correlates. For example, the development of a highly organized microvillous border is temporally associated with the appearance of many brush border enzymes including alkaline phosphatase (17,30,33,37) leucine aminopeptidase (22,37), numerous disaccharidases (3,4,17), dipeptidases (4,39,58), and tripeptidases (28). Similarly, the presence of lysosomal elements parallels the detection of acid phosphatase, nonspecific esterases, and other acid hydrolytic enzymes by 12 weeks of gestation (3,22,37).

At the time of their appearance, the columnar cells in proximal and distal intestine are morphologically similar. By 16 weeks, however, differentiation of the intracellular organelles results in distinct regional differences. Two organelle systems in particular, the apical tubular system (ATS) and the meconium corpuscle system (MCS), first appear at the beginning of the second trimester and undergo dramatic sequential changes with increasing gestational age. The ATS is a membranous system characterized by invaginations of the apical plasma membrane, vesicular and tubular profiles, and occasional small vacuoles in the apical cytoplasm (Figs. 12–15). The membranes of these structures are similar in width and density to the apical plasma membrane and wider than the membranes surrounding other organelles. In some cells, especially in the distal intestine between 15 and 20 weeks, the inner leaflet of the membranes is characterized by an ordered array of electron-dense particles (Fig. 13). These particulate arrays, which are also occasionally seen along the plasma membrane at the base of the microvilli, resemble those described in the ATS of distal epithelial cells in suckling rodents (56,66). In this animal model these arrays are known to have n-acetyl-β-glucosaminidase activity (35).

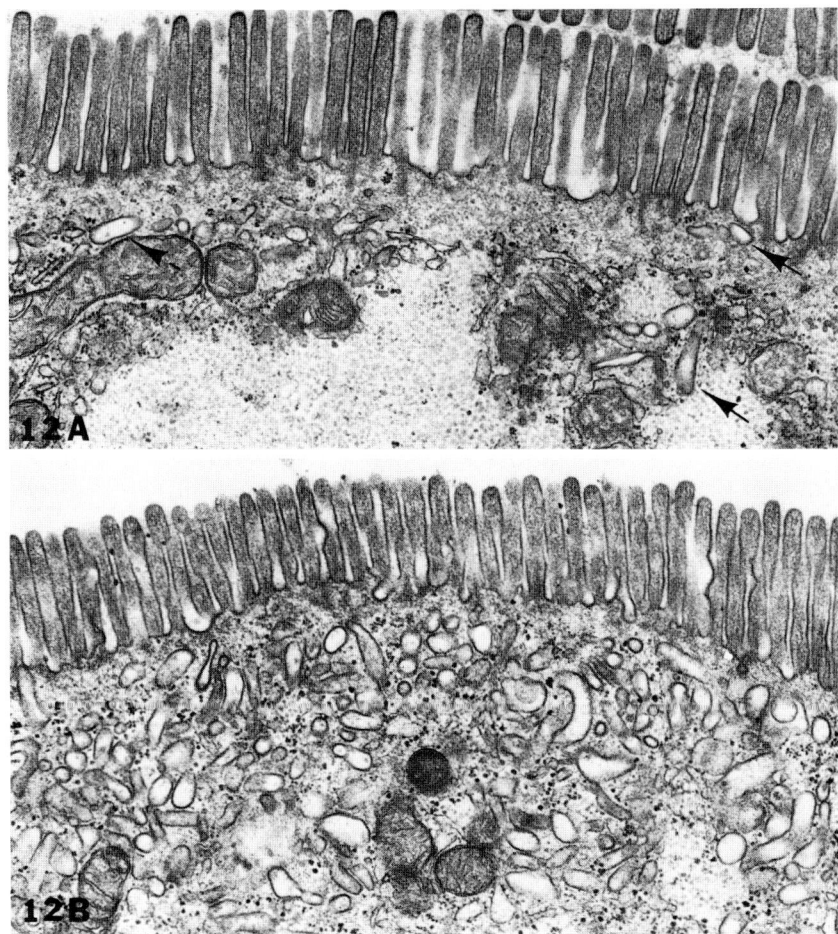

FIG. 12.A: The apical cytoplasm from the proximal intestine of a 15-week fetus contains few membrane-bound vesicles of the ATS (*arrows*) in the region subjacent to the microvilli. ×17,800. **B:** The apical cytoplasm of an absorptive cell from the distal intestine of the same fetus as in **A.** Here abundant tubules and vesicles of the ATS are evident. ×17,600. (From Moxey and Trier, ref. 44, with permission of the Wistar Institute Press.)

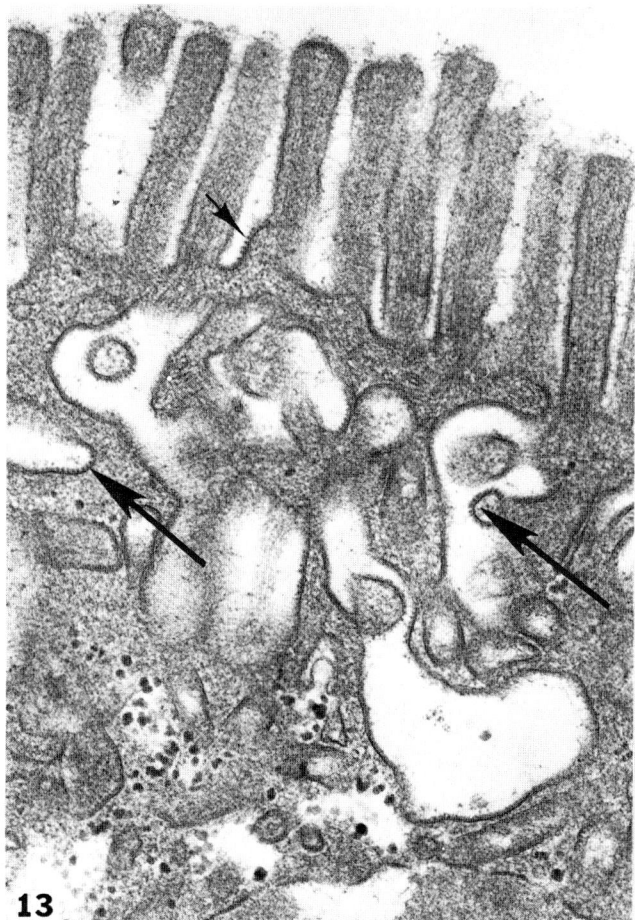

FIG. 13. The apical cytoplasm from an absorptive cell in the distal intestine of a 17–18-week fetus. Note the presence of an ordered array of particles (*long arrows*) on the inner membrane leaflet of some elements of the ATS, and along the apical plasma membrane at the base of a microvillus (*short arrow*). ×52,100. (From Moxey and Trier, ref. 44, with permission of the Wistar Institute Press.)

The second organelle system, the MCS, also appears in the apical cytoplasm of villous columnar cells early in the second trimester. The MCS is a membranous complex of vesicles and vacuoles comprising the lysosomal system. The term "meconium corpuscle" derives from the original observation of Schmidt (59). He described large, round, yellow inclusions in the human fetal intestine. Parat (52) noted that these structures were larger and more prevalent in the distal intestine, and that they increased in size and number with increasing age, reaching a peak at 6 months. Subsequent histologic and electron microscopic studies have demonstrated that the so-called meconium corpuscles are in fact lysosomal elements (2,8,44). It is still uncertain, however, if the original assumption that the meconium present in the intestinal lumen after the third month of gestation (17,30) is in fact actively taken up and concentrated in the MCS of the epithelial cells.

The degree of differentiation of both the ATS and MCS changes dramatically between 12 and 20 weeks of gestation. Initially (between 10 and 13 weeks), few elements of either membrane system are present and no regional differences are noted. Between 15 and 17 weeks there is a marked increase in the extent and complexity of both systems in the distal, but not the proximal, intestine (Figs. 12 and 14). After this peak, the structural elements of each system decrease, and in some proximal cells are undetectable by 22 weeks. Semiquantitative morphometric analyses has confirmed this morphological impression (44). This pattern of development with a peak at 15 to 17 weeks correlates with the peak in activity of n-acetyl-β-glucosaminidase activity in the distal intestine of 17- to 24-week fetuses (3). This activity may reflect the peak in the MCS, since it is a lysosomal enzyme, or in the ATS, since it may

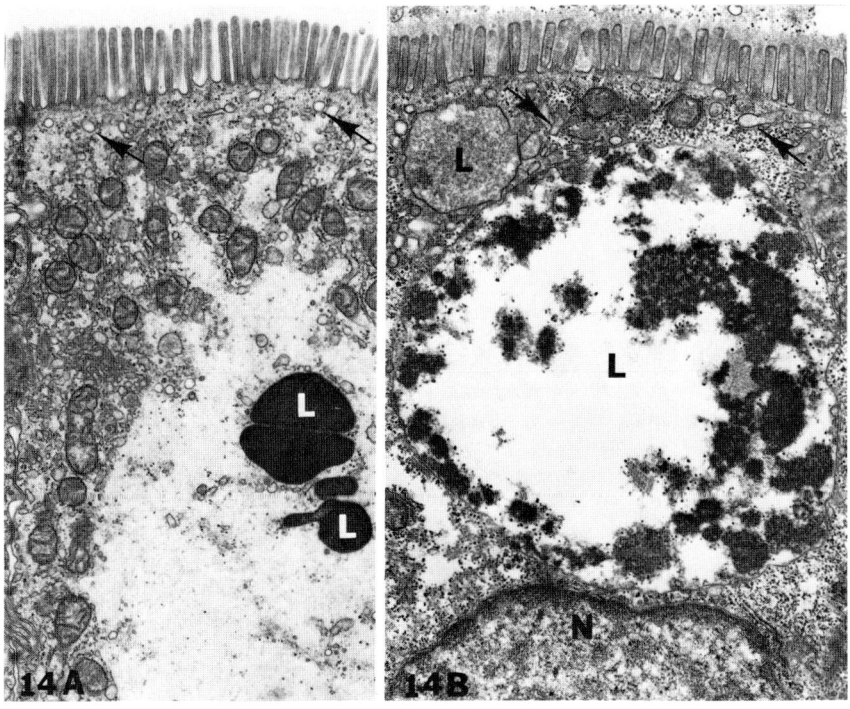

FIG. 14.A: The apical cytoplasm of an absorptive cell from the proximal intestine of a 16-week fetus. Few elements of the ATS (*arrows*) are present beneath the microvilli, though small irregular lysosomal elements (L) of the MCS are present in the supranuclear glycogen. ×9,500. **B:** The apical cytoplasm of an absorptive cell from the distal intestine of a 16-week fetus. The supranuclear region is dominated by highly heterogeneous elements of the lysosomal MSC (L) and vesicles of the ATS (*arrows*). N, nucleus. ×9,800.

be present in the particulate arrays as in the rodent (35), or it may represent a composite peak in both membranous systems.

In the developing small intestine of other mammals the morphological correlates of these two membranous systems, that is, the apical endocytic complex and the supranuclear vacuole and its associated lysosomes, are involved in the uptake of lumenal macromolecules (25,47,68). This uptake is common to most species studied, but the subsequent transport across the epithelium varies among species, ranging from nonspecific transport to a highly selective process (for review see Rodewald, ref. 57). There is general agreement that the initial uptake occurs via elements of the ATS and/or coated vesicles. The transport pathway is more controversial, but appears to be mediated by coated vesicles (for review see King, ref. 34). These coated vesicles may originate at the apical plasma membrane as coated pits or bud off from elements of the ATS. Macromolecules not enclosed within these coated vesicles are shuttled to the lysosomal system (MCS) for degradation. As in animal models, nonspecific uptake of macromolecules occurs in the human fetal intestine at the time when ATS and MCS are present, e.g., during the second trimester. Ferritin (44), and horseradish peroxidase (HRP) (36) can be demonstrated in elements of the ATS in absorptive cells of the human fetal intestine (Fig. 15) between 12 and 20 weeks of gestation. Neither of these substances is seen in the intercellular spaces or lamina propria, i.e., transport is not observed. In fact, the presence of some HRP in dense bodies resembling lysosomes suggests intracellular degradation. This would be consistent with findings in animal models where nonspecific macromolecules are degraded and only physiologically important substances are transported across the epithelium. For example, it is known that ferritin alone is not transported in neonatal rat intestine whereas ferritin-labeled IgG crosses readily (56). The possibility still exists, therefore, that the human fetal intestine may transport biologically important materials from the amniotic fluid into the fetal circulation. Indirect evidence supporting this concept include the observations that: (a) the fetus swallows amniotic fluid late in gestation (23,55), and (b) between 34 and 40 weeks proteins, including hormones and gamma globulin, are cleared from amniotic fluid (1–23). Clearly, further research is necessary to define the pathway and selectivity of this potential transport *in utero*.

THIRD PHASE OF DEVELOPMENT: MATURATION

As determined morphologically and morphometrically, both the ATS and the MCS decrease in extent and complexity between 18 and 22 weeks of gestation. This reduction proceeds in a craniocaudal direction with a consistent difference between the proximal and distal regions of the same fetus. In a single 22-week fetus, no profiles of either membranous system are detectable proximally, though elements of each are present distally. Indications of continued

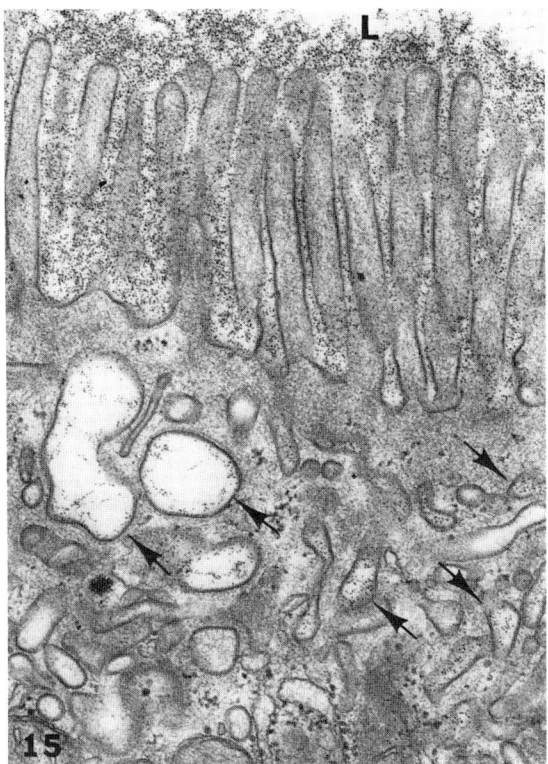

FIG. 15. An absorptive cell from the distal intestine of an 18-week fetus exposed to ferritin for 8 min prior to fixation. Ferritin is present in the lumen (L), between the microvilli, and within the vesicles and tubules of the ATS (arrows). ×34,300. (From Moxey and Trier, ref. 44, with permission of the Wistar Institute Press.)

differentiation in these proximal absorptive cells include a reduction in glycogen content and the appearance of accumulations of smooth endoplasmic reticulum (Fig. 16). These cells are, in fact, morphologically similar to those present in the adult mucosa. This transition to an adult-type epithelium marks the end of the second phase of intestine development, the period of cellular differentiation, and introduces the final phase of maturation. The term "maturation" has been arbitrarily applied to this period, but due to a lack of tissue there is no morphological data to confirm continued cellular differentiation and mucosal maturation. In fact, there are only limited data available concerning any aspect of this final period of intestinal development. It is largely speculative, therefore, that structural and functional maturation continue during the last trimester, though the normal birth-weight infant appears to differ significantly from the premature infant in both absorptive and digestive capacities (5,65,69).

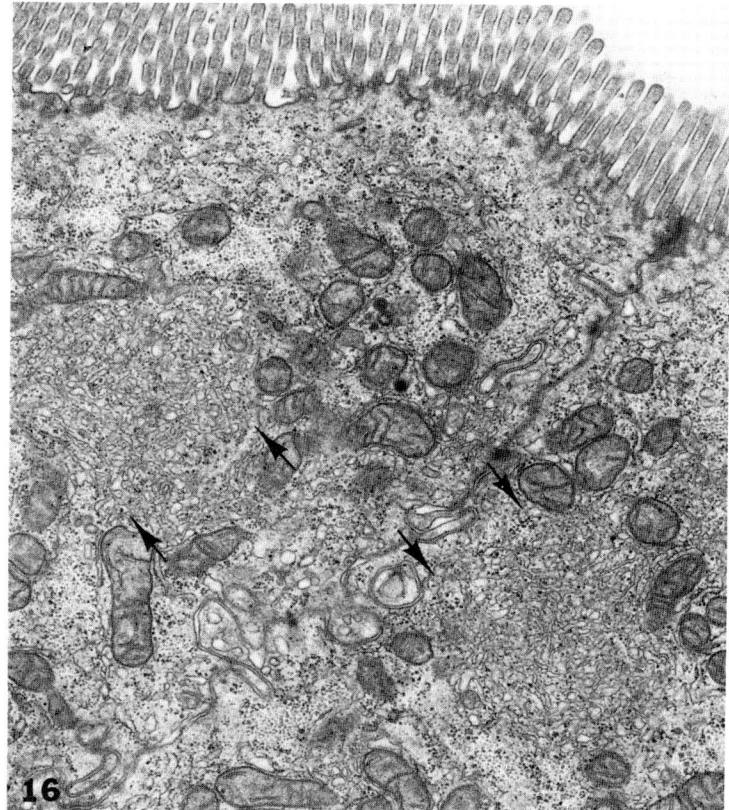

FIG. 16. Two adjacent cells from the proximal intestine of a 22-week fetus demonstrating the decrease in cytoplasmic glycogen and elements of the ATS and MCS, along with the concomitant increase in smooth endoplasmic reticulum (*arrows*). ×14,100.

CONCLUSIONS

In conclusion, it is possible to delineate at least three successive phases of human fetal intestinal development. The first trimester involves the formation of the primitive gut and is a period of cellular proliferation, growth, and morphogenesis. The second phase, the period of cellular differentiation, marks the appearance and structural differentiation of all the cell types common to the adult mucosa as well as several types that are unique to the fetus. Parallel development of functional capacity is indicated by biochemical studies. For example, adult-appearing endocrine cells differentiate during the second trimester and there is a simultaneous appearance of at least eight regulatory peptides as determined by immunocytochemistry and radioimmunoassay (11). It is interesting that most of these peptides have an adult pattern of distribution by 20 to 24 weeks of gestation. Similarly, many of the digestive enzymes associated with the villous absorptive cell appear early in development and attain adult levels and patterns of distribution by the end of the second trimester (4; for review see Grand et al., ref. 24). By 22 weeks, therefore, the fetal intestinal mucosa morphologically resembles the adult and has many of the same functional capacities. Though data are limited, the last third of gestation is presumably one of enhanced functional development. It appears that this final period of "maturation" involves not only the intestinal tract but also the accessory organs. For example, fat digestion is less efficient in the newborn than in the adult. This reduced functional capacity reflects loss of bile salts from the intestinal tract due to inadequate ileal active transport of bile salts (18), as well as low pancreatic lipase and bile acid levels (26). Clearly, additional research on the structural and functional processes of maturation will assist in the understanding of the digestive, absorptive, and barrier functions of the newborn intestinal tract.

REFERENCES

1. Abbas, J. M., and Tovey, J. E. (1960): Protein of the liquor amnii. *Br. Med. J.,* 1:476–478.
2. Andersen, H., Bierring, F., Matthiessen, M., Egeberg, J., and Bro-Rasmussen, F. (1964): On the nature of the meconium corpuscles in human fetal intestinal epithelium: II. A cytochemical study. *Acta Pathol. Microbiol. Scand.,* 61:377–393.
3. Antonowicz, I., Chang, S. C., and Grand, R. J. (1974): Development and distribution of lysosomal enzymes and disaccharidases in human fetal intestine. *Gastroenterology,* 67:51–58.
4. Auricchio, D., Stellato, A., and Devizia, B. (1981): Development of brush border peptidases in human and rat small intestine during fetal and neonatal life. *Pediatr. Res.,* 15:991–995.
5. Barness, L. A. (1981): Nutritional requirements of the full-term neonate. In: *Textbook of Pediatric Nutrition,* edited by R. M. Suskind, pp. 21–28. Raven Press, New York.
6. Behnke, O., and Moe, H. (1964): An electron microscopic study of mature and differentiating Paneth cells in the rat, especially of their endoplasmic reticulum and lysosomes. *J. Cell Biol.,* 22:633–652.
7. Berry, J. M. (1900): On the development of the human intestine. *Anat. Anz.,* 17:242–249.
8. Bierring, F., Andersen, H., Egeberg, J., Bro-Rasmussen, F., and Matthiessen, M. (1964): On the nature of the meconium corpuscles in human fetal intestinal epithelium. I. Electron microscopic studies. *Acta Pathol. Microbiol. Scand.,* 61:365–376.
9. Bockman, D. E., and Cooper, M. D. (1973): Pinocytosis by epithelium associated with lymphoid follicles in the bursa of Fabricius, appendix, and Peyer's patches. *Am. J. Anat.,* 136:455–478.
10. Boquist, L., and Falkmer, S. (1969): In: *The Structure and Metabolism of the Pancreatic Islets,* edited by S. Falkmer, B. Hellman, and E. B. Taljedal, pp. 25–35. Pergamon Press, New York.
11. Bryant, M. G., Buchanan, A. M. J., Gregor, M., Chatei, M. E., Polak, J. M., and Bloom, S. R. (1982): Development of intestinal regulatory peptides in the human fetus. *Gastroenterology,* 83:47–54.
12. Cho, D. (1931): Histological investigation of the digestive tract of the human fetus. II. Development of small intestine. *Jpn. J. Obstet.,* 14:324–330.
13. Christina, M. L., Lehy, T., and Peranzi, G. (1978): Étude ultrastructurale des cellules endocrines dans le colon humain foetal. Ontogenèse et distribution. *Gastroenterol. Clin. Biol.,* 2:1011–1023.
14. Colony, P. C., and Neutra, M. (1981): Cytochemical and ultrastructural differentiation of the fetal rat colon. *Anat. Rec.,* 199:57A.
15. Colony, P. C., and Neutra, M. R. (1983): Epithelial differentiation in the fetal rat colon. I. Membrane phosphatase activities. *Devel. Biol.,* 97:349–363.
16. Cornes, J. S. (1965): Number, size and distribution of Peyer's patches in the human small intestine. I. The development of Peyer's patches. *Gut,* 6:225–229.
17. Dahlquist, A., and Lindberg, T. (1966): Fetal development of the small intestinal disaccharidase and alkaline phosphatase activities in the human. *Biol. Neonate,* 9:24–32.
18. de Belle, R. C., Vaupshas, V., Bitullo, B. B., Haber, L. R., Shaffer, E., Mackie, G. G., Owen,

H., Little, J. M., and Lester, R. (1979): Intestinal absorption of bile salts: Immature development of neonate. *J. Pediatr.,* 94:472–476.
19. Eastwood, G. L., and Trier, J. S. (1974): Epithelial cell proliferation during organogenesis of the rat colon. *Anat. Rec.,* 179:303–310.
20. Eberl-Rothe, G., and Langegger, P. A. (1953): Uber die entwicklung der Peyerschen platten. *Z. Anat. Entwick. Gesch.,* 117:26–35.
21. Falkmer, S., and Patent, G. J. (1972): Comparative and embryological aspects of the pancreatic islets. In: *Handbook of Physiology, Vol. 1,* edited by D. G. Steiner and N. Freinkel, pp. 1–23. Waverly Press, Baltimore.
22. Garbarsch, C. (1969): Histochemical studies on the early development of the human small intestine. *Acta Anat.,* 72:357–375.
23. Gitlin, D., Junate, J., Morales, C., Noriega, L., and Arevalo, N. (1972): The turnover of amniotic fluid protein in the human conceptus. *Am. J. Obstet. Gynecol.,* 113:632–645.
24. Grand, R. J., Watkins, J. B., and Torri, F. M. (1976): Development of the human gastrointestinal tract: A review. *Gastroenterology,* 70:790–810.
25. Graney, D. O. (1968): The uptake of ferritin by ileal absorptive cells in suckling rats: An electron microscopic study. *Am. J. Anat.,* 123:227–254.
26. Hamosh, M. (1979): Fat digestion in the newborn-role of lingual lipase and preduodenal digestion. *Pediatr. Res.,* 13:615–622.
27. Helander, H. F. (1975): Enzyme patterns and protein absorption in rat colon during development. *Acta Anat.,* 91:330–349.
28. Heringová, A., Koldovský, O., Jirsová, V., Uher, J., Noack, R., Friedrich, M., and Schenk, G. (1966): Proteolytic and peptidase activities of the small intestine of human fetuses. *Gastroenterology,* 51:1023–1027.
29. Hermos, J. A., Mathan, M., and Trier, J. S. (1971): DNA synthesis and proliferation by villous epithelial cells in fetal rats. *J. Cell Biol.,* 50:255–258.
30. Jirásek, J. E., Uher, J., and Koldovský, O. (1965): A histochemical analysis of the development of the small intestine of human fetuses. *Acta Histochem. (Jena),* 22:33–39.
31. Johnson, F. P. (1910): The development of the mucous membrane of the esophagus, stomach and small intestine in the human embryo. *Am. J. Anat.,* 10:521–561.
32. Johnson, F. P. (1912): The development of the mucous membrane of the large intestine and vermiform process in the human embryo. *Am. J. Anat.,* 14:187–233.
33. Kelley, R. O. (1973): An ultrastructural and cytochemical study of developing small intestine in man. *J. Embryol. Exp. Morphol.,* 29:411–430.
34. King, B. F. (1982): A freeze fracture study of the guinea pig yolk sac epithelium. *Anat. Rec.,* 202:221–230.
35. Knutton, D., Limbrick, A. R., and Robertson, J. D. (1974): Regular structures in membranes. I. Membranes in endocytic complex of ileal epithelial cells. *J. Cell Biol.,* 62:679–694.
36. Lev, R. (1977): Correlative studies of function and morphology. In: *Gastrointestinal Development and Neonatal Nutrition. Proceedings of the 72nd Ross Conference on Pediatric Research,* pp. 24–27. Ross Laboratories, Ohio.
37. Lev, R., Siegel, H. I., and Bartman, J. (1972): Histochemical studies of development of human fetal small intestine. *Histochemie,* 29:103–119.
38. Lev, R., and Weisberg, H. (1969): Human foetal epithelial glycogen: A histochemical and electron microscopic study. *J. Anat.,* 105:337–349.
39. Lindberg, T. (1966): Intestinal dipeptidases: Characterization, development, and distribution of intestinal dipeptidases of the human foetus. *Clin. Sci.,* 30:505–515.
40. Madara, J. L., Trier, J. S., and Neutra, M. R. (1980): Structural changes in the plasma membrane accompanying differentiation of epithelial cells in human and monkey small intestine. *Gastroenterology,* 78:963–975.
41. Mathan, M., Moxey, P. C., and Trier, J. S. (1976): Morphogenesis of fetal rat duodenal villi. *Am J. Anat.,* 146:73–92.
42. Moxey, P. C., and Trier, J. S. (1977): Endocrine cells in the human fetal small intestine. *Cell Tissue Res.,* 183:33–50.
43. Moxey, P. C., and Trier, J. S. (1978): Specialized cell types in the human fetal small intestine. *Anat. Rec.,* 191:269–286.
44. Moxey, P. C., and Trier, J. S. (1979): Development of villous absorptive cells in the human fetal small intestine: A morphological and morphometric study. *Anat. Rec.,* 195:463–482.
45. Nabeyama, A., and LeBlond, C. P. (1974): Caveolated cell characterized by deep surface invaginations and abundant filaments in mouse gastrointestinal epithelia. *Am. J. Anat.,* 140:147–166.

46. Nakamura, M., and Motoyoshi, Y. (1971): Ultrastructural studies on the islets of Langerhans of the carp. *Z. Anat. Entwick. Gesch.*, 134:61–72.
47. Orlic, D., and Lev, R. (1973): Fetal rat intestinal absorption of horseradish peroxidase from swallowed amniotic fluid. *J. Cell Biol.*, 56:109–119.
48. Orlic, D., and Lev, R. (1977): An electron microscopic study of intraepithelial lymphocytes in human fetal small intestine. *Lab. Invest.*, 37:554–561.
49. Owen, R. L. (1977): Sequential uptake of horseradish peroxidase by lymphoid follicle epithelium of Peyer's patches in the normal unobstructed mouse intestine: An ultrastructural study. *Gastroenterology*, 72:440–451.
50. Owen, R. L., and Jones, A. L. (1974): Epithelial cell specialization within human Peyer's patches: An ultrastructural study of intestinal lymphoid follicles. *Gastroenterology*, 66:189–203.
51. Owen, R. L., and Jones, A. L. (1974): Scanning Electron Microscopy. *Proceedings of the Workshop on Advances in Biomedical Applications of the SEM*, pp. 697–704. Chicago IIT Research Institute, Chicago.
52. Parat, M. (1922): Contribution a l'histo-physiologie des organes digestifs de l'embryon. *C. R. Soc. Biol.*, 87:1273–1275.
53. Patzelt, V. (1931): Die feinese Ausbildung des menschlichen Darmes von der fünften Woche bis zur Geburt. *Z. Mikrosk. Anat. Forsch.*, 27:269–518.
54. Patzelt, V. (1936): Der Darm. In: *Handbuch der mikroskopischen Anatomie des Menschen, Vol. 5*, edited by W. von Mollendorff, pp. 1–448. Springer Verlag, Berlin.
55. Pritchard, J. A. (1965): Deglutition by normal and anencephalic fetuses. *Obstet. Gynecol.*, 25:289–297.
56. Rodewald, R. (1973): Intestinal transport of antibodies in the newborn rat. *J. Cell Biol.*, 58:189–211.
57. Rodewald, R. (1980): Immunoglobulin transmission in mammalian young and the involvement of coated vesicles. In: *Coated Vesicles*, edited by C. J. Ocklefore and A. Whyte, pp. 60–101. Cambridge University Press, Cambridge.
58. Rubino, A., Pierro, M., Toretta, G. L., Vetrella, M., Martino, D., and Auricchio, S. (1969): Studies on intestinal hydrolysis of peptides. II. Dipeptidase activity toward L-glutaminyl-L-proline and glycyl-L-proline in the small intestine of the human fetus. *Pediatr. Res.*, 3:313–319.
59. Schmidt, J. E. (1905): Beiträge zue normalen und pathologischen Histologie einiger Zellarten der Schleimhaut des menschlichen Darmkanales. *Arch. Mikrosk. Anat.*, 66:12–40.
60. Staehelin, L. A. (1974): Structure and function of intercellular junctions. *Int. Rev. Cytol.*, 39:191–283.
61. Staley, M. W., and Trier, J. S. (1965): Morphologic heterogeneity of mouse Paneth cell granules before and after secretory stimulation. *Am. J. Anat.*, 117:365–384.
62. Varkonyi, T., Gergely, G., and Varo, V. (1974): The ultrastructure of the small intestinal mucosa in the developing human fetus. *Scand. J. Gastroenterol.*, 8:495–500.
63. von Rosen, L., Podjaski, B., Bettmann, I., and Otto, H. (1981): Observations on the ultrastructure and function of the so-called 'microfold' or 'membranous' cells (M cells) by means of peroxidase as a tracer. An experimental study with special attention to the physiological parameters of resorption. *Virchows Arch. [Pathol. Anat.]*, 390:289–312.
64. Walker, W. A., Cornell, R., Davenport, L. M., and Isselbacher, K. J. (1972): Macromolecular absorption. Mechanism of horseradish peroxidase uptake and transport in adult and neonatal rat intestine. *J. Cell Biol.*, 54:195–205.
65. Watkins, J. B. (1979): Infant nutrition and the development of gastrointestinal function. In: *Pediatric Nutrition Handbook*, pp. 58–69. American Academy of Pediatrics, Evanston, Ill.
66. Wissig, S. L., and Graney, D. R. (1968): Membrane modifications in the apical endocytic complex of ileal epithelial cells. *J. Cell Biol.*, 37:564–579.
67. Wolf, J. L., Rubin, D. H., Finberg, R., Kauffman, R. S., Sharpe, A. H., Trier, J. S., and Fields, D. B. (1981): Intestinal M cells: A pathway for entry of retrovirus into the host. *Science*, 212:471–472.
68. Worthington, B. B., and Graney, D. O. (1973): Uptake of adenovirus by intestinal absorptive cells of the suckling rat. II. The neonatal jejunum. *Anat. Rec.*, 175:63–76.
69. Ziegler, E. E., Biga, R. L., and Foman, S. J. (1981): Nutritional requirements of the premature infant. In: *Textbook of Pediatric Nutrition*, edited by R. M. Suskind, pp. 29–39. Raven Press, New York.

DISCUSSION

Dr. Ferguson: I would like to ask you a question about the follicle associated epithelium in which the M cells are present. Have you any information that suggests that the first thing to appear is the lamina propria alterations associated with an aggregation of lymphocytes and associated as cells, and then the epithelium becomes specialized, or is it the other way round?

Dr. Colony: It is not possible to answer this question based on the limited number of older foetuses available to me. The lymphocytes don't start accumulating in the lamina propria until about 18 to 20 weeks of gestation so that you are dealing with a later time period than most of my material. It appears, however, that there are more accumulations of lymphocytes than dome regions with M cells forming. I would assume, therefore, that the lymphocytes accumulate first, and then there is differentiation of the superficial epithelial cells, though I don't have the data to confirm this.

Dr. Kretchmer: Do you know of any experiments where the oesophagus has been tied off, say in the rat foetus, and the development of the intestine followed with the swallowing of the amniotic fluid? There are similar human situations with oesophageal atresia, and I just wonder if the circulation of the amniotic fluid was shown to have any effect on the development of the intestine?

Dr. Colony: There are cases of oesophageal atresia in humans where the authors have claimed that the infant had a particularly low birth weight, but this seems to be somewhat controversial. I am not aware of any reports in animal species.

Dr. Zetterström: As regards Dr. Kretchmer's question, I can tell you that we are conducting studies on the intestinal function in cases of intestinal congenital atresia. We have observed morphological changes in those cases; after a period of about 4 to 6 weeks following surgical correction, there is a sudden development. So there is retardation in the physiological development of the factors in cases of high intestinal atresia.

Dr. Jacquot: I am very impressed by the fact that, apparently, the differentiation of the digestive tract proceeds simultaneously in its various parts—at the same time as the intestine is differentiating, the liver and the endocrine and exocrine pancreas are differentiating. This is true of both humans and rodents. There might be a synchronization mechanism for the whole digestive tract, and this might be one of the functions of the cells you describe as endocrine on a morphological basis with no known function as yet. They might be synchronizers for the differentiation of the digestive tract and of its annexes; i.e. the liver and pancreas.

You also stated that some cells undergo differentiation and later on regress in differentiation as far as granules and lysosomes are concerned. It would be very interesting to know if it is the same cell that regresses or if it is a new cell population because of cellular migration. In terms of cellular biology it makes a great difference. It would be very surprising that cells with well-developed organelles would lose them later on.

Dr. Colony: In the human being the cellular changes I have discussed occur over a 6 to 8 week time period. Even though the migration rate might be slower in the developing human foetus, as in the developing rat intestine, I would be very surprised if this is the same cell population.

Dr. Jacquot: Is there any indication of changes in intercellular junctions according to time of development?

Dr. Colony: Studies on junctions in fetal rat small intestine have been reported, and I have investigated the changes in the fetal rat colon. Surprisingly, even in the stratified epithelium, the superficial cells always have well-developed tight junctions as determined by electron microscopy and freeze fracture. The number and complexity of the strands of these occluding junctions do not appear to change significantly as a function of age. No studies in human fetal intestine are available.

Nutritional Adaptation of the Gastrointestinal Tract of the Newborn, edited by N. Kretchmer and A. Minkowski. Nestlé, Vevey/Raven Press, New York © 1983.

Anchoring and Biosynthesis of Small-Intestinal Sucrase–Isomaltase

Giorgio Semenza

Laboratorium für Biochemie der ETH, ETH-Zentrum, CH-8092 Zürich, Switzerland

The present chapter summarizes some recent and less recent work on the positioning, anchoring and biosynthesis of the small-intestinal sucrase–isomaltase (SI) complex, which is the most abundant integral protein of the brush border membrane; it then discusses the implications of the results as to the possible mechanisms underlying human sucrose–isomaltose malabsorption.

I became interested in this enzyme some years ago because (a) it plays a central role in the digestion of starch (accounting for approximately 80% of the small-intestinal maltase activity); (b) it is the major integral protein of the brush border (accounting for approximately 10% of the proteins in the membrane); (c) there is a simultaneous absence or lack of activity of isomaltase (I) and sucrase (S) in sucrose malabsorption; and (d) it has some interesting properties, which will be discussed below. This chapter will first consider the following: (a) the similarities in properties of the two subunits of the SI complex; (b) their common or related biological control mechanism; and (c) the mode of anchoring of the SI complex in the brush border membrane.

PROPERTIES OF THE SUBUNITS OF THE SI COMPLEX

Most work has been carried out on the SI complex of the rabbit small intestine. Whenever available, the information obtained on the SI from other species indicates that the SIs from other mammals are very similar to the rabbit enzyme. The SI complexes from the various species cross-react immunologically.

As obtained from Triton-solubilized SI complex, the I subunit has a molecular weight of approximately 140,000 and the S subunit one of approximately 120,000 (11). Both are glycoproteins composed of a single polypeptide chain (15), and both have one active site each (48). Their large size has discouraged sequencing. There are strong indications, however, that they have at least some degree of homology: (a) the (limited) sequence of part of the known active sites (49) is identical in S and I; (b) fingerprints of the tryptic digests of the SI complex yield only a few more peptides as there are Lys +

Arg residues (15); (c) S and I have an extensive overlapping in substrate specificities, maltose, maltitol, (55) and a number of aryl-α-glucopyranosides (16) being split by both subunits. The major differences in substrate specificities are: sucrose, which is not split by I, and the 1,6-α-glucopyranoside bonds in isomaltose and some limit dextrins, which are not split by S; (d) S and I have an extensive overlapping in their fully competitive inhibitors: common to both are D-glucose (30,61), the tris-hydroxy-methyl-amino-methane, lanthanides, D-1:5 gluconolactone (16), nojirimycin and deoxynojirimycin (28). Competitive inhibitors discriminating between S and I are: acarbose, which does not inhibit I, and dextran, which does not inhibit S (38); (e) the same compound, conduritol-B-epoxide, acts as an active-site-directed irreversible inhibitor of both S and I (48); (f) the secondary deuterium effect is approximately as large in S and I (16); (g) the values of the coefficients in the Hensch–Hammett equation are nearly the same in both subunits (16); (h) pK_a- values of the groups in the active sites involved in catalysis and/or substrate binding, as deduced from double-logarithmic Dixon plots, are approximately the same in S and I (23,28,71); (i) both enzymes are activated by Na^+; (j) both enzymes have the same kinetic mechanism (30,61); (k) both enzymes have the same minimum catalytic mechanism (16).

A COMMON OR RELATED BIOLOGICAL CONTROL MECHANISM(S) OF S AND I

This is supported by the following observations: (a) simultaneous appearance during development, both in man (in whose intestine both activities appear during intrauterine life (20) and in species in which both activities appear after birth, e.g., the rat (51), and the mouse (3); (b) simultaneous response to the stimulation by sugars and/or corticosteroids *in vivo* (40; see also for review, ref. 37); (c) simultaneous absence or lack of activities in sucrose–isomaltose malabsorption (8,17,22,25,26,47,60,65), which is a monofactorial genetic disease (32,46,50); (d) constant ratios between S and I activities in random samples of human peroral biopsies (9).

These observations, while not allowing the identification of the common step(s) in the control of biosynthesis and/or membrane insertion of S and I, do nevertheless indicate that these processes in the subunits of the SI complex are mutually related.

THE MODE OF ANCHORING OF THE SI COMPLEX IN THE BRUSH BORDER MEMBRANE

The SI complex is an integral membrane protein, as shown by the failure of neutral buffers of high or low ionic strength to bring it into solution. Solubilization can be achieved either by controlled proteolytic treatment, as for instance with papain (6,62), or elastase (1,41), or with detergents, such as

Triton X-100 (62,69). Most of the information on the positioning and anchoring of SI in the brush border membrane is derived from studies on the mechanism of solubilization with papain and Triton, and by comparing the characteristics of the SI forms thereby obtained.

When sealed (35) brush border membrane vesicles are subjected to limited papain digestion from the luminal side, SI activity is totally solubilized, although the permeability and transport properties of the vesicles remain unchanged (70). Thus, most of the SI complex can be removed from the luminal side without disrupting the membrane fabric. Also, opening up of the vesicles with detergent does not lead to any apparent increase in S activity (33). By negative staining "lollipops" can be visualized on the luminal surface of the brush border membrane; at least some of them have been identified with the SI complex (44). Ferritin-labeled antibodies have also localized the SI complex at the luminal surface of the brush borders (18). It seems, therefore, that the SI complex is anchored in the membrane in such a way as to protrude from its luminal side, and that only a small part of the protein mass directly interacts with the membrane fabric.

Solubilization by papain is likely to be related to the hydrolysis of one or more peptide bond(s), whereas Triton solubilization is not likely to be. Triton-solubilized SI, but not papain-solubilized SI, easily forms aggregates upon removal of the detergent and can interact with phosphatidyl choline, yielding regularly shaped proteoliposomes (12). Triton-solubilized SI, but not papain-solubilized SI, has (a) hydrophobic segment(s), as detected by charge-shift electrophoresis (72). The irreversible solubilization by papain is accompanied by the loss of one or more hydrophobic segments, which are necessary for the interaction of SI with either natural or artificial membranes. Indeed, papain treatment of isolated Triton-solubilized SI or of Triton-SI-proteoliposomes leads to a protein indistinguishable from papain-solubilized SI plus a rather short highly hydrophobic peptide (11).

This hydrophobic "anchor" is likely to be localized at the N-terminal region of the I subunit (Fig. 1) since papain solubilization does not lead to any change in (a) the C-terminal regions of either subunit, (b) the N-terminal of sucrase, or (c) the apparent molecular weight of S. Papain solubilization, however, produces covalent changes in the N-terminal region of I, since it leads to (a) a decrease (by ~20,000 daltons) of its apparent molecular weight and (b) a change of its N-terminal with appearance of heterogeneity (the substrate specificity of papain is rather broad). The conclusion appears therefore to be that (a) the SI complex is anchored to the brush border membrane via a hydrophobic segment located at the N-terminal region of the I subunit; (b) neither S nor the C-terminal region of I are inserted in the brush border membrane; and (c) since papain solubilizes SI by acting from the *luminal* side without modifying the C-terminal regions of S or I, or the N-terminal region of S, these polypeptide segments must not span the membrane: these C- and N-termini must therefore be located at the *luminal* side of the membrane (Fig. 1) (11).

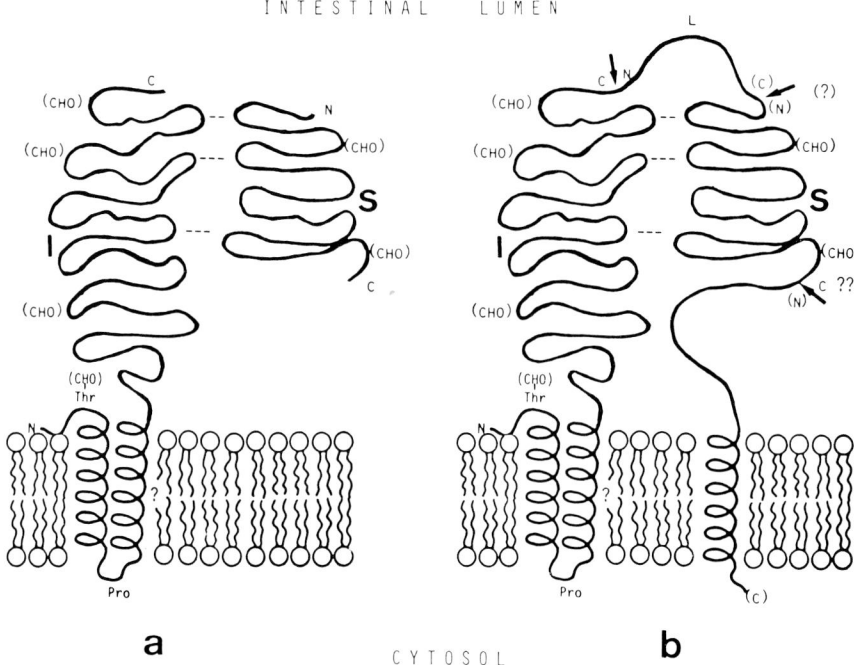

FIG. 1. Positioning of the SI complex **(a)** and suggested positioning and possible structure of ProSI **(b)** in the small-intestinal brush border membrane. The drawings are not to scale and are meant to convey the major features only. L, Pancreatic (and other?) protease(s) at the point(s) indicated by *arrows* (it is not known whether this loop includes a hydrophobic segment and whether it is split at one or more points); N and C, N- and C-termini, respectively, of SI and ProSI; (CHO), carbohydrate chains; ?, the chain between Thr-11 and the bulk of the protein mass either does not cross the hydrophobic layer or crosses it twice (the latter seems at the moment more probable); ??, it is not known whether this extracellular C-terminus is the product of post-translational proteolysis or not; ↓, site of proteolytic attack. (From Semenza, ref. 58, with permission.)

Sequencing of the N-terminal of I reveals, as expected, a highly hydrophobic sequence—probably the most hydrophobic one ever reported (Fig. 2) (24,64). Some points in this sequence are worth discussing.

Residue 11 is glycosylated (24,64). The neutral sugars galactose, glucose and fucose are associated with this amino acid residue in approximately 1:1:1 molar ratios. Since glycosylation is confined to the luminal compartment of the endoplasmic reticulum and of the Golgi membranes (for reviews see refs. 27,52,53), these observations indicate that residue 11 is located on the extracellular side of the membrane. Since the 1–11 sequence, even if stretched, could barely cross the membrane (and many of its residues are charged) it seems unlikely that Ala-1 is located on the side of the membrane opposite to residue 11.

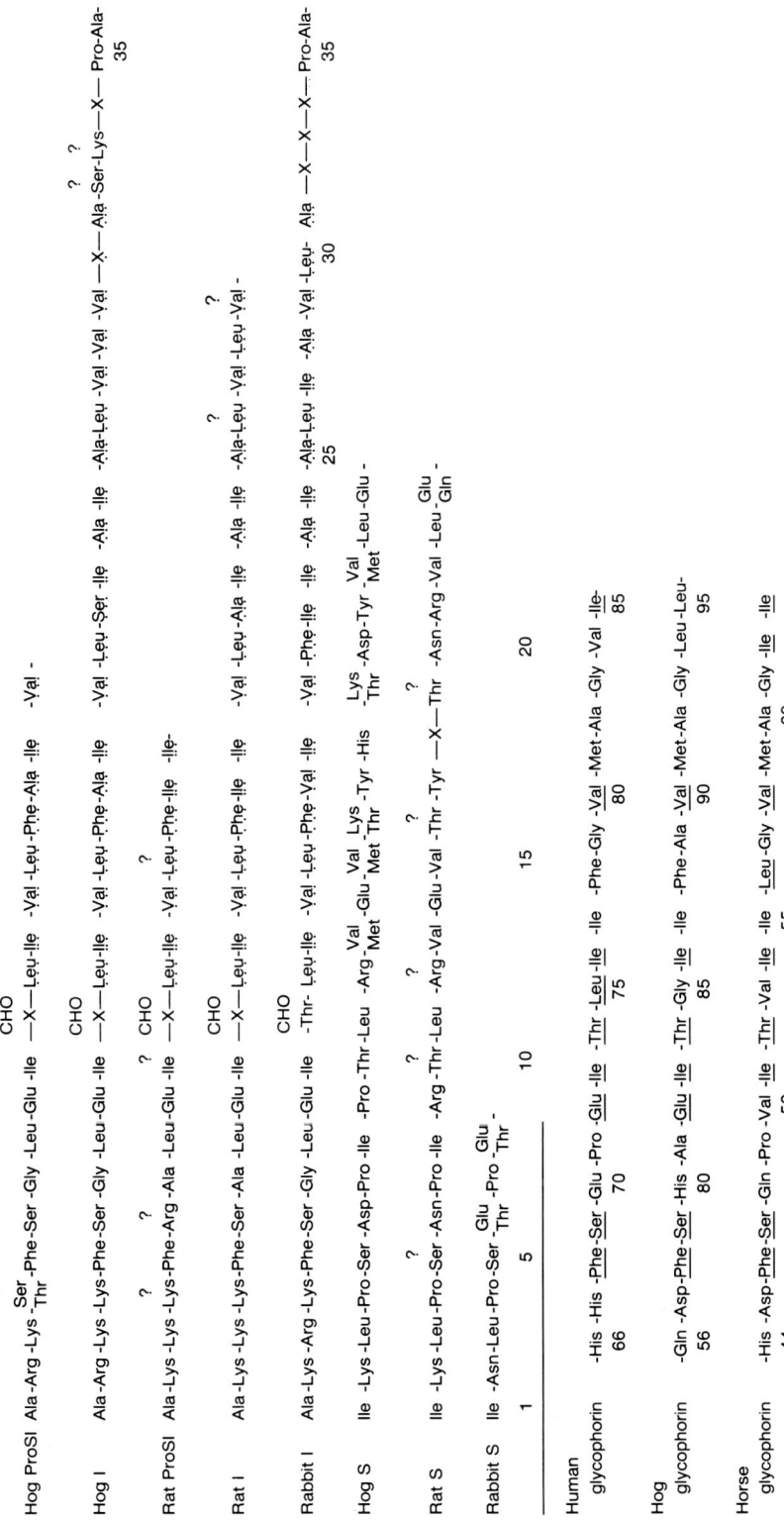

FIG. 2. Partial N-terminal sequences of ProSI and IS polypeptides. (From Hauri et al., ref. 29, and Sjöström et al., ref. 64, with permission.)

The N-terminal of I is located on the luminal side: direct evidence for this has been provided recently by the use of a new, little permanent acetimidate (3-[dimethyl-2-(acetimidoyethyl)ammonio]-propane-sulfonic acid, DAP) (14). The degree of modification of the I N-terminal (Ala) by this reagent is the same, irrespective of whether the reaction is carried out on right-side out brush border membrane vesicles (35) or on membrane fragments obtained by deoxycholate extraction (36). Ala-1 is as easily accessible to DAP acting on the luminal side only as to DAP acting on both sides. It must, therefore, be located at the luminal side. Similar results have been obtained with Ile-1 (the N-terminal of the sucrase subunit), which we know from other evidence to be located at the luminal side (11). If the isomaltase polypeptide chain has both termini at the luminal side, it must either not cross the membrane fabric or cross it an *even* number of times. In order to make a statement on these points, the following data on the I anchor have to be collected.

The hydrophobic anchor is some 60 amino acid residues long. A highly hydrophobic photolabel has been developed by Dr. J. Brunner in the author's laboratory (trifluoromethyl-3-(m-[^{125}I]iodophenyl)-diazirine, TID) (13). With the use of this reagent it can be shown that the anchoring segment of I is indeed confined to its N-terminal region (66). The isolated anchor is approximately 60 amino acid residues long and has a helical configuration, interrupted around residue 35 (a Pro) by a β turn. The most likely conformation of the anchor and its interaction with the membrane core is, therefore, that indicated in Fig. 1.

BIOSYNTHESIS AND MEMBRANE INSERTION OF THE SI COMPLEX

In order to explain the positioning of the two subunits (Fig. 1), their homologies, and their common or related biosynthetic control mechanism, the author suggested in 1979 (56,57) that SI is synthesized and inserted in the membrane as a single very long (260,000 daltons at least) polypeptide chain ("pro-sucrase-isomaltase" (ProSI)) which is processed into the "final" two-subunit complex by (extracellular) proteolysis. Since then, direct evidence has been obtained for the existence of an immunologically cross-reacting precursor and of a fully active ProSI in brush borders not previously exposed to pancreatic protease(s) (21,29,43,63,64). Subsequently, other brush border two-subunit enzymes have been shown to be likewise synthesized as a single-chain proform (renal γ-glutamyl-transpeptidase), intestinal glucoamylase, and the β-glycosidase complex (Sjöström et al., *personal communication*).

In vitro cell-free translation of ProSI has been achieved recently (73). This protein is the largest identified membrane polypeptide chain successfully translated thus far in a cell-free system from total RNA. In addition to providing further evidence that SI is synthesized as a one-chain precursor, the cell-free *in vitro* translation will hopefully help to solve problems related to the detailed mechanism of biosynthesis and membrane insertion. Prior to this, however, the following questions on the positioning and structure of ProSI have to be answered.

1. Does ProSI begin with the I or the S portion? Figure 2 shows the N-terminal sequences of rat (29), and hog (64) ProSIs. Clearly, they are *identical* (not merely homologous!) to those of the corresponding I subunits. This identity strongly indicates that the I portion corresponds to the N-terminal part of ProSI (Fig. 1).

2. How many hydrophobic segments (and thus potential anchors) does ProSI carry? In the original suggestion (Fig. 1) (56,57) no mention was made as to the possible existence of a hydrophobic segment at the C-terminal region and/or in the "loop". The latter possibility can now be ruled out, at least for the ProSI found in the brush border membrane prior to its processing by pancreatic proteases. As a matter of fact, in addition to the amphipathic (Triton-solubilized) ProSI, a water-soluble, nonamphipathic form can be prepared. This form, which shows no charge shift in the electrophoresis in detergents, has an apparent molecular weight *only slightly* smaller than the amphipathic form: thus, the loop (if it exists at all) between the I and the S portions does not contain any detectable hydrophobic sequence (H. Sjöström et al., *personal communication*).

PHYLOGENETIC CONSIDERATIONS

From a survey of the literature on the occurrence of disaccharidase activities in vertebrates (55), it is clear that I activity is found in all species investigated; this is not the case for S, which in mammals is not found in Pinnipedia [Otarioidea or Phocoidea (31,39,68)], nor in a few species of Marsupiala and Monotremata, and, in birds, in some penguins. In general, S activity is found in terrestrial species feeding on fruits and vegetables. The scattered data do not allow a phylogenetic pedigree to be put forward. No species, however, has been reported as having S but no I activity (which, incidentally, makes physiological sense). This is the reason why the author suggested that the product of the original partial gene duplication would be a "double I" rather than a "double S". The author has therefore investigated whether the small-intestinal I of a species not endowed with S activity, the sea lion (*Zalophus californianus*), has two active sites per polypeptide chain and thus mimics the phylogenetic precursor of ProSI (or is a phylogenetic "dead end" thereof) (Table 1).

Sea lion maltase-isomaltase has been isolated by detergent solubilization and immunoabsorption using antibodies directed against final rabbit SI. With the exception of sucrose, which it does not attack, sea lion I has the same substrate specificity as rabbit SI. It has two active sites (shown by labeling with the substrate-site-directed irreversible inhibitor conduritol-B-epoxide) per poly-

TABLE 1. *A hypothetical scheme of part of the phylogenesis and of the biosynthesis of small-intestinal I and S in mammals*

	Major characteristics of the enzyme(s)	Possible example
Early gene	One polypeptide chain with *one* active site splitting both maltose and I	None found thus far
By (partial?) gene duplication	One long polypeptide chain with *two* identical active sites, each splitting both maltose and I	(Sea lion I may be a *model* of this original double I. See text)
By mutation(s) producing a change in the substrate specificity of one of the sites (i.e., isomaltose → sucrase	One polypeptide chain with *two* similar (but no more identical) active sites, one splitting maltose and I, the other splitting maltose and sucrose	ProSI found in transplants of fetal rat small intestine and in the small intestine of adult hogs, whose pancreas had been disconnected from the duodenum 3–4 days before sacrifice
By splitting of the single polypeptide chain by pancreatic protease(s)	*Two* polypeptide chains with *one* active site each, one site splitting maltose and I, the other splitting maltose and sucrose	The SI complex from the small intestine of most mammals; the bands arising from ProSI upon treatment with pancreatic protease(s) *in vitro*

peptide chain of approximately 250,000 molecular weight. The active sites are identical, each of them splitting maltose, isomaltose, and palatinose, with no sign of deviation from Michaelis behavior (72).

It is still premature, however, to take sea lion I as an exact copy of the hypothetical double I. In fact, S activity is found both in species which have branched off from the phylogenetic tree prior to the Otarioidea (the "eared seals", to which the Californian sea lion belongs), and in others which have branched off later on. As a result, additions to the simplistic scheme must be considered. For example, (a) the "one-chain SI" (i.e., fully active ProSI) may have back-mutated to a double I in Otarioidea, in penguins and possibly in other species; (b) a mutation in the one-chain SI may have led to inactivation or loss of S. Subsequent protein fusion (and modification?) would have produced a pseudo-double I in the sea lion. No obvious advantage seems to be connected with events (a) or (b). (c) The appearance of S activity (that is, the mutation presumed to have transformed the hypothetical double I into the single-chain ProSI) may have occurred more than once. SI in phylogenetically remote species would thus be the product of convergent evolution, perhaps owing to the advantage of including sucrose-containing foodstuff in the diet of land animals feeding on vegetables and fruits. Pending further information on these points, sea lion I should be regarded only as an interesting possible analogy to the hypothetical double I in the phylogenetic and ontogenetic pedigree of the usual SI complex (Table 1).

Polypeptides carrying more than one enzymatically active site are rare, particularly among eukaryotes (for reviews see refs. 10,34,67). In general, enzymes associated in the same polypeptide chain catalyze a sequence of different reactions belonging to the same metabolic pathway, which may be an advantage in eukaryotes (67). It is, however, quite exceptional for two similar or identical active sites (acting "in parallel", rather than "in series") to occur on the same polypeptide chain. The only other example in addition to ProSI and sea lion I is probably the ATPase of myosin filaments. What evolutionary advantage, if any, may be associated with two-enzyme one-chain structure in the case of the intestinal carbohydrases is not apparent at present.

SUCROSE–ISOMALTOSE MALABSORPTION

Sucrose–isomaltose malabsorption was identified in 1960–1961 (2,46,74,75). It is less rare than it was originally thought to be: it may occur in as many as 0.2% of North Americans (45) and 10% of Greenland Eskimos (4,42). It is characterized by a complete, or almost complete, lack of S activity, a very strong reduction of I activity and a decrease of maltase activity to about one-third of the normal level (8). In the clinical history the intolerance to sucrose is usually prominent. The tolerance to starch is also reduced (5), more so than to palatinose (isomaltulose). Thus, the clinical picture is that expected if the subunits of the SI complex were both either absent or inactive. In the Sephadex chromatography of the disaccharidase activities of a small-intestinal biopsy from a patient, the peaks of S, I and maltase activities of the SI complex are not found (59). The residual I and maltase activities are likely to be due, in most cases, to the "heat-stable" maltases, i.e., to the maltase-glucoamylases (4) and/or to an I devoid of S activity (25,65).

Sucrose-maltose malabsorption is an hereditary, autosomic (46), monofactorial recessive condition (32,50). The actual enzyme defect underlying this disease, however, is not quite clear. In view of what is known on the positioning and anchoring of the SI complex in the brush border membrane, and of the possible existence of precursors, the following possibilities should be considered: (a) an "operon mutation", or (if S and I arise from two contiguous, fused genes) an extensive deletion of the two-cistron unit; (b) formation of an unstable or ineffective messenger RNA; (c) failure to respond to the hormonal stimulation during development, located at the translational or at a later step; (d) point mutation in the I gene, with loss (or perhaps strong reduction) of I activity and lack of capacity of I to keep S attached; (e) point mutation in the "precursors" with defective activation and/or insertion in the membrane; (f) point mutation (e.g., in I) making the SI complex abnormally susceptible to intracellular proteases or to those of the intestinal lumen. Other possibilities may also exist.

Preiser et al. (47) conclusively demonstrated the absence of SI and of any additional abnormal band in the SDS-polyacrylamide gel electrophoresis patterns of brush border membranes from some patients, and Gray et al. (26) failed to detect by a very sensitive radioimmunoassay any cross-reacting material in the intestinal homogenates or in the brush border membranes of other patients. It thus appears that in these patients mechanisms (d) and (e) alone are unlikely.

The existence in the cytosol of the small intestine of patients with sucrose-isomaltose malabsorption of an enzymatically inactive protein with an apparent molecular weight (by SDS-polyacrylamide gel electrophoresis under nondenaturing conditions) of approximately 220,000 has recently been reported. This observation would be compatible with mechanism (e) above. Characterization of this extra protein occurring in the cytosol could provide decisive evidence on whether or not it qualifies as an intracellular precursor of brush border SI.

Other mechanism(s), i.e., (d) and/or (e) above, are suggested by the observations of other authors. Dubs et al. (22), reported the presence of catalytically inactive, immunologically cross-reactive material in the brush border region of biopsies from sucrose–isomaltose-intolerant patients (by immunofluorescence). Freiburghaus et al. (25) and Skovbjerg and Krasilnikoff (65) found that the residual I activity in some patients has an electrophoretic mobility different from that of the normal SI complex. Changes involving other brush border enzymes were also observed. Furthermore, Cooper et al. (17) have found in three cases, using a highly sensitive fluorogenic assay, that both S and I, although very severely reduced, were nevertheless detectable. In density-gradient centrifugations of the homogenates, S activity of the patients sedimented at the same location as normal S, which indicated that the patient's S was located in the same organelle as the enzyme from normal tissue.

Summing up, it is difficult to draw conclusions which should be valid for all cases of sucrose–isomaltose malabsorption. Rather, it seems most likely that this syndrome may not be genetically homogeneous and that different mechanisms may be operative in the various pedigrees. Examination of the same patients by the various techniques may shed additional light in the future.

ACKNOWLEDGMENTS

I want to thank most heartily my co-workers—they are the ones who have actually carried out the experimental work and have contributed significantly to our ideas. It is a pleasure to thank those clinicians and physiopathologists with whom we shared our problems. This study was partially funded by the SNSF, Berne and by Nestlé Alimentana, Vevey.

REFERENCES

1. Alpers, D. H., and Tedesco, F. J. (1975): The possible role of pancreatic proteases in the turnover of intestinal brush border proteins. *Biochim. Biophys. Acta,* 401:28–40.
2. Anderson, C. M., Messer, M., Townley, R. R. W., and Freeman, M. (1963): Intestinal sucrase and isomaltase deficiency in two siblings. *Pediatrics,* 31:1003–1010.
3. Arthur, A. B. (1968): Development of disaccharidase activity in the small intestine of suckling mouse. *N. Z. Med. J.,* 67:614–616.
4. Asp, N. G., Berg, N. O., Dahlqvist, A., Gudmand-Høyer, E., Jarnum, S., and McNair, A. (1975): Intestinal disaccharidase in Greenland Eskimos. *Scand. J. Gastroenterol.,* 10:513–519.
5. Auricchio, S., Ciccimarra, F., Moauro, L., Rey, F., Jos, J., and Rey, J. (1972): Intraluminal and mucosal starch digestion in congenital deficiency of intestinal sucrase-isomaltase activities. *Pediatr. Res.,* 6:832–839.
6. Auricchio, S., Dahlqvist, A., and Semenza, G. (1963): Solubilization of the human intestinal disaccharidases. *Biochim. Biophys. Acta,* 73:582–589.
7. Auricchio, S., Rubino, A., Landolt, M., Semenza, G., and Prader, A. (1963): Isolated intestinal lactase deficiency in the adult. *Lancet,* 324:2–6.
8. Auricchio, S., Rubino, A., Prader, A., Rey, J., Jos, J., Frézal, J., and Davidson, M. (1965): Intestinal glucosidase activities in congenital malabsorption of disaccharidases. *J. Pediatr.,* 66:555–564.
9. Auricchio, S., Rubino, A., Tosi, R., Semenza, G., Landolt, M., Kistler, H., and Prader, A. (1963): Disaccharidase activities in human intestinal mucosa. *Enzym. Biol. Clin.,* 3:193–208.
10. Bisswanger, H., and Schmincke-Ott, E. (1980): *Multifunctional Proteins.* John Wiley, New York.
11. Brunner, J., Hauser, H., Braun, H., Wilson, K. J., Wacker, H., O'Neill, B., and Semenza, G. (1979): The mode of association of the enzyme complex sucrase-isomaltase with the intestinal brush border membrane. *J. Biol. Chem.,* 254:1821–1828.
12. Brunner, J., Hauser, H., and Semenza, G. (1978): Single bilayer lipid-protein vesicles formed from phosphatidylcholine and small intestinal sucrase-isomaltase. *J. Biol. Chem.,* 253:7538–7546.
13. Brunner, J., and Semenza, G. (1981): Selective labeling of the hydrophobic core of membranes with 3-(trifluoromethyl)-3-(m-(^{125}I)iodophenyl)diazirine, a carbene-generating reagent. *Biochemistry,* 20:7174–7182.
14. Bürgi, R., Brunner, J., and Semenza, G. (1983): Use of an impermeant imidoester for determining the sideness of the N-termini of the small-intestinal sucrase-isomaltase. *J. Biol. Chem.* (in press).
15. Cogoli, A., Eberle, A., Sigrist, H., Joss, C., Robinson, E., Mosimann, H., and Semenza, G. (1973): Subunits of the small-intestinal sucrase-isomaltase complex and separation of its enzymatically active isomaltase moiety. *Eur. J. Biochem.,* 33:40–48.
16. Cogoli, A., and Semenza, G. (1975): A probable oxocarbonium ion in the reaction mechanism of small intestinal sucrase and isomaltase. *J. Biol. Chem.,* 250:7802–7809.
17. Cooper, B. T., Candy, D. C. A., Harries, J. T., and Peters, T. J. (1979): Subcellular fractionation studies of the intestinal mucosa in congenital sucrase-isomaltase deficiency. *Clin. Sci.,* 57:181–185.
18. Cummins, D. L., Gitzelmann, R., Lindenmann, J., and Semenza, G. (1968): Immunochemical study of isolated human and rabbit intestinal sucrase. *Biochim. Biophys. Acta,* 160:396–403.
19. Dahlqvist, A., Hammond, J. B., Crane, R. K., Dunphy, J. V., and Littman, A. (1963): Intestinal lactase deficiency and lactose intolerance in adults: Preliminary report. *Gastroenterology,* 45:488–491.
20. Dahlqvist, A., and Lindberg, T. (1966): Development of the intestinal disaccharidase and alkaline phosphatase activities in the human foetus. *Clin. Sci.,* 30:517–528.
21. Danielsen, E. M., Sjöström, H., and Norén, O. (1981): Biosynthesis of intestinal microvillar proteins. Putative precursor forms of microvillus aminopeptides and sucrase-isomaltase isolated from Ca^{2+}-precipitated enterocyte membranes. *FEBS Lett.,* 127:129–132.
22. Dubs, R., Steinmann, B., and Gitzelmann, R. (1973): Demonstration of an inactive enzyme antigen in sucrase-isomaltase deficiency. *Helv. Paediatr. Acta,* 28:187–198.

23. Flückinger, R. (1973): Untersuchungen über den Reaktionsmechanismus der Isomaltase. Diplomarbeit an der ETH, Zürich.
24. Frank, G., Brunner, J., Hauser, H., Wacker, G., Semenza, G., and Zuber, H. (1978): The hydrophobic anchor of small-intestinal sucrase–isomaltase. N-terminal sequence of the isomaltase subunit. *FEBS Lett.*, 96:183–188.
25. Freiburghaus, A. U., Dubs, R., Hadorn, B., Gaze, H., Hauri, H. P., and Gitzelmann, R. (1978): The brush border membrane in hereditary sucrase–isomaltase deficiency: Abnormal protein pattern and presence of immunoreactive enzyme. *Eur. J. Clin. Invest.*, 7:455–459.
26. Gray, G. M., Conklin, K. A., and Townley, R. R. W. (1976): Sucrase-isomaltase deficiency. Absence of an inactive enzyme variant. *N. Engl. J. Med.*, 294:740–753.
27. Hanover, J. A., and Lennarz, W. J. (1981): Transmembrane assembly of membrane and secretory glycoproteins. *Arch. Biochem. Biophys.*, 211:1–19.
28. Hanozet, H., Pircher, H. P., Vanni, P., Oesch, B., and Semenza, G. (1981): An example of enzyme hysteresis. The slow and tight interaction of some fully competitive inhibitors with small intestinal sucrase. *J. Biol. Chem.*, 256:3703–3711.
29. Hauri, H. P., Wacker, H., Rickli, E. E., Bigler-Meier, B., Quaroni, A., and Semenza, G. (1982): Biosynthesis of sucrase–isomaltase. Purification and NH_2-terminal amino acid sequence of the rat sucrase–isomaltase precursor (pro-sucrase-isomaltase) from fetal intestinal transplants. *J. Biol. Chem.*, 257:4522–4528.
30. Janett, M. (1974): Identifikation der durch Saccharase und Isomaltase gespaltenen Bindung im Substrat. Steady-state Kinetik der Isomaltase. Diplomarbeit an der ETH, Zürich.
31. Kerry, K. R., and Messer, M. (1968): Intestinal glycosidases of three species of seals. *Comp. Biochem. Physiol.*, 25:437–446.
32. Kerry, K. R., and Townley, R. R. W. (1965): Genetic aspects of intestinal sucrase-isomaltase deficiency. *Aust. Paediatr. J.*, 1:223–235.
33. Kessler, M., Acuto, O., Storelli, C., Murer, H., Müller, M., and Semenza, G. (1978): A modified procedure for the rapid preparation of efficiently transporting vesicles from small intestinal brush border membranes. *Biochim. Biophys. Acta*, 506:136–154.
34. Kirschner, K., and Bisswanger, H. (1976): Multifunctional proteins. *Annu. Rev. Biochem.*, 45:143–166.
35. Klip, A., Grinstein, S., and Semenza, G. (1979): Transmembrane disposition of the phlorizin binding protein of intestinal brush borders. *FEBS Lett.*, 99:91–96.
36. Klip, A., Grinstein, S., and Semenza, G. (1979): Distribution of sulfhydryl groups in intestinal brush border membranes. Localization of side-chains essential for glucose transport and phlorizin binding. *Biochim. Biophys. Acta*, 558:233–245.
37. Koldovský, O. (1981): Developmental, dietary and hormonal control of intestinal disaccharidases in mammals (including man). In: *Carbohydrate Metabolism and its Disorders, Vol. 3*, edited by P. J. Randle, D. F. Steiner, and W. J. Whelan, pp. 481–522, Academic Press, N.Y.
38. Kolínská, J., and Semenza, G. (1967): Studies on intestinal sucrase and on intestinal sugar transport. V. Isolation and properties of sucrase–isomaltase from rabbit small intestine. *Biochim. Biophys. Acta*, 146:181–195.
39. Kretchmer, M., and Sunshine, P. (1967): Intestinal disaccharidase deficiency in the sea lion. *Gastroenterology*, 53:123–129.
40. Lebenthal, E., Sunshine, P., and Kretchmer, N. (1972): Effect of carbohydrates and corticosteroids on activity of β-glucosidases in the intestine of the infant rat. *J. Clin. Invest.*, 51:1244–1250.
41. Maestracci, D. (1976): Enzymic solubilization of the human intestinal brush border membrane enzymes. *Biochim. Biophys. Acta*, 433:469–481.
42. McNair, A., Gudmand-Høyer, E., and Jarnum, S. (1972): Sucrose malabsorption in Greenland. *Br. Med. J.*, 2:1921.
43. Montgomery, R. K., Sybicki, A. A., Forcier, A. G., and Grand, R. J. (1981): Rat intestinal microvillus membrane sucrase–isomaltase is a single high molecular weight protein and fully active enzyme in the absence of luminal factors. *Biochim. Biophys. Acta*, 661:346–349.
44. Nishi, Y., Yoshida, T. O., and Takesue, Y. (1968): Electron microscope studies on the structure of rabbit intestinal sucrase. *J. Mol. Biol.*, 37:441–444.
45. Peterson, M. L., and Herber, R. (1967): Intestinal sucrase deficiency. *Trans. Assoc. Am. Physicians*, 80:275–283.
46. Prader, A., Auricchio, S., and Mürset, G. (1961): Durchfall infolge hereditären Mangels an

intestinal Saccharaseaktivität (Saccharoseintoleranz). *Schweiz. Med. Wochenschr.,* 91:465–468.
47. Preiser, H., Menard, D., Crane, R. K., and Cerda, J. J. (1974): Deletion of enzyme protein from the brush border membrane in sucrase–isomaltase deficiency. *Biochim. Biophys. Acta,* 363:279–282.
48. Quaroni, A., Gershon, E., and Semenza, G. (1974): Affinity labeling of the active sites in the sucrase–isomaltase complex from small intestine. *J. Biol. Chem.,* 249:6424–6433.
49. Quaroni, A., and Semenza, G. (1976): Partial amino acid sequences around the essential carboxylate in the active sites of the intestinal sucrase–isomaltase complex. *J. Biol. Chem.,* 251:3250–3253.
50. Rey, Y., and Frézal, J. (1967): Les anomalies des disaccharidases. *Arch. Fr. Pediatr.,* 24:65–101.
51. Rubino, A., Zimbalatti, F., and Auricchio, S. (1964): Intestinal disaccharidase activities in adult and suckling rats. *Biochim. Biophys. Acta,* 92:305–311.
52. Sabatini, D. D., and Kreibich, G. (1976): Functional specialization of membrane-bound ribosomes in eukaryotic cells. In: *The Enzymes of Biological Membranes,* edited by A. Martonosi, pp. 531–579. John Wiley, New York.
53. Sabatini, D. D., Kreibich, G., Morimoto, T., and Adesnik, M. (1982): Mechanism for the incorporation of proteins in membranes and organelles. *J. Cell. Biol.,* 92:1–22.
54. Schmitz, J., Preiser, H., Maestracci, D., Ghosh, B. K., Cerda, J. J., and Crane, R. K. (1973): Purification of the human intestinal brush border membrane. *Biochim. Biophys. Acta,* 323:98–112.
55. Semenza, G. (1968): Intestinal oligosaccharidases and disaccharidases. In: *Handbook of Physiology: Alimentary Canal, V,* Chap. 119, pp. 2543–2566. American Physiological Society, Washington, D. C.
56. Semenza, G. (1979): The mode of anchoring of sucrase–isomaltase to the small intestinal brush-border membrane and its biosynthetic implications. In: *Proceedings of the 12th FEBS Meeting, Vol. 53,* Dresden, 1978, edited by S. Rapaport and T. Schewe, pp. 21–28. Pergamon Press, Oxford, New York.
57. Semenza, G. (1979): Mode of insertion of the sucrase–isomaltase complex in the intestinal brush border membrane: Implications for the biosynthesis of this stalked intrinsic membrane protein. In: *Development of Mammalian Absorptive Processes,* Ciba-Foundation Series 70 (new series), pp. 133–146. Elsevier-North-Holland, Amsterdam.
58. Semenza, G. (1981): Molecular pathophysiology of small-intestinal sucrase-isomaltase. In: *Clinics in Gastroenterology,* Vol. 10, pp. 691–706. W. B. Saunders, Philadelphia.
59. Semenza, G., Auricchio, S., and Rubino, A. (1965): Multiplicity of human intestinal disaccharidases. I. Chromatographic separation of maltases and of two lactases. *Biochim. Biophys. Acta,* 96:487–494.
60. Semenza, G., Auricchio, S., Rubino, A., Prader, A., and Welsh, J. D. (1965): Lack of some intestinal maltases in a human disease transmitted by a single genetic factor. *Biochim. Biophys. Acta,* 105:386–389.
61. Semenza, G., and v. Balthazar, A. K. (1974): Steady state kinetics of rabbit small intestinal sucrase: Kinetic mechanism, Na^+-activation, inhibition by Tris(hydroxymethyl)-amino-methane at the glucose subsite, with an appendix on "interactions between enzyme inhibitors: A kinetic test for some simple cases". *Eur. J. Biochem.,* 41:149–162.
62. Sigrist, H., Ronner, P., and Semenza, G. (1975): A hydrophobic form of the small intestinal sucrase–isomaltase complex. *Biochim. Biophys. Acta,* 406:433–446.
63. Sjöström, H., Norén, O., Christiansen, L., Wacker, H., and Semenza, G. (1980): A fully active, two-active-site, single-chain-sucrase-isomaltase from pig small intestine. *J. Biol. Chem.,* 255:11332–11338.
64. Sjöström, H., Norén, O., Christiansen, L. A., Wacker, H., Spiess, M., Bigler-Meier, B., Rickli, E. E., and Semenza, G. (1982): Membrane anchoring and partial structure of small intestinal pro-sucrase-isomaltase. A possible biosynthetic mechanism. *FEBS Lett.,* 148:321–325.
65. Skovbjerg, H., and Krasilnikoff, P. A. (1981): Immunoelectrophoretic studies on human intestinal brush border proteins. The residual isomaltase in sucrose intolerant patients. *Pediatr. Res.,* 15:214–218.
66. Spiess, M., Brunner, J., and Semenza, G. (1982): Hydrophobic labeling, isolation and partial characterization of the NH_2-terminal membranous segment of sucrase–isomaltase complex. *J. Biol. Chem.,* 257:2370–2377.

67. Stark, G. R. (1977): Multifunctional proteins: One gene-more than one enzyme. *Trends Biochem. Sci.*, 2:64–66.
68. Sunshine, P., and Kretchmer, N. (1964): Intestinal disaccharidase: Absence in two species of sea lions. *Science,* 144:850–851.
69. Takesue, Y., Yoshida, T. O., Akaza, T., and Nishi, Y. (1973): Localization of sucrase in the microvillus membrane of rabbit intestinal mucosal cells. *J. Biochem. (Tokyo),* 74:415–423.
70. Tannenbaum, C., Toggenburger, G., Kessler, M., Rothstein, A., and Semenza, G. (1977): High-affinity phlorizin binding to brush border membranes from small intestine: Identity with (a part of) the glucose transport system, dependence on the Na^+-gradient, partial purification. *J. Supramol. Struct.,* 6:519–533.
71. Tellier, C., Bertrand-Triadou, N., and Alvarado, F. (1979): Determination of the catalytic groups of intestinal brush border sucrase by pH-variation studies. *Trans. Biochem. Soc.,* 7:1071–1072.
72. Wacker, H., Aggeler, R., Kretchmer, N., Takesue, Y., and Semenza, G. (1983): A two-active site one-polypeptide enzyme: The isomaltase from sea-lion small intestinal brush border membrane. Its possible phylogenetic relationship with sucrase–isomaltase (*in preparation*).
73. Wacker, H., Jaussi, R., Sonderegger, P., Dokow, M., Ghersa, P., Hauri, H. P., Christen, P., and Semenza, G. (1981): Cell-free synthesis of the one-chain precursor of a major intrinsic protein complex of the small intestinal brush border membrane (pro–sucrase–isomaltase). *FEBS Lett.,* 136:329–332.
74. Weijers, H. A., van de Kamer, J. H., Dicke, W. K., and Ijsseling, J. (1961): Diarrhoea caused by deficiency of sugar splitting enzymes. *Acta Paediatr.,* 50:55–71.
75. Weijers, H. A., van de Kamer, J. H., Mossel, D. A. A., and Dicke, W. K. (1960): Diarrhoea caused by deficiency of sugar-splitting enzymes. *Lancet,* ii. 296–297.

DISCUSSION

Dr. Ribadeau Dumas: Unless I missed it, you did not mention any data supporting the hypothesis you choose for anchoring in the membrane. Also, did you get confirmation of cell-free translation of signals?

Dr. Semenza: It seems likely that the NH_2 terminus of pre-proteins is initially located at the cytosolic rather than at the cisternal surface of the rough endoplasmic reticulum membrane, and that the growing polypeptide chain crosses the bilayer folded as a "loop" or "helical hairpin"; the first hydrophobic helix of the hairpin would pull the polar portions of the polypeptide chain as a second helix into and across the membrane. The first half of the hairpin (i.e., the first hydrophobic helix) would be the pre-piece (the "signal"). Along these lines it has been suggested that ProSI is synthesized as pre-ProSI and inserted into the membrane as follows. The first hairpin establishing the first insertion would be composed of a hydrophobic helix (the pre-piece, not demonstrated yet), followed by a β-turn which encompasses the short hydrophilic sequence 1 to 11 of ProSI; this hydrophilic sequence is extruded until the hydrophobic sequence which follows terminates the extrusion process. A second hydrophobic–hydrophilic hairpin would follow immediately, and the rest of ProSI could be synthesized and extruded either completely or up to another hydrophobic segment situated close to the COOH terminus. Signal peptidase would split the loop between the two helices of the first hairpin, thus creating a secondary (extracellular) NH_2 terminus and producing the final positioning of ProSI. Some of the predictions made by the helical hairpin hypothesis still lack experimental confirmation. (a) Is ProSI originally translated with a pre-piece? *In vitro* translation of the message should give an answer. (b) Following the hydrophobic sequence which is to span the membrane should be a second hydrophobic piece which enables the anchor to loop back. A proline residue found in position 35 of rabbit I could indicate this "turning point".

Nutritional Adaptation of the Gastrointestinal
Tract of the Newborn, edited by N. Kretchmer
and A. Minkowski. Nestlé, Vevey/Raven
Press, New York © 1983.

Effect of Variation of Dietary Intake of Starch and Sucrose on the Activity of Sucrase and Lactase in Jejunum of Adult Rats

Otakar Koldovský, Sergio Bustamante,
Toshinao Goda, and Kazuhiko Yamada

Departments of Pediatrics and Physiology, University of Arizona Health Sciences Center, Tucson, Arizona 85724

The problem of the regulation of activity of intestinal disaccharidases, especially lactase, has attracted the attention of researchers for many years (6,8); there are still many unresolved questions. This chapter, which deals with the authors' recent experiments with rats, summarizes data concerning (a) the effect of variation of carbohydrate intake on the activity of sucrase and lactase, (b) the mechanisms involved in changes of the activity of disaccharidases as influenced by the variation of carbohydrate intake, and (c) the locus of the first expression of the effect of the variation of carbohydrate intake along the height of the crypt–villus columns.

METHODS

Rats born in our animal facilities were weaned at 30 days of age and fed a standard laboratory chow (Lab Blox, Allied Mills, Inc., Chicago, Ill.) until 11 to 12 weeks of age. They were then fed isocaloric synthetic diets. (For detailed composition of diets, see refs. 3,14.) The low-carbohydrate diet provided 5% cal. from starch, 21% cal. from protein, and 73% cal. from corn oil. The high-carbohydrate diets contained 72%, 23%, and 5% cal., respectively.

All rats were fed *ad libitum* and had unrestricted access to water. Fresh food was given every second day. Food intake was measured by weighing the food every morning. Rats were sacrificed by decapitation between 9 and 10 a.m. in a fed state. The entire small intestine was removed, the duodenum was discarded, the jejunoileum was divided into three equal parts along its length, flushed with cold saline solution, and frozen at $-20°C$. before the assays of activity for disaccharidases and determinations of protein were performed. This chapter summarizes data related only to the proximal third of the jejunum.

Sucrase activity was determined according to Dahlqvist (4), and lactase according to Koldovský et al. (7). The lactase assay mixture contained *p*-chloromercuribenzoate [(PCMB) Aldrich Chemical Company, Milwaukee, Wisc.] in order to inhibit any residual lysosomal acid β-galactosidase activity (7). Assays of enzyme activity were performed under the condition of linearity of reaction with time and amount of homogenate used. Protein was determined according to Lowry et al. (10). Enzyme activity was expressed as μmoles of substrate split per mg of tissue protein (specific activity) or per total intestinal segment (total activity). Since specific activity is a ratio between enzyme activity and tissue protein, a change in the value can be caused by a change either of the numerator, or of the denominator (tissue protein or other parameter, e.g., DNA). The denominator can change not only quantitatively, but also qualitatively, i.e., changes in tissue protein other than the structures carrying the hydrolases studied can occur. Expressing the data as total activity removes the possibility of an artifact when data are related to protein, DNA, etc.

To assay the activity of disaccharidases at different levels of the villus, a 5 × 5-mm segment of jejunum was sectioned within a cryostat at −18°C, as previously described (2). Horizontal sections were cut 10 μm thick. A section at a given depth into the villus–crypt unit was mounted on a microscope slide for immediate inspection of histology under a phase-contrast microscope. The tissue blocks were sectioned through the submucosa into the muscular layer. Every 10 consecutive sections were combined and homogenized in 0.5-ml distilled water by vortex shaking.

When cell migration was studied, the technique as described by Ulshen and Grand (13) was used. Simultaneously with the initiation of sucrose feeding, animals received 100 μCi [methyl-^{3}H]thymidine intraperitoneally. From an approximately 10 × 10-mm segment of jejunum, 10 slices of 10 μm thick per tube were prepared using cryostat sectioning. These were solubilized in protosol (New England Nuclear, Boston, Mass.) to which a standard toluene-PPO-POPOP mixture, liquifluor (New England Nuclear) was added. Samples were counted in a Beckman liquid scintillation spectrometer (LS-230). With this technique, similar data to those of Ulshen and Grand (13) were obtained.

RESULTS

Variation of Carbohydrate Intake

Two models were used: (a) starvation, i.e., complete deprivation of carbohydrate and all other sources of energy, and (b) variation of carbohydrate content in isocaloric diets. As already indicated, the protein content of the isocaloric diets remained practically constant; carbohydrate was replaced by fat and vice versa.

Effects on Sucrase

Starvation as well as the decrease of carbohydrate intake leads to a decrease of sucrase specific activity (Fig. 1). Within three days, the specific activity decreases more in the animals fed isocaloric diets than in the starved ones. Also, when the data are expressed as total activity per jejunal segment, the decrease in the high-fat low-carbohydrate diet group is more pronounced than in the starved animals (Fig. 2). Feeding the starved animals or the animals fed the low-carbohydrate diet with a high-carbohydrate (starch or sucrose) diet leads to a rapid increase of specific and total sucrase activities (Figs. 1 and 2).

Effects on Lactase

In starved animals, the specific activity of lactase increases (Fig. 1b). This increase is only "apparent" and the total activity of lactase (Fig. 2b) does not change; thus, this effect obviously occurs because of "preservation" of lactase activity together with the loss of other unspecific intestinal proteins.

Whereas during starvation sucrase and lactase activities tend to diverge, changes in the carbohydrate content of isocaloric diets are followed by changes of lactase activity that parallel those of sucrase activity (3,14). Refeeding of starved animals leads to an apparent decrease of specific lactase (Fig. 1b) ac-

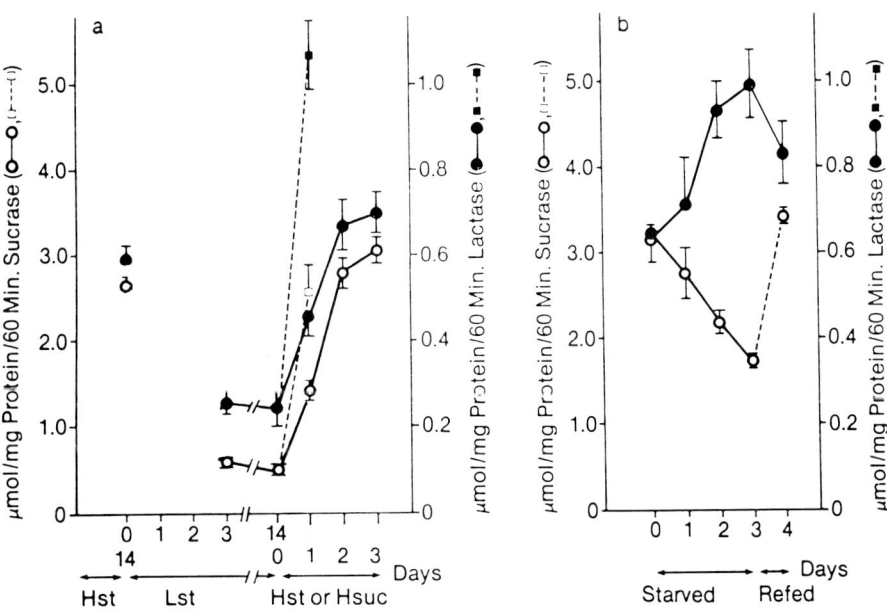

FIG. 1. Effect of variation of carbohydrate intake on the specific activity of sucrase and lactase in adult rat jejunum. **a:** *Symbols not connected,* rats fed 2 weeks a high-starch diet. Animals were then fed 14 days a low-starch high-fat diet (Lst), and then were fed a high-starch low-fat diet (Hst) or a high-sucrose low-fat diet (Hsuc). *Solid line* represents high-starch diet; *broken lines,* sucrose diet. **b:** Rats fed laboratory chow (Lab Blox) were starved for 3 days and then fed for 24 hr a high-sucrose, low-fat diet. Mean (5–6 animals) and 2 SEM are given. (Constructed from data from refs. 3 and 14.)

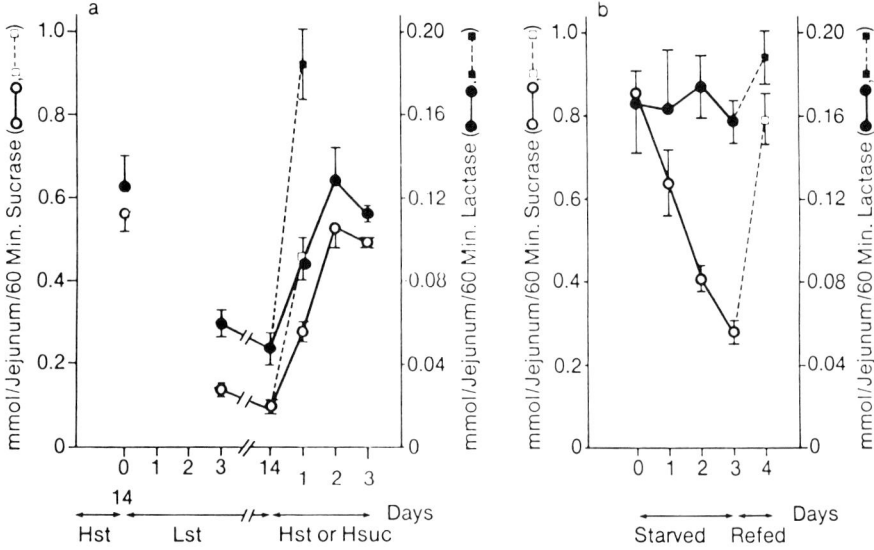

FIG. 2. Effect of variation of carbohydrate intake on the total activity of sucrase and lactase in adult rat jejunum. (Same arrangement as in Fig. 1.)

tivity with no change of total lactase activity (Fig. 2b). Feeding a high-carbohydrate (starch or sucrose) diet to a low-carbohydrate-fed animal leads to an increase of lactase activity parallel to the changes of sucrase activity (specific and total) (Figs. 1a and 2a).

Studies of animals fed isocaloric diets have thus shown a surprising similarity of the reactivity of sucrase and lactase activity in adult rats to the variation of carbohydrate intake. It is noteworthy that the increase of both lactase and sucrase activity is observed in animals fed high-carbohydrate diets containing either sucrose or starch, that is, the variation in lactase activity is independent of lactose, and changes of activity are affected by α-glucosides.

This finding has led to several other experiments testing the specificity of the sugars involved in the increase of these two disaccharidases activities. Ongoing experiments in our laboratory show that both sucrase and lactase activities increase in jejunal homogenates in animals that have been fed a low-carbohydrate diet for 14 days and then switched for the next 24 hr to high-carbohydrate diets containing either sucrose, fructose, galactose, or lactose.

Another large group of experiments explores the *locus where first changes* of enzyme activity on the *villus–crypt columns* are expressed after an introduction of a high-sucrose diet to animals that were previously fed a low-carbohydrate diet. Since the work of Leblond and Stevens (9), it has been recognized that the enterocytes mature both morphologically and biochemically while migrating from the crypts to the villus. Activity of sucrase and lactase is absent from the crypt cells and increases as the enterocytes migrate toward the tip of the villus (2,11). This leads to a logical question: At which level of the villus, that is, at what time during their lifespan, are the enterocytes capable of responding to a dietary change with an alteration in disaccharidase activity? For sucrase this question has recently been explored by two laboratories (12,13). Both studies have shown that in adult rats, when the sucrase activity is lowered by starvation, feeding with sucrose leads to an increase of sucrase activity in the cells of the crypt. The sucrase activity increases as enterocytes move toward the villus tip.

The results of our experiments with starving rats are in agreement with the previously quoted observations, namely, the increase is first seen in cohorts

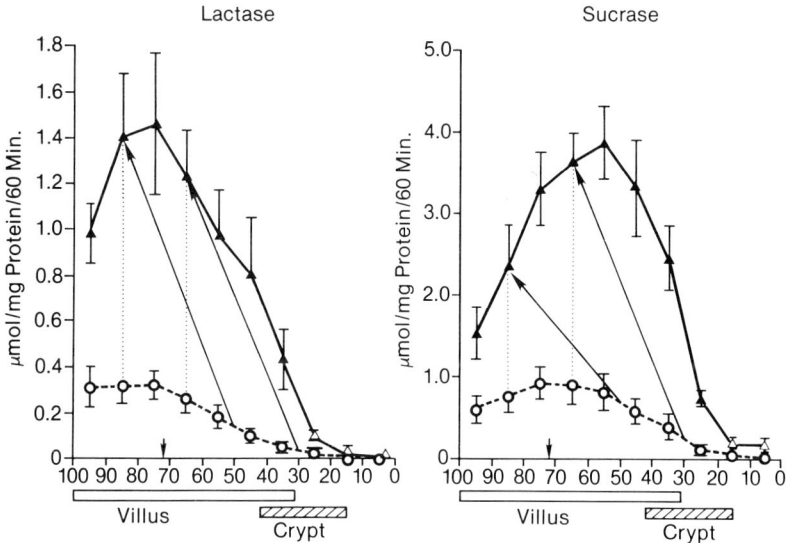

FIG. 3. Lactase and sucrase activity along villus–crypt columns in jejunum of rats that were fed 14 days a low-carbohydrate diet and then for 24 hr a high-sucrose diet. *Abscissa* depicts total height of the intestinal wall with 100% representing the top part of the villus and 0% representing the bottom of the serosal side. Villus and crypt portions are depicted with rectangles; the overlapping area is the crypt–villus transition (mix) zone. Mean and 2 SEM are given; number of animals per group = 5. *Circles,* Control group fed low-starch, high-fat diet; *triangles,* experimental group fed high-sucrose, low-fat diet for 24 hr. *Solid symbols* depict significantly different values from the low-carbohydrate diet group ($p < 0.025$) at the same location. The rate of cell migration within 24 hr was the same in both groups and is indicated by the arrow on the *abscissa.* The *arrows from dotted line to solid line* indicate that the cohorts of cells present at the start of the high-carbohydrate diet at the level of 30% of the height of the intestinal wall (still in crypt) or at the level of 50% (already in villus) migrate to the levels of 65% and 85% of the height, respectively. Comparison thus shows that the increase of sucrase and lactase during migration occurred in enterocytes that were in crypts and also in the lower villus at the time of the introduction of the high-sucrose diet. (Modified from ref. 15.)

of cells that are in the villus–crypt region at the time of beginning of sucrose feeding. A different situation exists in rats where the activity of lactase and sucrase is lowered by feeding a low-carbohydrate diet the preceding two weeks and then switching to a high-sucrose diet. In this case, the sucrase activity is increased *along the entire* height of the villus [i.e., both in the cells that are in the crypts at the time of the start of the new dietary regimen, and in the cells that are "out" of the villus (Fig. 3)]. Lactase activity exhibits a similar change; its activity increases along the entire height of the villus.

CONCLUSION

The data summarized above, as well as other studies from our laboratory (3), clearly show that the activity of sucrase and of lactase depends, in adult rats fed isocaloric diets, on the carbohydrate content of these diets. The effect of carbohydrate intake on sucrase activity is well-established in the literature (1,5,6), but the effect of carbohydrates not containing β-linkage on lactase activity is rather new (3,14,15). Whereas, in the latter case, sucrase and lactase exhibit a close linear correlation (3,14), during short-term starvation they react differently: sucrase activity decreases, but lactase activity does not change.

Feeding starved animals with a high-sucrose diet influences only the sucrase activity of enterocytes present in the crypts. On the other hand, feeding a high-carbohydrate diet to rats previously fed a low-carbohydrate isocaloric diet is followed by an increase of sucrase and lactase activity along the entire height of the villus. Further experiments are needed to analyze the dependency of the reaction of villus cells on the nutrition state of the animal.

The question of functional significance of this dietary manipulation on disaccharidase activity is being explored in studies on absorption capacity of these rats for sucrose and lactose. Furthermore, present studies on adult rats will be followed by studies designed to evaluate the adaptation capability of disaccharidases in suckling rats.

ACKNOWLEDGMENT

This work was supported by NIH grant AM 27624.

REFERENCES

1. Blair, D., Yakimets, W., and Tuba, J. (1963): Rat intestinal sucrase. II. The effect of rat age and sex and of diet on sucrase activity. *Can. J. Biochem. Physiol.,* 41:917.
2. Boyle, J., Celano, P., and Koldovský, O. (1980): Demonstration of a difference in expression of maximal lactase and sucrase activity along the villus in the adult rat jejunum. *Gastroenterology,* 79:503.
3. Bustamante, S., Gasparo, M., Kendall, K., Coates, P., Brown, S., Sonawane, B., and Koldovský, O. (1981): Increased activity of rat intestinal lactase due to increased intake of α-saccharides (starch, sucrose) in isocaloric diet. *J. Nutr.,* 111:943.
4. Dahlqvist, A. (1964): Method for assay of intestinal disaccharidases. *Anal. Biochem.,* 7:18.

5. Deren, J., Broitman, S., and Zamcheck, N. (1967): Effect of diet upon intestinal disaccharidases and disaccharide absorption. *J. Clin. Invest.*, 46:186.
6. Koldovský, O. (1981): Developmental, dietary and hormonal control of intestinal disaccharidases in mammals (including man). In: *Carbohydrate Metabolism and Its Disorders, Vol. 3*, edited by Randle et al., p. 482. Academic Press, New York.
7. Koldovský, O., Asp, N. G., and Dahlqvist, A. (1969): A method for the separate assay of "neutral" and "acid" β-galactosidase in homogenates of rat small-intestinal mucosa. *Anal. Biochem.*, 27:409.
8. Kretchmer, N. (1972): Lactose and lactase. *Sci. Am.*, 227:71.
9. Leblond, C., and Stevens, C. (1948): Constant renewal of intestinal epithelium in albino rat. *Anat. Rec.*, 100:357.
10. Lowry, O., Rosebrough, N., Farr, A., and Randall, R. (1951): Protein measurement with the Folin phenol reagent. *J. Biol. Chem.*, 193:265.
11. Nordström, C., Dahlqvist, A., and Joseffson, L. (1968): Quantitative determination of enzymes in different parts of the villi and crypts of rat small intestine. Comparison of alkaline phosphatase, disaccharidases and dipeptidases. *J. Histochem. Cytochem.*, 15:713.
12. Raul, F., Simon, P., Kedinger, M., Grenier, J., and Haffen, K. (1980): Effect of sucrose refeeding on disaccharidase and aminopeptidase activities of intestinal villus and crypt cells in adult rats. Evidence for a sucrose-dependent induction of sucrase in the crypt cells. *Biochim. Biophys. Acta*, 630:1.
13. Ulshen, M., and Grand, R. (1979): Site of substrate stimulation of jejunal sucrase in the rat. *J. Clin. Invest.*, 64:1097.
14. Yamada, K., Bustamante, S., and Koldovský, O. (1981): Time and dose dependency of intestinal lactase activity in adult rat on starch intake. *Biochim. Biophys. Acta*, 676:108.
15. Yamada, K., Bustamante, S., and Koldovský, O. (1981): Dietary induced rapid increase of rat jejunal sucrase and lactase activity in all regions of the villus. *FEBS Letts.*, 129:89.

DISCUSSION

Dr. Jacquot: Did you measure the actual food intake after changing the diet?
Dr. Koldovský: Yes, we did. The diet is prepared with agar as a caloric diluter.
Dr. Jacquot: So the rats did not change their alimentary habits—they continued eating the foodstuff. The second point I should like to bring up is that I have no idea about the accessibility of lactase as compared to sucrase for pancreatic enzymes. I mean, are they buried in the same way inside the cell membrane or not? I am concerned with the changes in pancreatic exocrine secretion and in changes in the enzymatic digestion of those brush border membranes.
Dr. Kretchmer: I have one statement and one question to make. The statement is related to what Professor Jacquot brought up. I think it is fairly accepted, at least in a hypothetic sense, that pancreatic proteolytic enzymes participate in one or two phases of the biology of the disaccharidases: one phase would probably be the activation of sucrase in the membrane, and the other phase might be the participation of pancreatic enzymes in the degradation of the disaccharidases. The one most studied has been sucrase, lactase being more difficult to study, especially in these age groups that you are dealing with. So that when you manipulate the diet, you have to think of the effects in terms of the two parts of the digestive tract; the effects, whatever they may be, on the degradation or synthesis of a particular disaccharidase or peptidase, or whatever enzyme you want to study, and, two, the effects on the exocrine secretions of the pancreas which might participate in the degradation of the particular enzyme, either slowing it down or speeding it up, which would, of course, affect the activity of the enzyme as you would measure it. It is really, I think, more complex than it is presented.
My question is as follows: one of the conclusions that you gave was that you had evidence to show that the substrate affected the activity—that's what you measured—of the enzyme in the cell after the cell was on the villus, in other words, after the cell had left the crypt. What evidence do you have for that statement?

Dr. Koldovský: The question first. One of the slides (Fig. 3) shows that the changes of intestinal disaccharidases also occur beyond the 24-hr migration point of enterocytes. As I said, using labeled thymidine, we have measured the rate of migration of the enterocytes; in agreement with data in the literature, the migration time from the crypt to villus is around 48 hr. It is not influenced by the dietary manipulations.

As far as your statement is concerned, I will make another statement in answer. I agree with what you and Professor Jacquot have said, but—as I have stressed—we have measured the *activity*. Only further experiments will clarify *what mechanisms* are influencing these changes. The role of pancreatic proteases involved in the regulation of intestinal brush border disaccharidases is quite important [Alpers, D. H., and Tedesco, F. J. (1975): *Biochim. Biophys. Acta,* 401:28]. We tried to minimize their role in our experiments by using diets in which we did not vary the content of the protein. This, of course, does not exclude the possibility that proteases might have been influenced. Therefore, one of the experiments to be done in the near future is a study under conditions that will exclude pancreatic secretion. The question of changes of activity versus changes of amount of enzymes is one which we can actually begin to answer with the results of experiments that we have done in the last year with Sunshine and Tsuboi from Stanford. Using their technique, we have measured immunochemically the amount of these disaccharidases (namely sucrase, lactase and maltase), their synthesis, and compared those with the synthesis of total mucosal protein. Our experiments indicate that the increase of carbohydrate intake is not only reflected in the increase of disaccharidases activities, but also in their rate of synthesis as well as in the amount of specific enzyme protein.

Dr. Strang: It does seem very surprising that these enzymes should respond nonspecifically. Have you tried sugars that are nonmetabolizable—do they have an effect? Have you tried things that are simply an osmotic load or simply something that produces a mechanical effect, like undigestible cellulose?

Dr. Koldovský: Some of the experiments that you are suggesting are those we intend to perform in the near future. At the present time, we have some other supporting data that indicate that this is an effect of sugars. (a) Since the intake of isocaloric low- and high-starch diets by the animals and body weight changes are equal, we are not dealing in these experiments with the effect of caloric deprivation, etc. (b) The animals do not exhibit any diarrhea. (c) Furthermore, we have shown the dose-dependent effect of carbohydrate content of the diets on disaccharidase activity [Yamada et al. (1981): *Biochim. Biophys. Acta,* 676:108]. (d) As far as the sucrase and maltase activity are concerned, the activity changes are in the expected way, that is, the increase of carbohydrate intake is followed by an increase of their activity. (e) The situation which affects the activity of sucrase and lactase differently is starvation. In starved animals the sucrase activity (total and specific) goes down, but lactase activity does not change; (total) specific activity exhibits an increase [Yamada et al. (1983): *Am. J. Physiol.,* 244:G449].

Dr. Greene: I have just been trying to reconcile the data that you presented with the data that Dr. Rosenweig presented in the early 1970s, and I wonder if part of it might not be the method of expression. He expressed his data first in terms of milligrams of protein and decided that this was an inappropriate method of measuring it because of the biopsy technique in which he took various levels of the lamina propria, so that enzyme activity per milligram protein might not have been so much the epithelial cell protein, but many of the supporting structures. For that reason then, when he found no difference in the lactase activity with the various diets, he decided that it might be better to express it in terms of one enzyme activity versus the enzyme that didn't appear to change (in that instance lactase). Most of his data presented thereafter were the sucrase or maltase activity per unit lactase. I wonder, if he had been able to express the data in the same way—that is, per epithelial cell—do you think he would have had the same findings as you showed?

Dr. Koldovský: This question has to be answered in several parts. The first is simple. The Rosenweig data you quoted are on man, and our work is on the rat; so there is one possible difference. Furthermore, the number of volunteers was relatively small. Now let us examine the methodology. First I will speak about our methodology which uses the total intestinal mucosa of intestinal segments (jejunum, ileum). Thus, we can express our data not only per protein, but also as total activity per animal. The range of mean lactase activity was (in the mid-jejunum) in different groups between 0.5 and 1.75 μmoles/mg protein/hr. This range was similar for the activity of sucrase which was 1.5–4.5 μmoles/mg protein/hr [Bustamante et al. (1981): *J. Nutr.,* 111:943]. The degree of correlation between activity of sucrase and lactase in these dietary experiments [Bustamante et al. (1981): *J. Nutr.,* 111:943; Yamada et al. (1981): *Biochim. Biophys. Acta,* 676:108] is very high in all intestinal segments. Second, I stress that when we expressed the data either per protein, per DNA or mucosa wet weight, or per total intestinal mass, we always got the same results. So in our experiments the data are not a result of changes of the denominator, for example, protein. Finally, the data generated together with Sunshine and Tsuboi showing the increase of amount of disaccharidases and their synthesis provide another independent support.

Now, concerning the expression of the data using the ratio of sucrase activity per lactase activity in biopsy specimen: Rosenweig and co-workers assumed that activity of sucrase and lactase are distributed along the height of the villus in a parallel fashion—and this is not true. We have extended in rats [Boyle, Celano, and Koldovský (1980): *Gastroenterology,* 79:503] the original observation on a human biopsy specimen [Nordström and Dahlqvist (1973): *Scand. J. Gastroenterol.,* 8:407] that sucrase to lactase ratio along the height of the villus is not identical. Sucrase activity increases along the height of the villus *earlier* than lactase. Lactase "needs more time" to express its maximal activity. If you have a ratio of sucrase to lactase in the upper villus of about three, then this value is around five in the lower villus [Boyle et al. (1980): *Gastroenterology* 79:503]. The risk involved in expressing sucrase to lactase data in biopsies depends on the fact that activity of sucrase and lactase do not exhibit on all heights of the villus the same ratio.

Dr. Guesry: Since we may expect quite a large change of enzyme activity with a change of diet, do you have any data on much younger animals—suckling rats, weaning rats, or even suckling babies?

Dr. Koldovský: There are several data from the literature. One of them is from Kretchmer's laboratory [Lebenthal, E., Sunshine, P., and Kretchmer, N. (1972): *J. Clin. Invest.,* 51:1244]. The other group that studied this is F. Raul, P. M. Simon, M. Kedinger, J. F. Grenier, and K. Haffen. [*Biol. Neonate* (1978): 33:100]. From their data, the conclusion can be reached that in suckling animals an increased intake of carbohydrates is followed by an increase of the activity of disaccharidases. The question is what are the mechanisms involved; are they the same as in adults or are they different?

Dr. Ransome-Kuti: What I understood is that if you give an experimental rat substance like fructose or sucrose you could increase the activity of lactase. Is this true? Because from all the evidence that we have, we have not been able to increase the activity of lactase in the human being when we have administered lactose itself, so it is a bit puzzling to hear that in adult rats, if you give them a disaccharide which is absolutely unrelated to the enzyme, you could increase the activity of the enzyme. I would like Dr. Koldovský to confirm that this is what he is finding and comment on whether this has got any relationship whatsoever to what we have observed in the human being. I think he must also know about a Thai experiment in which they fed Thai children with milk and some without milk—they did not find any increase in lactase activity after the absorption of lactose by these children.

Dr. Koldovský: According to the literature, lactase is probably an adaptive enzyme in the adult mammals, but the question of the specificity of the substrate that will influence lactase activity is not clear. Experiments have been done so far where the effect on the lactase activity was tested by studying lactose, as a substrate and as an inducer of the activity, and glucose, galactose and sucrose were used as control sugars. In our studies in rats, in adult rats, we have clearly shown that sucrose and starch are equal in their effect on sucrase and lactase activity in animals. The problem that I probably did not state sufficiently is that we are operating, as Dr. Kretchmer also stated, in a range allowed by genetic background or age. For example, in the suckling animal, the specific activity of lactase is between one and two units, and in the adult animal it is between 0.2 and one unit depending on the part of the small intestine and age of the animal that you study. So, within that range, the lactase activity in the adult animal is affected by quantitative changes of carbohydrates—we have clear data on this as far as the effects of sucrose, starch, and glucose are concerned. These are the sugars where we have both quantitative and time-dependent types of responses and these are practically the same. The story is open as far as other monosaccharides which might be affecting this activity. The changes in the sucrase and the lactase activity may be the result of changes of the total glycoprotein synthesis in the small intestine. Maybe the variations of carbohydrate intake affect the total glycoprotein content of the brush border. If we call the changes depending on the intake of some substrate adaptation, we are operating in a given range that is genetically controlled. In other words, this is not an approach that can increase or overcome a genetic deficiency of lactase in mammals, including man.

Dr. Kretchmer: The one question that Dr. Ransome-Kuti asked was what is the functional significance of your findings?

Dr. Koldovský: The enzymatic activity changes in a ratio of 1 to 5, so there probably will be.

Dr. Kretchmer: Yes, but 1 to 5 when you start at a very low level.

Dr. Koldovský: If I change it, for example, for an adult animal, it has 100% activity, and I can vary this from 150% to 30% in that range.

Dr. Kretchmer: So, it is your speculation that there will be a functional effect.

Dr. Guthrie: I think Dr. Ransom-Kuti gave us a very important piece of information. I just would like to ask him if he checked to see if by giving lactose he could induce increased lactase activity in these children.

Dr. Ransome-Kuti: What we found was that by the age of 2 to 4 years, the children in Lagos did have a low lactase activity as shown by lactose tolerance tests. Now, the evidence that the lactase activity could not be increased by giving lactose was established by trying it on our medical students: they were fed lactose for about a month, and they were tested before and after with the lactose tolerance test. We found that they did not reactivate their lactase. Similar experiments have been carried out in Thailand where subjects were also fed milk for very long periods, and we have found that there was no reactivation of lactase activity. Even South African Bantus, who regularly drank milk and were able to tolerate large amounts of milk, were found to have very low lactase activity when they were tested. Of course, there was some type of adaptation going on in these individuals in South Africa, but this adaptation was not as a result of lactase activity in the intestine.

Fetal Forms of Enzymes of Intestinal Brush Border

S. Auricchio

Clinica Pediatrica II Facoltà di Medicina e Chirurgia di Napoli, Naples, Italy

The surface membrane of the small intestine comes into contact with luminal nutrients, organisms, drugs and foreign antigens. The natural frontier between the body and the intestinal content is represented by the glycoproteins of the brush border membrane, which act as receptors, carriers and hydrolytic enzymes. Developmental variability of these glycoproteins may therefore regulate intestinal functions during the first part of life.

In various mammalian species the pre- and postnatal developmental pattern of digestive enzymes has been extensively studied with regard to the level of enzyme activity as well as its distribution along the intestine and along the crypt–villus axis at different ages.

The author has also studied the developmental pattern, in human fetal intestine, of the various brush border peptidases and has found that all brush border peptidases, with the single exception of aminopeptidase A, have already reached the adult stage by the end of the third month of gestation (2).

A further interesting developmental aspect of the intestine involves the presence, during fetal and neonatal life, of brush border enzymes structurally different from those which are present during adult life: these will be indicated as fetal and adult forms of these enzymes, respectively.

The best example of a fetal form of enzyme in human and animal intestine is alkaline phosphatase. The pioneer studies of Moog and his group demonstrated the presence in the duodenum of the mouse of fetal forms of alkaline phosphatase differing from the adult forms as regards kinetic, chromatographic and electrophoretic properties. The adult forms appear in the mouse duodenum during the third postnatal week (13–16).

Various authors have found that in the rat and in the human small intestine the alkaline phosphatase is also different from the adult form because of a quicker anodal electrophoretic mobility, lower isoelectric point and different patterns of enzymatic protein bands (10,12,17,20,23).

The molecular basis of the difference between fetal and adult enzymes is largely unknown. The studies of Moog (14,15) suggest that in the mouse and in the rat alkaline phosphatase differentiation may reflect the posttranslational modification of a core material. The electrophoretic differences between the adult and the fetal enzymes disappear totally in rats, partially or totally in humans after neuraminidase digestion (10,12,17); this suggests that the fetal and adult enzymes differ in their sialic acid content.

A fetal form of γ-glutamyltranspeptidase may be differentiated in the rat intestine from the adult form using the lectin Concanavalin-A, which binds the adult type but not the fetal one (8,9). The binding pattern of glycoproteins to lectins depends on the carbohydrate part of these proteins. Binding of the fetal type to Concanavalin-A was obtained after neuraminidase digestion, this suggesting that in this case also the fetal type is a sialic acid rich enzyme.

A further difference between brush border enzymes of adult and newborn rats is the presence in the ileum of the suckling animal of large quantities of some brush border enzymes in the cytosol as soluble enzymes. This has been demonstrated for the alkaline phosphatase and the glucamylase (4,5,19,24). The soluble enzymes are identical in many enzymatic and immunological aspects with the membrane enzymes, but their carbohydrate content appears to be quite different.

In the human intestine, many enzymes are structurally different during the fetal life and at birth from the adult enzymes. The enzymes the author has studied (1) are sucrase and two peptidases, oligoaminopeptidase and dipeptidyl-aminopeptidase IV. They were solubilized by papain or Triton from brush border prepared from adult intestine or human fetuses during the third month of gestation and from particles obtained from the first meconium of prematures. The oligoaminopeptidase was purified from these meconial particles (3). The human meconium is, in fact, a very good source of oligoaminopeptidase and also contains dipeptidylaminopeptidase and sucrase.

After Triton solubilization and ammonium sulfate precipitation, the enzyme was absorbed on a column of DEAE Sephacel in 5 mM Tris–HCl at pH 8. The column was developed first by changing the pH and a first enzyme was eluted. A second oligoaminopeptidase was eluted by developing the column with a double pH and NaCl gradient. The second enzyme which was still contaminated by the dipeptidylaminopeptidase IV was then further purified; after gel filtration on Sephadex G-200, the separation of the two peptidases was obtained by polyacrylamide gel electrophoresis. A similar procedure may be utilized for the purification of dipeptidylaminopeptidase IV. The final oligoaminopeptidase II showed a specific activity of about 11 units/mg of protein.

The aminopeptidase II was considered pure on the basis of the following criteria:

1. Practically no activity on substrates of other brush border hydrolases.
2. One band of protein on polyacrylamide gel electrophoresis, which was a little bit large but coincident with the band of enzyme activity as revealed by staining on the gel.
3. On isoelectric focusing three bands of proteins, each coincident with a band of enzyme activity: the isoelectric points ranged between 4.9 and 4.5.

The molecular weight on Sephadex G-200 column is approximately 240,000.

The following studies (2,3) on crude fetal and meconial sucrase and peptidases, as well as on the purified oligoaminopeptidase, have demonstrated that these enzymes are different from the adult ones.

1. Polyacrylamide gel electrophoresis and agar gel electrophoresis of papain solubilized meconial and adult enzymes, as well as that of enzymes prepared from brush border of fetal intestine and of purified meconial peptidase, reveal that the fetal and meconial enzymes have a quicker electrophoretic mobility than the adult enzymes; furthermore, this difference is clearly evident in a mixture of fetal and adult enzymes.

2. The meconial and the fetal peptidases have more acidic isoelectric points than the adult peptidases. This confirms that there is a charge difference between adult and fetal human brush border hydrolases.

3. Crossed immunoelectrophoresis of the brush border enzymes of fetuses of 16th week of gestation and the Ouchterlony electrophoresis of adult and fetal enzymes against immunoglobulins of rabbit immunized with adult human brush border membrane demonstrate that the adult and fetal enzymes have the same specific activity as well as immunological similarities (or identity).

4. The pattern of binding of the fetal and meconial enzymes to columns of *Helix pomatia* lectin–Sephadex is quite different from that of the adult enzymes. Most of the meconial and fetal enzymes are not adsorbed, but most of the adult enzymes are adsorbed on the column and eluted by N-acetylgalactosamine. Furthermore, various differences can be demonstrated when meconial and adult enzymes are adsorbed on columns of other lectins, such as Concanavalin-A and lentil–lectin. These results suggest that the charge difference responsible for the difference in the electrophoretic mobility, as well as in the isoelectric point, between adult and fetal enzymes is probably caused, at least in part, by differences in the carbohydrate composition of these glycoproteins.

The observed differences between fetal and adult forms of human brush border enzymes may represent age-dependent variations of the posttranslational modifications of these enzymes. This may be due to changes in the activity of enzymes involved in the intracellular processing of the carbohydrate moiety of these glycoproteins, or to age-dependent variations of luminal agents capable of modifying brush border glycoproteins, such as bacterial glycosidases or pancreatic enzymes.

It is unknown if the presence on the brush border of fetal forms of enzymes has any meaning in terms of gastrointestinal function during the first period of extrauterine life.

As the sucrase and the peptidases (6,11,18,22) protrude into the lumen from the external surface of the brush border membrane, it is possible that the age-dependent variations of the carbohydrate structure of the glycoproteins alter the hydrophylic groups emerging from the bilayer (7).

On the other side, evidence is accumulating that cell surface carbohydrates play a direct role in certain recognition phenomena that occur at the plasma membrane (21).

Alterations of the carbohydrate part of the brush border glycoproteins may therefore not interfere with the digestive properties of this membrane, but may alter their recognition properties, such as those involved in bacterial, or virus, or more generally, antigen enterocyte interaction, as well as absorption and transport functions.

REFERENCES

1. Auricchio, S., Caporale, C., Santamaria, F., and Skovbjerg, H. (1983): "Fetal" forms of oligoaminopeptidase, dipeptidylaminopeptidase IV and sucrase in human intestine and meconium. *J. Pediatr. Gastroenterol. Nutr.* (*in press*).
2. Auricchio, S., Stellato, A., and De Vizia, B. (1981): Development of brush border peptidases in human and rat small intestine during fetal and neonatal life. *Pediatr. Res.*, 15:991–995.
3. Caporale, C., Fontana, P., Fontanella, A., Murolo, E., Santamaria, F., and Auricchio, S.: Isolation and characterization of two particle bound oligoaminopeptidases from human meconium, which are different from the oligoaminopeptidase of the adult small intestine (*in preparation*).
4. Forstner, G., and Forstner, J. (1979): Segmental distribution of soluble neutral maltase activity in suckling rat intestine. *Biochim. Biophys. Acta*, 586:250–257.
5. Galand, G., and Forstner, G. (1974): Soluble neutral and acid maltases in the suckling rat intestine. *Biochem. J.*, 144:281–292.
6. Gitzelmann, R., Bachi, T., Binz, H., Lindenmann, J., and Semenza, G. (1970): Localization of rabbit intestinal sucrase with ferritin–antibody conjugates. *Biochim. Biophys. Acta*, 196:20–28.
7. Jacobs, L. R., and Gray, G. M. (1979): Intestinal brush border membrane proteins. Orientation in intact intestine. *Gastroenterology*, 76:1159 (abstract).
8. Köttgen, E., and Lindinger, G. (1976): Nachweis molekularer varianten der γ-glutamyltransferase mit differenter Concanavalin-A affinität. *Hoppe-Seyler's Z. Physiol. Chem.*, 357:1439–1442.
9. Köttgen, E., Reutter, W., and Gerok, W. (1976): Two different gamma-glutamyl-transferases during development of liver and small intestine: A fetal (sialo-) and an adult (asialo-) glycoptorein. *Biochim. Biophys. Res. Commun.*, 72:61–66.
10. Lafont, J., and Rozière, J. (1973): Heterogeneity dependent on age of intestinal alkaline phosphatase in the rat. *Comp. Biochem. Physiol.*, 54b:135–143.
11. Louvard, D., Maroux, S., and Desnuelle, P. (1975): Topological studies on the hydrolases bound to the intestinal brush border membrane. II. Interactions of free and bound aminopeptidase with a specific antibody. *Biochim. Biophys. Acta*, 389:389–400.
12. Miki, K., Suzuki, H., Inio, S., Hoda, T., Hirano, K., and Sugiura, M. (1977): Human fetal intestinal alkaline phosphatase. *Clin. Chim. Acta*, 79:21–30.
13. Moog, F. (1961): Regional differences in the alkaline phosphatases of the small intestine of the mouse from birth to one year. *Dev. Biol.*, 3:153–174.
14. Moog, F. (1964): Intestinal phosphatase activity: Acceleration of increase by puromycin and actinomycin. *Science*, 144:441–446.
15. Moog, F. (1966): The regulation of alkaline phosphatase activity in the duodenum of the mouse from birth to maturity. *J. Exp. Zool.*, 161:353–386.
16. Moog, F., Etzler, M. E., and Grey, R. D. (1969): The differentiation of alkaline phosphatase in the small intestine. *Ann. N.Y. Acad. Sci.*, 166:447–461.
17. Mulivor, R. A., Hannig, V. L., and Harris, H. C. (1978): Developmental change in human intestinal alkaline phosphatase. *Proc. Natl. Acad. Sci. USA*, 8:3909–3912.
18. Nishi, Y., and Takesue, Y. (1975): Localization of rabbit intestinal sucrase on the microvilli membrane with nonlabeled antibodies. *J. Electron. Microsc.*, 24:203–213.

19. Seetharam, B., Yeh, K. Y., Moog, F., and Alpers, D. H. (1977): Development of intestinal brush border membrane proteins in the rat. *Biochim. Biophys. Acta,* 470:424–436.
20. Simon, P. M., Kedinger, M., Raul, F., Grenier, J. M., and Haffen, K. (1979): Developmental pattern of rat intestinal brush border enzymatic proteins along the villus–crypt axis. *Biochem. J.,* 178:407–413.
21. Stanley, P., and Sudo, T. (1981): Microheterogeneity among carbohydrate structure at the cell surface may be important in recognition phenomena. *Cell,* 23:763–769.
22. Takesue, Y., and Nishi, Y. (1978): Topographical studies on intestinal microvillus leucine-β-naphthylamidase on the outer membrane surface. *J. Membr. Biol.,* 39:285–296.
23. Uezato, T., Ohta, H., and Fujita, M. (1981): Developmental change in rat intestinal alkaline phosphatase. *J. Biochem. Int.,* 2:561–566.
24. Young, G. P., Yedlin, S. T., and Alpers, D. H. (1981): Distribution of soluble and membranous forms of alkaline phosphatase in the small intestine of the rat. *Biochim. Biophys. Acta,* 676:257–265.

DISCUSSION

Dr. Kretchmer: Can you estimate the molecular weight of the fetal sucrase versus the molecular weight of the adult sucrase?

Dr. Auricchio: We have not measured the molecular weight of the fetal sucrase, because we were interested in the purification of peptidase. We measured the molecular weight of the three forms of oligoaminopeptidase, the fetal forms, 1 and 2, and the adult form: they all have the same molecular weight.

Dr. Metcalf: Do you have any idea of the ontogeny of the fetal form with respect to gestational age?

Dr. Auricchio: We found fetal forms of enzymes in the meconium and in the small-intestinal mucosa of fetuses during the third month of gestation. We have not examined older fetuses. We suppose that these forms are present in the brush border up to birth.

Dr. Colony: Were you not surprised that the forms you found in the meconium were comparable to those which you found in the epithelium, considering the presence of so many hydrolitic enzymes in the meconium itself?

Dr. Auricchio: We have studied enzymes of meconium: these have the same electrophoretic mobility and the same binding pattern to lectin of fetal brush border enzymes. This does not mean that they have identical structures.

Nutritional Adaptation of the Gastrointestinal Tract of the Newborn, edited by N. Kretchmer and A. Minkowski. Nestlé, Vevey/Raven Press, New York © 1983.

Influence of Lymphocytes and of Cell-Mediated Immunity on the Epithelial Cell Kinetics in the Intestine

Anne Ferguson, Allan McI. Mowat, and Stephan Strobel

Gastrointestinal Unit, Western General Hospital and University of Edinburgh, Edinburgh EH4, United Kingdom

Ontogeny of the intestinal immune system is relevant to infant nutrition in many ways. Not only are lymphocytes and lymphoid tissues integral components of the stomach, small intestine, and colon, but immune responses in these organs also influence the nature of the commensal gut flora, confer protective immunity against pathogenic microorganisms and parasites, and contribute, via hypersensitivity mechanisms, to intestinal diseases, including malabsorption. Studies of human neonatal intestinal immunology have not been performed, and, indeed, clinical investigation of the gastrointestinal lymphoid apparatus in man has been confined almost exclusively to studies of secretory antibodies and to counts of mucosal lymphoid cells. We have directed our attention to the lymphocytes of the small intestine, and to induction of cell-mediated immunity (CMI) in the intestinal mucosa. To date, most of their research has been performed in experimental animals. This chapter briefly reviews recent information on the nature of mucosal T-cells and their traffic and on the effects of a mucosal CMI reaction on the small intestinal epithelium. It also outlines a hypothesis of the various roles which mucosal T-cells may play in gastrointestinal physiology and pathology.

T-LYMPHOCYTES IN THE INTESTINES

There are T-lymphocytes in the organized gut-associated lymphoid tissues, such as Peyer's patches and mesenteric lymph nodes (MLNs) and many T-cells are scattered within the mucosae of the gastrointestinal tract.

Peyer's Patch Lymphocytes

The majority of Peyer's patch T-cells are present in the thymus-dependent areas under the epithelium and around the post-capillary venules. Studies of

---

Dr. Mowat's current address is Department of Bacteriology and Immunology, Western Infirmary, Glasgow, U. K.

lymphocyte traffic, which involve tracing of isotope-labeled lymphocytes by autoradiography and liquid scintillation counting, show that there is a traffic of small T-lymphocytes from blood to the thymus-dependent areas of Peyer's patches, but that small T-lymphocytes do not enter the mucosa (21). It is still not known whether or not there are two distinct pools of recirculating small T-lymphocytes, intestinal and peripheral. Certainly, gut-associated immune reactions often occur independently of systemic immunity, but the cellular basis of this may be the separate traffic of intestinal and peripheral activated T lymphoblasts rather than of small T-cells.

Mucosal T-Cells

Lymphocytes, mainly medium-sized, are found within the epithelium (intraepithelial, IE lymphocytes) (4) as well as in the lamina propria of the gut (LP lymphocytes). Although the small-intestinal mucosa has been most extensively studied, similar IE and LP lymphocytes are present, although in smaller numbers, in gastric and colonic mucosae. The first evidence that many of these mucosal lymphocytes are thymus-dependent came from the findings of low IE lymphocyte counts in animals depleted of T-cells in various ways (7,9). Recent work, in rodents and in man, using antisera directed against T-cell antigenic determinants, has confirmed that most IE lymphocytes are T-cells (10,14,24). By using the OKT antiserum, the majority of IE T-lymphocytes have been found to be of the suppressor/cytotoxic phenotype (staining with OKT8 antiserum) (23).

Studies of lymphocyte traffic have shown that, just as in the case of B-cells, T-immunoblasts derived from lymph or from MLNs home to the gut mucosa, where most can later be identified as IE cells (10). Further, elegant experiments involving local irradiation of Peyer's patches or MLNs have confirmed that the route of T-cell traffic is from Peyer's patches via MLN and lymph back to the IE site in the small intestinal mucosa (14).

An important additional source of T-cells in the gut has been demonstrated by Rose and her colleagues (22) in their studies of T-immunoblast migration. They found that in normal animals mesenteric T-immunoblasts migrated back to the intestine, and peripheral T-immunoblasts migrated to inflamed peripheral tissues. However, peripheral T-immunoblasts were also found to home to the gut, but only if it was the site of inflammation, for example, as a result of infection with a nematode. Thus, it is likely that in situations of intestinal inflammation components of the systemic immune apparatus, such as serum proteins, may gain access to mucosal tissues, and local disease will also lead to recruitment of systemic T-lymphocytes into the gut.

ANIMAL MODELS OF INTESTINAL MUCOSAL CMI

The small-intestinal mucosa is a continuously changing organ, and, in addition to the considerable amounts of fluid which cross the epithelium in both directions, the epithelial and connective tissue cells are regularly renewed by cell division in the crypts and exfoliation from the surface. Since CMI reactions take a day or more to evolve, it could be argued that conditions will rarely be appropriate for a CMI reaction to occur in this organ. However, the authors and others have successfully produced mucosal CMI reactions in a number of experimental situations, including graft-versus-host (GvH) disease, rejection of transplanted allografts of intestine, parasite infections (comparing normal and T-cell depleted hosts), and, recently, mucosal challenge with antigen in animals immunized orally or systemically.

The primary objective of our series of experiments in animals has been to establish the features of intestinal pathology and/or changes in function which mark the presence of a local CMI reaction, and which can allow measurement of the magnitude of a CMI reaction in experimental conditions and in man.

Effects of Allograft Rejection on Small-Intestinal Mucosa

The models which we have studied most thoroughly have been rejection of heterotransplanted grafts of fetal intestine in mice, and GvH disease in adult and neonatal F_1 mice. Experiments with mice which have been thymectomized, irradiated, and bone marrow reconstituted (8) and studies of the humoral immune response to allografts of fetal small intestine (3) confirm that the tissue damage in allograft rejection is thymus-dependent and cell-mediated. The effects of allograft rejection on the small-intestinal mucosa have been studied by conventional histopathology with subjective grading of the abnormality, by morphometry of paraffin sections, and by counts of IE lymphocytes. We have also used a stathmokinetic technique to measure crypt cell production rate and scanning and transmission electron microscopy to study epithelial changes (5,8,11,12).

The sequence of events observed in small-intestinal allograft rejection are infiltration of the LP by lymphocytes, which are also found within the epithelium; greatly increased mitotic activity in the epithelial cells of the crypts of Lieberkuhn with, later, flattening of the villi, exfoliation of surface enterocytes, and, finally, ulceration and destruction of the mucosa. The pathology of allograft rejection is very similar to that of the jejunal mucosa in celiac disease, and in helminth parasite infections of man and animals.

By using various strain combinations, and neonatal and adult hosts, a spectrum of intestinal pathology (as assessed subjectively) has been demonstrated, ranging from apparently completely normal histology to subtotal villous atrophy with crypt hyperplasia (Table 1). However, studies of the cytokinetics of the absorptive epithelium (the technique used involved injection of colchicine to block mitosis in metaphase, microdissection, measurements of villi and crypts, and counts of crypt metaphases) (12) have shown that even when conventional histological appearances are normal, there is an increase in ep-

TABLE 1. *Subjective grading of small-intestinal pathology in animal models of CMI in the small-intestinal mucosa*

Model	Strains	Pathology of small intestine[a]	
		(1 week)	(2 weeks)
Rejection of heterotopically transplanted allograft	CBA–BALB/c	SVA	Destroyed
Rejection of heterotopically transplanted allograft	CBA–C3H	Normal	PVA
GvH disease (neonatal host)	CBA–C3H	PVA	PVA
GvH disease (adult host)	CBA–BALB/c		Normal
GvH disease (adult host)	CBA–C3H		Normal

[a] PVA, partial villous atrophy with crypt hyperplasia; SVA, subtotal villous atrophy with crypt hyperplasia.

ithelial cell proliferation rate, accompanied by increased lymphocyte infiltrate of the tissue, the two features which are found in the early stages of allograft rejection.

Evolution of Intestinal Mucosal Changes in GvH Reaction

A series of experiments have been conducted in order to define the speed of onset of effects on epithelial cell kinetics in the graft–versus–host reaction (GvHR) and, further, to examine the hypothesis that mucosal changes occur by direct effect of T-cells on the crypts rather than via preliminary damage to villus cells (6,16,18). A GvHR was induced in neonatal F_1 hybrid mice (CBA $\times$ BALB/c)F_1, by intraperitoneal injection of spleen cells from adult CBA strain mice. Control littermates were injected with either F_1 spleen cells or medium alone. GvHR was induced between 5 and 7 days after birth, and, at intervals after transfer of parental cells, recipient mice were killed, weighed, their spleens removed and weighed, and the magnitude of the GvHR measured by a spleen index, being mean relative spleen weight (mg/10 g body weight) in GvHR mice divided by mean relative spleen weight in controls (Fig. 1). Measurements of jejunal villi and crypts were performed in Feulgen-stained preparations, by a microdissection technique, and crypt cell production rate by a stathmokinetic technique using colchicine. Tissue was also processed for routine histological examination and IE lymphocyte counts carried out on H & E stained sections; mucosal mast cell counts were performed in Carnoy-fixed, astra blue safranin-stained sections. Groups of animals were studied between one and 62 days after induction of GvHR.

There was no reduction in villus length in animals with GvHR; however, both crypt length (Fig. 2) and crypt cell production rate increased significantly within 3 days of induction of the GvHR, and there was significant correlation between crypt length and spleen index ($r = 0.76$, $p < 0.01$) and between cell production rate and spleen index ($r = 0.74$, $p < 0.01$). IE lymphocyte count

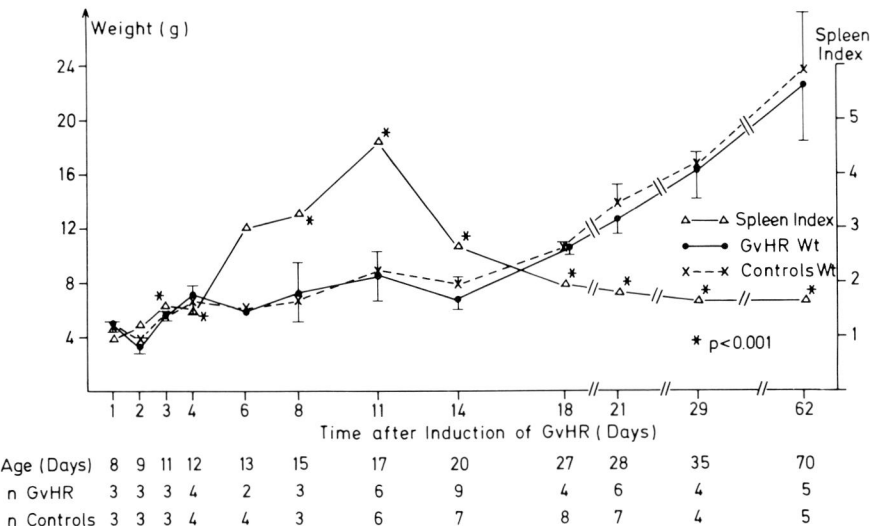

FIG. 1. Progress of the GvHR in neonatal CBA × BALB/c F_1 mice. Spleen indices in mice with GvHR, and growth rates of GvHR and control mice. Bars represent mean ± 1 SD. The *lower panel* gives details of the number of mice per group and age at time of death. (From Mowat et al., ref. 18, with permission.)

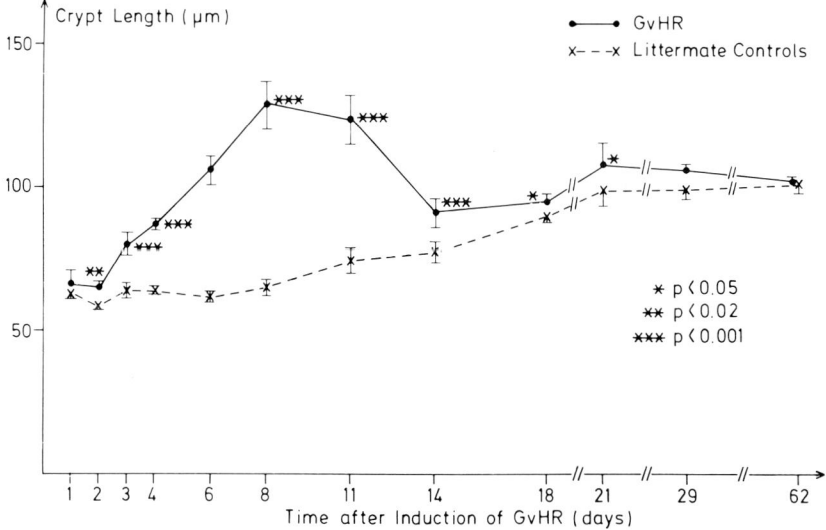

FIG. 2. Crypt lengths in neonatal CBA × BALB/c F_1 mice with GvHR and in littermate controls, at intervals after transfer of parental cells. Mean ± 1 SD for each age group. (From Mowat et al., ref. 18, with permission.)

(Fig. 3) was also significantly correlated with spleen index ($r = 0.86$, $p < 0.01$) but the mucosal mast cell count, although it did rise, did not parallel the GvHR.

Phases of Intestinal Mucosal CMI Reactions

The experiments reported above confirm our previous hypothesis that both crypt cell production rate and the IE lymphocyte count provide evidence, in animal experiments, of a local CMI reaction. We have suggested that these features, when found in a jejunal biopsy from a patient with intestinal infection or inflammatory disease, may indicate that T-cell-mediated responses are taking place within the mucosa.

It is clear that the effects of local CMI reactions on epithelial cell kinetics occur in two stages (6):

Phase 1 appears normal to conventional histopathological examination, for the villi are of normal length, but there is an increase in mitotic activity of the crypts, and, when compared with normals, the enterocytes move more rapidly up the sides of the villi and have a shorter lifespan.

Phase 2 crypt hyperplasia persists with a high mitotic rate, but villi are short or absent, and, on the basis of electron microscopic studies of the enterocytes (5), it seems likely that this effect is due, not to direct damage of villus entero-

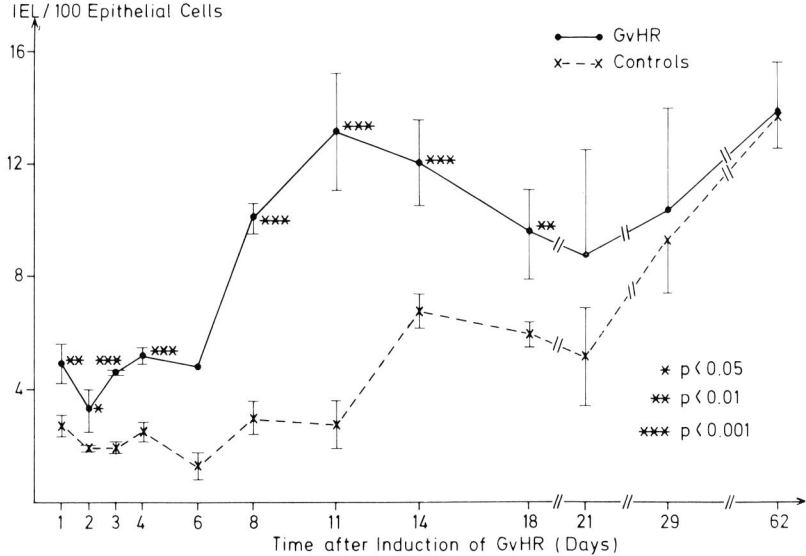

FIG. 3. IE lymphocyte counts in neonatal CBA × BALB/c F_1 mice with GvHR and in littermate controls. Mean ± 1 SD for each age group. (From Mowat et al., ref. 18, with permission.)

cytes, but to an effect of the underlying immune reaction on the adhesion of epithelial cells to one another and to the underlying tissues.

Mechanism of T-Cell-Mediated Damage to the Intestine

The traffic of activated T-cells from Peyer's patches via lymph back to the intestinal mucosa has been discussed above. Thus, within a few days of the ingestion of a new antigen, or infection of the intestinal mucosa with a newly encountered agent, the potential for any of a variety of T-cell-mediated immune reactions will be presented within the mucosa. As illustrated in Fig. 4, there are a number of ways in which the presence of antigen, together with the presence of a population of antigen-specific T-cells, could lead to mucosal damage. These include the spectrum of antibody-mediated immune reactions (including reaginic hypersensitivity and immune complex hypersensitivity) via helper T-cell effects; direct cytotoxicity due to cytotoxic T-cells in the LP or epithelium; and/or the effect of various humoral factors secreted by activated T-lymphocytes, lymphokines. Although we by no means exclude cytotoxic T-cell effects, and effects of humoral antibody, we consider that there is now good evidence that the features of intestinal mucosal damage described above are the result of secretion of lymphokines by activated T-cells, rather than by direct cytotoxicity. We initially made these proposals in view of the absence of evidence of cytotoxicity by the IE lymphocytes, as assessed by electron microscopy. However, support for the existence of humoral enteropathic factors in GvH disease has been provided by the work of Elson et al. (2). These workers produced GvH disease in mice, the animals previously having had implants of fetal small intestine. The objective of their experiments was to determine whether the intestine was injured in the GvHR as a direct antigenic target of immunocompetent cells or as an "innocent bystander" to the donor-

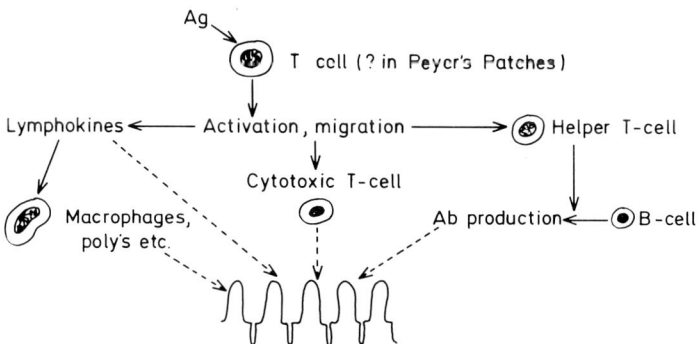

FIG. 4. Possible mechanisms for T-cell-mediated intestinal mucosal damage—including direct cytotoxicity, enteropathic lymphokines, and antibody-mediated hypersensitivity, indirectly induced via helper T-cells.

TABLE 2. Effects of GvHR on intestinal tissues of CBA × BALB/c F_1 mice with heterotopic grafts of intestine

Experimental group	Tissue	Villus height (μm)	Crypt mitoses (per hr; mean)	IEL count (per 100 enterocytes; mean)
Control (F_1 cells)	Host jejunum	484.5	6.1	9.9
GvH (CBA cells)	Host jejunum	536.1	10.6 ($p < 0.02$)	16.0 ($p < 0.001$)
Control (F_1 cells)	Grafted small intestine	288.5	3.1	3.7
GvH (CBA cells)	F_1 graft	284.7	8.6 ($p < 0.01$)	6.9 ($p < 0.001$)
	CBA graft	290.3	6.2 ($p < 0.05$)	7.2 ($p < 0.001$)

host lymphoid interaction. Results of their experiments supported the latter explanation.

We tested our hypothesis that mitotic activity of the crypts of Lieberkuhn and infiltration of the tissue with lymphocytes were markers of the presence of CMI in the intestinal mucosa by using Elson's graft-versus-host model (16). The protocol is outlined in Table 2. Both CBA × C3H and CBA × BALB/c strain combinations were examined, and similar results were obtained for both. Heterotopic grafts of fetal small intestine were transplanted under the kidney capsules of adult F_1 hosts. In half of the animals, the transplanted tissue was F_1 fetal gut, and, in the others, transplanted tissue was of the parental strain CBA. Four weeks later GvHR was induced in the hosts by the intraperitoneal injection of 60×10^6 CBA spleen cells. Two weeks later the animals were injected with colchicine, killed at intervals over the next 2 hr, and measurements made of mucosal structure and epithelial cell proliferation in the crypts of Lieberkuhn, together with counts of IE lymphocytes. Measurements of spleen weight confirmed the presence of GvH disease in the adult F_1 hosts. Results for the CBA × BALB/c strain combination are summarized in Table 2. Subjective examination of intestinal histology in the host intestine showed no difference between controls and GvH animals. Objective measurements, however, confirmed that, although villus height was similar in the two groups, crypt cell production rate and IE lymphocyte count were both significantly higher in the GvH animals when compared with the controls.

Studies of the grafts showed that, as in previous experiments, villus height and IE lymphocyte counts were lower in isografts than in normally sited intestine, but, in both types of grafts implanted in animals with GvH reaction, crypt cell production rate and IE lymphocyte count were significantly higher than for isografts. Thus, in a GvH reaction induced in CBA × BALB/c F_1 hosts by the injection of CBA cells, crypt hyperplasia and IE lymphocyte infiltration have been produced in a graft of CBA fetal intestine. These results confirm the "innocent bystander" phenomenon in this GvH disease model and support the hypothesis that crypt cell production and IE lymphocyte counts are markers of this local CMI reaction.

INDUCTION OF INTESTINAL CMI TO A FED ANTIGEN

Tolerance and Suppressor Mechanisms

Feeding of antigen induces a secretory antibody response, but little is known of the factors which will induce CMI to fed antigens. We failed in a number of previous attempts to induce CMI to fed antigens using a variety of antigen dosage, regimes, and routes of administration. In retrospect, these failures can be explained by recent evidence that oral administration of antigen induces the specific immune reaction of tolerance for CMI as well as humoral immunity (15). The fact that feeding of protein antigen to mice results in reduced humoral

TABLE 3. Effects of mucosal immune reaction to ovalbumin on intestinal tissues

Induction	Challenge	Migration index for MLN cells[a]	Villus height (μm)	Crypt mitoses (per hr)	IEL count (per 100 enterocytes)
Cyclophosphamide	—	1.12	680.7	6.6	15.8
Ovalbumin, 2 mg	Ovalbumin 0.1 mg (×10)	1.00	638.8	8.4	14.5
Cyclophosphamide	Ovalbumin 0.1 mg (×10)	0.63 ($p < 0.01$)	686.5	12.0[a] ($p = 0.025$)	25.9[a] ($p < 0.005$)

[a] Cultured in presence of 1 mg/ml ovalbumin. As positive control popliteal and auxiliary LN cells from animals immunized by footpad injection were similarly studied; these gave migration index of 0.70.

and CMI responses when that antigen is subsequently presented is probably associated with the ability of the gut-associated lymphoid tissues to generate suppressor T-cells in response to orally administered antigen (13,20).

We have, by using BALB/c mice, confirmed the results of others that prefeeding of mice with ovalbumin subsequently renders the mice tolerant to induction both of humoral and CMI responses to ovalbumin when given parenterally. We reasoned that if we treated animals with an agent which reduced or eliminated suppressor cell activity, it might be possible to alter the nature of the immune response to fed antigen, and thereby induce CMI. Administration of cyclophosphamide to mice in the dose of 100 mg/kg enhances CMI reactions via suppressor cell inhibition without an appreciable effect on antibody synthesis (1), so we used the following regime. BALB/c mice were treated with cyclophosphamide alone (100 mg/kg), oral ovalbumin alone (2 mg), or cyclophosphamide followed by oral ovalbumin. Four weeks later they were challenged with ovalbumin in drinking water at a dose of 0.1 mg daily for 10 days. At the end of this time the animals were killed and, in some, evidence of gut-associated CMI to ovalbumin was sought by using direct migration inhibition of MLN cells in the presence of ovalbumin (19), whereas in others crypt cell production rate and IE lymphocyte counts were made (17) to measure the mucosal CMI reaction. Results are summarized in Table 3. It can be seen that, with the migration inhibition technique, the positive control of draining lymph nodes from mouse footpad showed significant migration inhibition; animals which had been fed ovalbumin alone, or which had been given cyclophosphamide alone, had no significant migration inhibition, but the combination of cyclophosphamide and ovalbumin resulted in the presence of lymphoid cells, positive in the test described, in the MLNs. Furthermore, significant changes in crypt cell production rate and IE lymphocyte counts were obtained only in the cyclophosphamide/ovalbumin group.

These preliminary experiments indicate that there is probably a spectrum in the CMI reaction to dietary antigens which ranges from the induction of a population of sensitized T-cells, on the one hand, to the induction of specific tolerance, associated with a population of suppressor cells, on the other. This and similar animal models should allow elucidation of the factors which influence mucosal CMI responses and may be of value in establishing the pathogenesis of food allergic diseases.

ACKNOWLEDGMENTS

We acknowledge the skilled technical help of the staff of the Animal Unit, Western General Hospital, Edinburgh. This work has been supported by grants from the Medical Research Council of the U. K. and the Deutsche Forschungsgemeinschaft. Dr. Mowat was in receipt of the Allan Fellowship of the University of Edinburgh.

REFERENCES

1. Askenase, P. W., Hayden, B. J., and Gershon, R. K. (1975): Augmentation of delayed type hypersensitivity by doses of cyclophosphamide which do not affect antibody responses. *J. Exp. Med.,* 141:697–702.
2. Elson, C. O., Reilly, R. W., and Rosenberg, I. H. (1977): Small-intestinal injury in the GvHR: An innocent bystander phenomenon. *Gastroenterology,* 72:886–889.
3. Elves, M. W., and Ferguson, A. (1975): Effects of local hypersensitivity reactions in the small intestine. I. Thymus dependence of experimental "partial villous atrophy". *Gut,* 16:114–117.
4. Ferguson, A. (1977): Intraepithelial lymphocytes of the small intestine. *Gut,* 18:921–937.
5. Ferguson, A., Carr, K. E., MacDonald, T. T., and Watt, C. (1978): Hypersensitivity reactions in the small intestine. 4. Influence of allograft rejection on small intestinal mucosal architecture: a scanning and transmission electron microscope study. *Digestion,* 18:56–63.
6. Ferguson, A., and MacDonald, T. T. (1977): Effects of local delayed hypersensitivity on the small intestine. In: *Ciba Foundation Symposium No. 46,* pp. 305–327. Elsevier North-Holland, Amsterdam.
7. Ferguson, A., and Parrott, D. M. V. (1972): Growth and development of "antigen-free" grafts of foetal mouse intestine. *J. Pathol.,* 106:95–101.
8. Ferguson, A., and Parrott, D. M. V. (1973): Histopathology and time-course of rejection of allografts of mouse small intestine. *Transplantation,* 15:546–554.
9. Fichtelius, K. E., Yunis, E. J., and Good, R. A. (1968): Occurrence of lymphocytes within the gut epithelium of normal and neonatally thymectomised mice. *Proc. Soc. Exp. Biol. Med.,* 128:185–188.
10. Guy-Grand, D., Griscelli, C., and Vassalli, P. (1974): The gut-associated lymphoid system: Nature and properties of the large dividing cells. *Eur. J. Immunol.,* 4:435–443.
11. MacDonald, T. T., and Ferguson, A. (1976): Hypersensitivity reactions in the small intestine. 2. Effects of allograft rejection on mucosal architecture and lymphoid cell infiltrate. *Gut,* 17:81–91.
12. MacDonald, T. T., and Ferguson, A. (1977): Hypersensitivity reactions in the small intestine. 3. The effects of allograft rejection and of graft-versus-host disease on epithelial cell kinetics. *Cell Tissue Kinet.,* 10:301–312.
13. Mattingly, J. A., and Waksman, B. H. (1978): Immunologic suppression after oral administration of antigen. 1. Specific suppressor cells formed in rat Peyer's patches after oral administration of sheep red cells, and their systemic migration. *J. Immunol.,* 121:1878–1883.
14. Meuwissen, S. G. M., Feltkamp-Vroom, T. M., de la Riviere, A. B., von den Borne, A. E. G. K., and Tytgat, G. N. (1976): Analysis of the lymphoplasmacytic infiltrate in Crohn's disease with special reference to identification of lymphocyte sub-populations. *Gut,* 17:770–780.
15. Miller, S., and Hanson, D. (1979): Inhibition of specific immune responses by feeding protein antigens. IV. Evidence for tolerance and specific active suppression of cell-mediated immune responses to ovalbumin. *J. Immunol.,* 123:2344–2350.
16. Mowat, A. McI., and Ferguson, A. (1981): Hypersensitivity reactions in the small intestine. 6. Pathogenesis of the graft-versus-host reaction in the small intestinal mucosa. *Transplantation,* 32:238–243.
17. Mowat, A. McI., and Ferguson, A. (1981): Hypersensitivity reactions in the small intestine. 5. Induction of cell-mediated immunity to a dietary antigen. *Clin. Exp. Immunol.,* 43:574–582.
18. Mowat, A. McI., and Ferguson, A. (1982): Intraepithelial lymphocyte count and crypt hyperplasia measure the mucosal component of the graft-versus-host reaction in mouse small intestine. *Gastroenterology,* 83:417–423.
19. Mowat, A. McI., and Ferguson, A. (1982): Migration inhibition of lymph node lymphocytes as an assay for regional cell mediated immunity in the intestinal lymphoid tissues of mice immunised orally with ovalbumin. *Immunology,* 47:365–370.
20. Ngan, J., and Kind, L. S. (1978): Suppressor T cells for IgE and IgG in Peyer's patches of mice made tolerant by the oral administration of ovalbumin. *J. Immunol.,* 120:861–865.
21. Parrott, D. M. V., and Ferguson, A. (1974): Selective migration of lymphocytes within the mouse small intestine. *Immunology,* 26:571–588.

22. Rose, N. L., Parrott, D. M., and Bruce, R. G. (1976): Migration of lymphoblasts to the small intestine. II. Divergent migration of mesenteric and peripheral immunoblasts to sites of inflammation—the mouse. *Cell. Immunol.,* 27:36–46.
23. Selby, W. S., Janossy, G., Goldstein, G., and Jewell, D. P. (1981): T lymphocyte subsets in human intestinal mucosa. *Clin. Exp. Immunol.,* 44:453–458.
24. Selby, W. S., Janossy, G., and Jewell, D. P. (1981): Immunohistological characterisation of intraepithelial lymphocytes of the human gastrointestinal tract. *Gut,* 22:169–176.

DISCUSSION

Dr. Guesry: It seems that the permeability of the gut to food antigen is increased in premature babies—and it also seems that they don't react as much as normal babies would. Do you think that this could be explained by a defect in the helper T-cells, or by some kind of immunological defect due to immaturity?

Dr. Ferguson: I am not as persuaded as you are of the evidence that there truly is increased permeability of the gut in the neonate. After all, the amount of antigen which reaches the intestine is profoundly influenced by nonimmunological factors, such as gastric acid. Animal experiments show that achlorhydria enormously increases the amount of antigen which reaches the small intestine. Furthermore, the mere existence of permeability to protein is not necessarily the cause of hypersensitivity diseases. We all experience continuous penetration of small amounts of protein across the intestinal epithelium to reach the immune system. The net effect of this on helper and suppressor mechanisms is likely to be influenced in part by the amount of protein, but also by its immunochemical nature. For example, the presence or absence of aggregation, whether the antigen is monovalent or multivalent. So the normal neonate may be protected from harmful effects of antigen absorption because it has not yet acquired helper T-cells for cell-mediated immunity. It does seem that in the first year of life suppressor mechanisms are likely to be very important in modulation of the immune response, so that perhaps relative deficiency of suppressor mechanisms is the explanation for milk protein sensitivity in infants. Older children and adults not only have a more mature digestive apparatus, but also are likely to have several suppressor mechanisms which regulate this important homeostatic property of the gut immune system.

Dr. Arnaud-Battandier: Do you think that the secretion of soluble factors, lymphokines, is a specialized function of the IE lymphocytes, or is it a property of T-cells in general, those confined to the LP, or even those in Peyer's patches?

Dr. Ferguson: I do not think IE lymphocytes are the cells responsible for the phenomena which we have shown. IE lymphocytes comprise at least two populations, and one group may not even be T-cells, for there is some evidence, including your own work, which shows them to be natural killer cells. Nevertheless, some IE lymphocytes have surface markers which suggest they are the suppressor/cytotoxic phenotype. In man, T-cells with the helper surface markers appear to be mainly in the LP, so that even within the intestinal mucosa there is a segregation of different T-cell subclasses. We think that the T-cells in the LP, clustered around the crypts, are likely to be those involved in T-cell hypersensitivity. As for the nature and function of cells within the epithelium, a great many groups are studying these. We have suggested that the function of IE lymphocytes may indeed be inertia, protecting the 30 μm deep layer lining the intestinal mucosa from harmful hypersensitivity reactions. [Mowat, A. M., and Ferguson, A. (1981): Induction and expression of mucosal cell-mediated immunity. In: *Current Topics in Veterinary Medicine and Animal Science,* edited by F. J. Bourne, pp. 107–129. Martinus Nijhoff, London.]

Dr. Arnaud-Battandier: I agree with you that probably many IE lymphocytes are not T-cells and that other populations are likely also to be present.

Dr. Sunshine: When you found crypt hyperplasia, was there also an increase in intestinal secretion? I have been bothered for a long time that in situations where there is crypt hyperplasia, there also seems to be an increase in the intestinal secretion going along with it.

Dr. Ferguson: I have not measured enzymes or transport function in these experimental models. Certainly we have confirmed our results by the stathmokinetic technique by limited experiments using autoradiography. Delphine Guy-Grand in Paris has similar results which confirm the existence of crypt hyperplasia in GvHR, with an accelerated rate of cell transit up the sides of the villi. Immature cells on the villi would be more likely to have impaired absorptive functions and even salt and water secretion. GvHR is an easy experimental model to reproduce, and would certainly be amenable to studies of the effects of intestinal CMI on absorptive and secretory functions.

Dr. Halikovski: Have you looked at vascular changes in the villi during the reaction you have described?

Dr. Ferguson: We used electron microscopy to study allograft rejection. This work was done with Dr. Carr in Glasgow, and, in the main, we concentrated on epithelial cells. We noticed that the epithelium seemed to strip readily from the LP and concluded that there were likely to be changes in the basal lamina and in LP, but our anatomical techniques did not detect any. So I am afraid I cannot answer your question.

Dr. Auricchio: Please comment on the absence of villous atrophy in these experimental models you use.

Dr. Ferguson: We are very interested in the state of crypt hyperplasia in the absence of villous atrophy. I have selected only a few of our experiments to illustrate the phenomena, but we have found a complete spectrum of appearances, from normal villi to mild, partial villous atrophy, and, in allograft rejection, a completely flat mucosa. I think that there are probably two separate effects of T-cell-secreted lymphokines in the small intestine. One is to stimulate crypt mitosis—and, since the LP is still there in normal amounts, villi remain of normal height, and cells merely move more rapidly up the sides of the villi. The second factor, which may exert its effect only when there is a vigorous CMI reaction, or may require a higher concentration, is truly toxic. We think that the villous atrophy occurs because the LP crumples, not because there is direct toxicity to epithelial cells. After all, even in celiac disease, for example, in patients undergoing gluten reintroduction, one often finds a state where there is crypt hyperplasia with high counts of crypt mitosis, but with villi remaining of normal length. I am convinced that, because of the dynamic nature of the gut epithelium, there is a stage where there is relative compensation for the early effects of intestinal CMI. Of course, sophisticated studies of function of rapidly proliferating enterocytes may well demonstrate subtle abnormalities in their functions.

Protein Digestion and Absorption

D. M. Matthews

Department of Experimental Chemical Pathology, Vincent Square Laboratories of Westminster Hospital, London SW1V 2RH, United Kingdom

About three-quarters of a century ago, Santayana wrote, "Those who cannot remember the past are condemned to repeat it." This somber dictum is splendidly illustrated by the history of the study of protein digestion and absorption over the same three-quarters of a century (12,13). This chapter begins with a summary of this history, since it provides a deeper understanding of the principles involved than a mere outline of present views accompanied by an account of the minutiae of recent advances in the field.

By the late 19th century, it was understood that protein digestion was initiated by pepsin and continued by the proteolytic activity ("trypsin") of the pancreatic juice, the result of this digestion being "peptones", e.g., mixtures of polypeptides of moderate size with a proportion of dipeptides and free amino acids (17). Since peptones could not be demonstrated in the portal blood after protein meals, and for other reasons, it became widely believed that they were resynthesised to plasma proteins in the intestinal wall. This "hypothesis of resynthesis" received the powerful support of Abderhalden.

The modern era in the study of protein absorption began at the turn of the century when a young medical graduate in the Department of Physiology in Heidelberg (a Department headed by Willy Kühne, who had investigated and named trypsin) set himself the task of verifying the hypothesis of resynthesis. This young man was Otto Cohnheim; his findings were of such importance, and his career, which ended in tragedy, so interesting, that I wrote a short biography of him (14). What Cohnheim found was that extracts of the intestinal mucosa, far from synthesizing peptones into larger molecules, broke them down completely to free amino acids. Without this demonstration, further advances in the fields of protein absorption and metabolism would have been impossible. Cohnheim named the enzyme(s) responsible "erepsin" from a Greek root meaning "to break down" (4). At first, Cohnheim was unable to say whether erepsin acted within the absorptive cells or within the intestinal lumen: "Ob das Erepsin intracellular wirkt, oder in das Darmlumen secernirt wird, kann ich noch nicht sagen". A year later, however, he *was* able to say— he had formed the view that erepsin was primarily an intracellular enzyme. It followed that peptides might be expected to enter the absorptive cells and be hydrolysed within them. By 1912, Van Slyke and Meyer had reported a rise in amino acid nitrogen in the portal blood following protein meals, and in 1914 Abel, Rowntree, and Turner described the isolation of several individual amino acids from portal blood. In the years immediately preceding the First World War, it had become generally accepted that the final stages of hydrolysis of protein digestion products to free amino acids took place in the intestinal wall as well as in the intestinal lumen. That is exactly the view of today.

The next phase in the history of the study of protein absorption began with the development of a gigantic error, commonly known as the "classical hypothesis of protein absorption". This stated that the products of gastric and pancreatic digestion of proteins were completely hydrolyzed to free amino acids within the intestinal lumen, by the action of erepsin in the "succus entericus", and taken up by the absorptive cells only in this form. Nobody knows how this idea originated—probably in the imagination of the writers of textbooks—but it dominated thinking for two generations. Since it was almost universally believed, at least in the English-speaking countries, for so long, it was eventually assumed to have been "proved". It was "known" that proteins were completely broken down to free amino acids within the intestinal lumen, for, from the 1930s or earlier to the 1970s, all the textbooks said so. Around 1950, the classical hypothesis appeared to have been finally vindicated by two new and important observations. In 1949 Dent and Schilling reported that the novel technique of paper chromatography showed that there was a large rise in nearly all the individual free amino acids of the portal blood of dogs following a protein meal, but no unequivocal evidence for any increase in peptides. This was taken as strong support for the classical hypothesis, since by this time the once familiar idea that protein digestion products might leave the lumen in peptide form and enter the blood as amino acids had been forgotten. Then, in 1951, Gerald Wiseman showed that amino acids were actively transported by the small intestine, which seemed to leave no reasonable doubt that the amino acid form was that in which protein digestion products were taken up. In 1955, when I prepared my Ph.D. thesis on amino acid absorption, though well aware of the possibility of peptide uptake from the intestinal lumen and even of entry of peptides into the blood, I was convinced that the classical hypothesis was essentially correct, and wrote "it would be remarkable for the body to possess an enzyme system capable of hydrolysing protein to amino acids, and a special mechanism for absorbing amino acids, if a large part at least of the ingested protein were not absorbed in the amino acid form". I still believe that this rather cautiously worded conclusion was fair comment at the time. It seemed to me quite unnecessary, indeed somewhat perverse, to invoke mucosal uptake of peptides in addition to uptake of free amino acids. Brought up with the classical hypothesis, and impressed by recent advances, I thought myself entitled to wield Occam's razor: "Entia non sunt multiplicanda praeter necessitatem". However, as my old teacher Professor David Smyth (2) once put it, "God does not always shave with Occam's razor".

It was at about the same time that R. B. Fisher (6) published a monograph which initiated a chain of events culminating in the downfall of the classical hypothesis some 15 years later. In it he launched a vigorous attack on this hypothesis, about which he had always been skeptical. Fisher pointed out that the evidence on which it was based was both shaky and insufficient. In particular, he stressed that *in vitro* the process of protein digestion to the final stage of free amino acids was probably far too slow to account for the rapid absorption of protein observed *in vivo*. His attack was a remarkable feat of armchair science. I use the term armchair science in no derogatory sense, as I believe that nowadays the ratio of experimentation ("work") to reading and reflection is far too high. This is possibly related to a certain contemporary adulation of industrial or quasiindustrial activity of a "productive" nature.

As a direct result of Fisher's criticisms, D. H. Smyth and H. Newey, in the Department of Physiology at Sheffield, began a fresh investigation of the form or forms in which protein digestion products were absorbed. The results were published between 1957 and 1962. Their conclusions were that there must be a "second mode" of protein absorption: entry of small peptides into the absorptive cells, followed by intracellular hydrolysis and entry into the blood as free amino acids. They were apparently quite unaware that this had been the view held in 1914. Unfortunately, though their investigations were painstaking and their conclusions correct, the results were unexciting and could almost all be dismissed as the effect of hydrolysis in the brush border—then very much at the center of attention owing to the work of R. K. Crane on the absorption of disaccharides. At the time, the work of Smyth and Newey had comparatively little impact, and no perceptible effect on American opinion. What was needed was a finding so positive and dramatic that it would shock other workers into paying attention. Such a finding was to come a few years later.

In 1966, with the findings of Newey and Smyth in mind, I began, with I. L. Craft, what I thought was a fairly pedestrian piece of clinical research—an investigation of whether the low levels of mucosal glycylglycine dipeptidase expected to exist in such conditions as adult celiac disease could be detected by means of oral tolerance tests using free glycine and diglycine. I had no idea that we were to obtain results which seemed quite extraordinary, and which initiated a series of investigations which, 17 years later, are still far from complete. At one stage our work even led my laboratory into plant physiology, when we showed for the first time that active transport of peptides occurred in germinating seeds. We naturally had to begin by obtaining control curves in normal volunteers. It was soon found (by the end of 1966) that absorption of glycine from equivalent solutions (i.e., solutions containing the same number of amino acid units) appeared to be more rapid from diglycine than from free glycine, and most rapid from triglycine (Fig. 1) (5). This could not possibly happen if complete intralumen hydrolysis preceded uptake, and was most readily interpreted by mucosal uptake of intact peptides followed by intracellular hydrolysis, as suggested by Newey and Smyth. At first these findings, which are now so familiar as to be commonplace, evoked frank incredulity

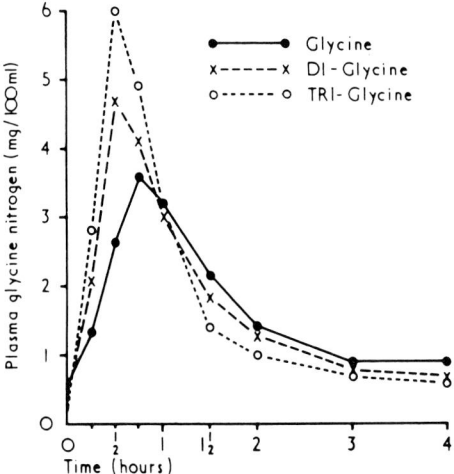

FIG. 1. The "crazy" results obtained in human volunteers. Plasma glycine nitrogen was measured in control subjects following equivalent oral doses of glycine (10 g/70 kg body wt), diglycine (8.8 g/70 kg) and triglycine (8.4 g/70 kg). The differences were unlikely to be due to differences in rates of stomach emptying after the different substances. (From Craft et al., ref. 5, with permission.)

in some quarters [the word "crazy" was used (18)], and I myself had moments of real uneasiness about them. However, the findings were easy to reproduce in animals and in other hands in a different laboratory, and similar results were soon obtained with mixed dipeptides—i.e., peptides composed of two different amino acids (Fig. 2). Furthermore, in the same year, confirmatory results obtained by intestinal perfusion of a mixed dipeptide in man were published by Siamak Adibi in Pittsburgh (1). Adibi had begun his work, which was entirely independent of ours, with no idea of the results he would obtain, and was initially as surprised and sometimes uneasy as we were. His findings too were first greeted with a very negative reaction, at once skeptical and

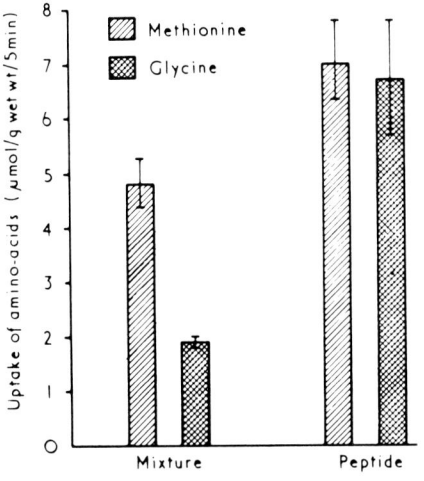

FIG. 2. Absorption from rat small intestine *in vivo* of an equivalent mixture of L-methionine and glycine (5 mmoles/liter of each) and the mixed peptide L-methionyl-glycine (5 mmoles/liter). The columns show means ± SEM. Note that the competitive inhibition of glycine absorption by methionine is avoided when the peptide is absorbed. (From Matthews, ref. 11, with permission.)

hostile. However, the publication in the same year of similar findings from independent laboratories separated by the Atlantic undoubtedly helped eventual acceptance of the results, especially in the United States. From 1968, the investigation of intestinal peptide uptake moved at a very rapid pace. The next really dramatic finding, obtained by M. D. Milne, myself, and our colleagues in 1969, was that patients with the inborn error of Hartnup disease, who cannot absorb neutral amino acids in the free form, can absorb them from dipeptides (Fig. 3). This explained the long-standing puzzle of how such patients avoided diarrhea and maintained their protein nutrition so well, and also provided some of the earliest and strongest evidence for intestinal uptake of amino acids and peptides by independent systems. Analogous findings were soon obtained in cystinuria, which affects dibasic amino acids and cystine. Another major advance came a few years later. For many years it had seemed an apparently impossible task to obtain firm evidence for active uptake of peptides by the small intestine, since this demanded a demonstration of their accumulation against an electrochemical gradient, and nearly all peptides underwent such rapid intracellular hydrolysis that they could not be found intact in the intestinal tissue even in traces. In 1972 and 1973, however, we obtained satisfactory evidence for active uptake of two dipeptides and a tripeptide by hamster small intestine by using peptides which are transportable but resistant to hydrolysis. This evidence seemed to convince most interested workers that intestinal transmembrane transport of small peptides by a special mechanism was a reality, and over the last decade its existence has never been seriously disputed. By the early 1970s, so much information on peptide absorption had accumulated that in 1975 I was able to publish a 70-page review of the subject with more than 240 references (12). Since then, a good deal more has been found out, so that at this point I shall have to abandon my narrative and attempt to summarize the salient features of protein digestion and absorption as they

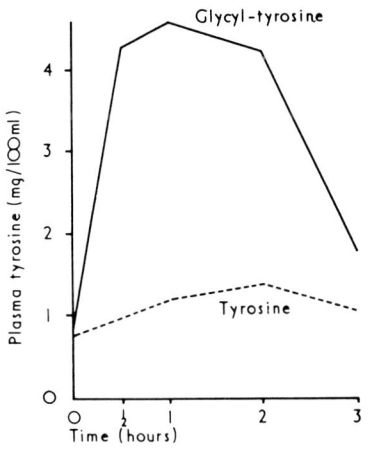

FIG. 3. Plasma tyrosine measured in a case of Hartnup disease following equivalent oral doses of free L-tyrosine and glycyl-L-tyrosine. Though absorption from the free amino acid is not totally absent, the difference between the two curves is very great. (From Matthews, ref. 11, with permission.)

appear today (Fig. 4). As above, in most cases original references, which are very numerous, are omitted where they are readily available in reviews and textbooks (see refs. 9–13,15–17,22).

PROTEIN DIGESTION

The usual "Western" intake of protein, as exemplified by the American diet, is 70 to 100 grams or more per day, though adults can survive on about 30 g of protein (ca. 0.4 g/kg body wt) per day. Much has been made of the magnitude of the contribution of "endogenous" protein to the total protein load for absorption—that is, protein derived largely from desquamated epithelial cells, but also from gastrointestinal secretions, and leakage of plasma proteins into the gut. Estimates of this endogenous protein load in man have been placed at 30 to 100 g or even 200 g/day, though there is reason to believe that the larger estimates may be unduly high. Relatively little protein-derived nitrogen escapes in the feces—perhaps 5 to 10% of the total exogenous load. It is not derived directly from dietary protein, but consists mainly of bacterial protein. In absolute terms, it amounts to 1 to 2 g nitrogen, equivalent to about 6 to 12 g protein.

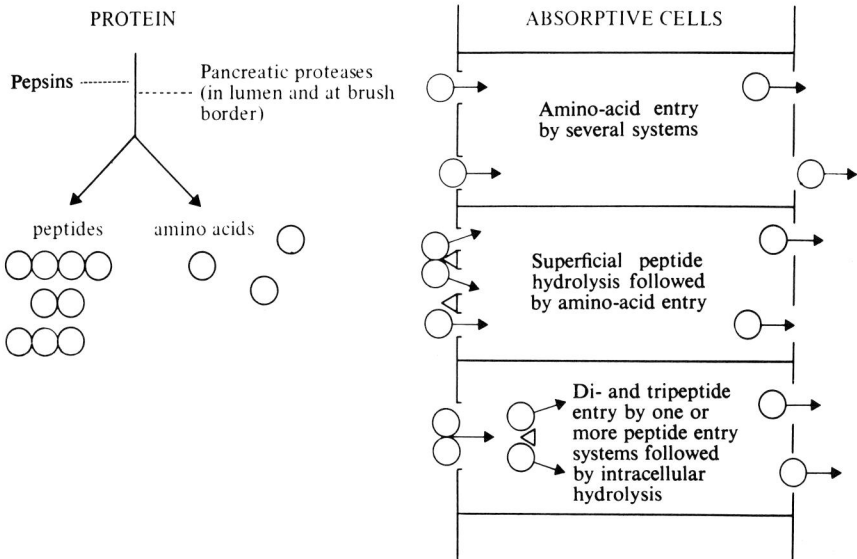

FIG. 4. Simplified scheme of protein digestion and absorption. Note that amino acid uptake following superficial peptide hydrolysis in the brush border occurs by the same systems which are utilized by amino acids liberated in the bulk phase of the fluid in the intestinal lumen. As the figure suggests, in addition to the native peptidases of the brush border, pancreatic proteases may be adsorbed in this region. (Modified from Matthews, ref. 10.)

Protein digestion is begun in the stomach by pepsin (strictly, perhaps one should say pepsins, since there are many isoenzymes) in the presence of hydrochloric acid, which produces the low pH necessary for peptic activity. The main products of gastric digestion are large polypeptides, with a small proportion of oligopeptides and free amino acids, and often some undigested or only very partially digested protein. Since (as patients with pernicious anemia or total gastrectomy and *in vitro* experiments show) protein digestion may be quite effectively initiated and continued to a very advanced stage by the proteolytic enzymes of the pancreas alone, one may well ask, in teleological terms, what is the "purpose" of gastric digestion of proteins. Probably there are three main reasons for it. The first is to aid mechanical reduction of such ingesta as lumps of tough meat into smooth paste. The second is to sterilize the gastric contents by killing and digesting microorganisms. The third is that the amino acids and peptides released trigger hormonal mechanisms stimulating gastric and pancreatic secretion; further, free amino acids influence the rate of gastric emptying. In fact some degree of malabsorption including malabsorption of protein nitrogen is frequent when gastric function is grossly disturbed.

The chief proteolytic enzymes of the pancreas are trypsin, chymotrypsin, carboxypeptidases and elastase, and as a result of their action the lumen of the small intestine contains, after a protein meal, a mixture of polypeptides, oligopeptides (small peptides of a few amino acids only) and free amino acids. In this mixture, oligopeptides are probably the major component. It is likely that what is presented to the brush border for further digestion and absorption is a mixture of oligopeptides of three to six amino acids and free amino acids, in which peptides predominate.

At the brush border, which is capable of hydrolysing peptides of up to at least six amino acids, further digestion of peptides takes place. Amino acids are removed sequentially from the N-terminal ends, and ultimately the resulting mixture of free amino acids and small peptides of two or three amino acids is taken up into the absorptive cells. Though the several peptidases of the brush border can hydrolyse most oligopeptides, activity against peptides of proline is absent from the brush border in at least two species—man and rat. The peptidases of the cytosol of the absorptive cells, which are probably many, with broad and overlapping specificities, are quite distinct from those of the brush border. In many cases they complete hydrolysis of peptides, which enter the blood largely in the form of amino acids. Cytosol peptidases are active mainly against di- and tripeptides. Some oligopeptides are markedly resistant to the action of both brush border and cytosol peptidases, being absorbed into the blood intact on a substantial scale, at least when given in large doses. These include peptides of proline and hydroxyproline (derived in large amounts from gelatin), carnosine (β-alanyl-methylhistidine) and glycylglycine. Peptides containing D-amino acids (which are not derived from a conventional diet) are very resistant to mucosal hydrolysis, but are also very poorly absorbed, so that they do not cross the mucosal barrier on a large scale.

ABSORPTION OF SMALL PEPTIDES

The absorption of amino acids has been studied intensively for more than 30 years, since it was shown that L-amino acids were actively transported by the small intestine, and the literature is very voluminous. The absorption of oligopeptides has been studied intensively for only about 15 years, since, in 1968, it was shown that peptides could be absorbed faster than the equivalent amino acids; consequently, the literature is not so great as that dealing with amino acids. However, this chapter will deal first with absorption of small peptides rather than that of free amino acids, as the former may well be the more important process in quantitative terms, despite the scant attention still paid to it in many textbooks [an honourable exception is the recent massive book on *Physiology of the Gastrointestinal Tract,* edited by Johnson (9)].

Small peptides (di- and tripeptides) are transported into the absorptive cells by an active mechanism. The process has definite structural requirements and is stereochemically specific (like the mechanisms for uptake of amino acids), preferring peptides containing L-amino acids and absorbing those containing D-amino acids very poorly. It is completely independent of the mechanisms responsible for taking up amino acids. The kinetics of peptide uptake are such that this is often more rapid than that of the equivalent amino acids. These statements will now be enlarged on.

Active Uptake of Small Peptides

The prime experimental criterion of active transport is transport against an electrochemical gradient. Until 1972, this could not be shown for intestinal uptake of peptides, since most are so rapidly hydrolyzed that they can be found in the absorptive cells only as the constituent amino acids. Then use was made of the hydrolysis-resistant dipeptide glycylsarcosine (this is equivalent to glycylglycine with a methylated peptide bond), which was already known to be accumulated intact by *Escherichia coli*. Rings of everted hamster small intestine took up glycylsarcosine against an apparent electrochemical gradient, uptake being inhibited by anoxia, metabolic inhibitors and sodium replacement. Subsequently the same was shown to be true of carnosine (β-alanyl-L-histidine), another hydrolysis-resistant dipeptide which is normally found in the diet (it is especially high in chicken meat) and the tripeptide glycylsarcosylsarcosine. The tetrapeptide glycylsarcosylsarcosylsarcosine was, however, taken up only very poorly. Since many other readily hydrolyzed peptides compete for uptake with the above three actively transported peptides, they, presumably, are also taken up by active transport. The uptake of ordinary peptides is also inhibited by anoxia and the presence of metabolic inhibitors—though the value of some of this indirect evidence for active uptake is not great, since these conditions cause rapid mucosal disintegration.

In recent years, some workers have cast doubt on the Na^+-dependence of intestinal peptide uptake (7). I have, however, little doubt that a substantial part at least of the uptake of di- and tripeptides against a concentration gradient by intact absorptive cells is, like that of amino acids, dependent on the presence of Na^+. In spite of this, the precise relationship between peptide transport and transport of Na^+ may be more complicated than previously supposed.

Structural Requirements for Active Uptake of Peptides

Peptide transport requires free terminal amino and carboxyl groups and an adjacent peptide bond or bonds. Nevertheless, a terminal imino group, as in prolyl peptides, is tolerated. The peptide linkage should preferably be an α-linkage. Peptides with a γ-linkage, such as glutathione (γ-L-glutamyl-L-histidyl-glycine) are very poorly transported. Stereochemical specifity is marked, peptides of L-amino acids (and glycine) being well absorbed, and peptides containing or made up of D-amino acids very poorly absorbed. Unlike the systems for uptake of free amino acids, the system(s) for peptide uptake appears indifferent to the charge on the side-chain. Thus basic, acidic and neutral peptides are all taken up by the same mechanism(s), and all compete with each other for uptake. Moreover, both di- and tripeptides appear to be taken up by the same mechanism(s). The reason for putting the plural "s" in brackets is that it is not yet certain whether there is one or more than one peptide uptake system. Some evidence, including recent results from my own laboratory suggests that there may be more than one system for uptake of dipeptides. Active transport of peptides is probably limited to peptides of not more than three amino acid residues.

Independence of Peptide and Amino Acid Uptake

The mechanism(s) responsible for taking up peptides are completely independent of those which take up free amino acids, though amino acids liberated in the brush border by partial hydrolysis of peptides will, naturally, compete for uptake with free amino acids, and vice versa. The independence of peptide and amino acid uptake is most clearly demonstrated by two pieces of evidence: (a) Using the hydrolysis-resistant peptides, glycylsarcosine, carnosine, and glycylsarcosylsarcosine, there is no doubt that peptide uptake is inhibited only by other di- and tripeptides and not by free amino acids; and (b) in the amino acid transport defects of Hartnup disease and cystinuria in man, "affected" amino acids are comparatively well absorbed from dipeptides. Even absorption of amino acid from a dipeptide composed only of an affected amino acid, such as phenylalanylphenylalanine in Hartnup disease, is almost normal. Additional evidence is provided by the observations that (c) in rodents the sites of maximal transport of amino acids and peptides along the length of the small intestine are different (see below), and (d) in rodents, peptide uptake is affected differently from amino acid uptake by adverse dietary conditions, and, in man, it is more resistant to the effects of intestinal disease.

Kinetics of Peptide Uptake

There are very many papers showing that, at one or more concentrations, di- and tripeptides are absorbed more rapidly than the equivalent amino acids. It was this phenomenon, which Smyth and Newey had failed to demonstrate, which aroused such interest in 1968. The phenomenon is partly associated with the avoidance of competition between free amino acids which occurs when peptides are absorbed (Fig. 2), but this is not the whole explanation. A contributory factor is that absorption of amino acids from many peptides involves some brush border hydrolysis, leading to uptake by at least two systems—the system(s) for free amino acids and the system(s) for intact peptides. More extensive investigation is needed before we can account for the phenomenon adequately. It is important to note that peptides are not invariably absorbed faster than the equivalent amino acids. There are several reports of slower absorption of peptides than of the equivalent amino acids, and in a recent study of uptake by hamster intestine *in vitro* of valine and valyl-valine (3), free valine was absorbed more rapidly than the equivalent peptide over a very wide range of concentrations. Further, an example is known of a peptide, lysyl-lysine, which is absorbed more rapidly than the equivalent amino acids at some concentrations and more slowly at others (25). Work in man has shown that, owing to the relatively rapid absorption of slowly absorbed amino acids when in peptide form, absorption of individual amino acids from a partial hydrolysate of protein consisting largely of peptides is far more "even" than it is from an equivalent amino acid mixture (Fig. 5). This effect, which has been shown for several proteins (23), could well be of nutritional importance, leading to improved protein synthesis through more simultaneous presentation of amino acids to the tissues—a point first made many years ago (10,17) and one which needs to be stressed, having been, as far as I know, completely ignored by workers in the field of protein nutrition. Many groups have found that amino acid mixtures simulating proteins are nutritionally less satisfactory than the proteins themselves, but have been unable to account for their results (17). Apart from this, the use of peptide-containing artificial diets for patients with intestinal disease in place of those containing mixtures of free amino acids has additional advantages. Such diets, which are now on the market, utilize the full absorptive capacity of the gut for protein digestion products, and they have a much lower osmolality than diets containing free amino acids, which helps to minimize the tendency to vomiting and diarrhea.

Site of Maximal Absorption of Peptides

In man, intestinal perfusion experiments suggest that both amino acids and peptides are most rapidly absorbed in the jejunum. In the rat and hamster, on the other hand, experiments *in vitro* and *in vivo* suggest that peptides are most rapidly absorbed in the proximal half of the small intestine and amino

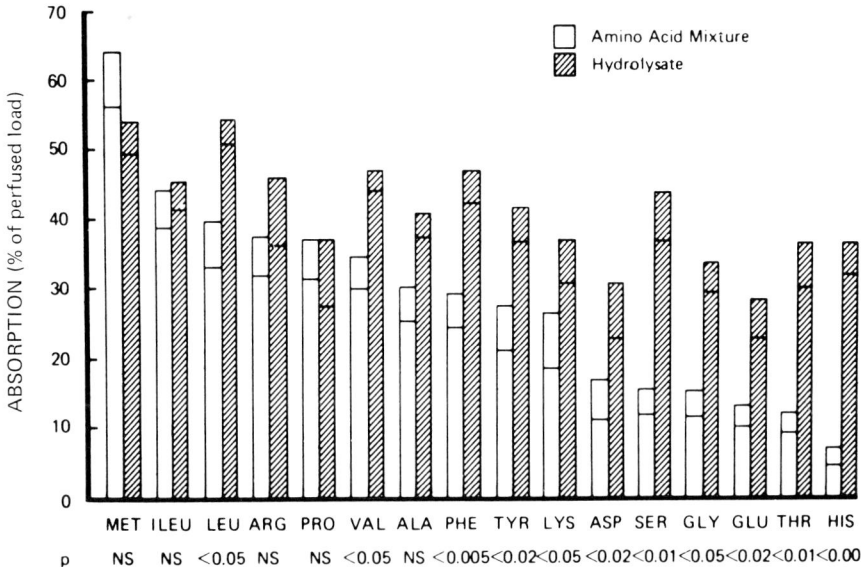

FIG. 5. Absorption, measured by jejunal perfusion in human volunteers, of amino acids from an amino acid mixture simulating lactalbumin and a partial hydrolysate of lactalbumin containing mainly small peptides. The columns represent means ± SEM. Notice how the "stepladder" effect seen with free amino acids is replaced by remarkably "even" absorption when the partial hydrolysate is absorbed. When the amino acid mixture is absorbed, the plasma concentration of a rapidly absorbed amino acid such as methionine is likely to reach an early, high peak. On the other hand, the plasma concentration of a slowly absorbed amino acid such as histidine is likely to rise to a delayed and lower peak. Such "temporal displacement", avoided when peptides are absorbed, could lead to inefficient protein synthesis. (From Silk et al, ref. 23, with permission.)

acids in the distal half. It has been suggested that the distal small intestine might "mop up" amino acids not completely absorbed in the proximal small intestine or amino acids which have back-diffused from peptides hydrolyzed in more proximal sites.

Factors Affecting Peptide Absorption

There is room for a great deal of work in this area. For example, nothing is known about the possible effects of hormones on peptide uptake by the small intestine. Little is known about the effects of sugars (which do affect amino acid absorption), apart from the results of a few experiments suggesting that glucose has no major effect on peptide uptake. Work has been done on the effects of dietary alterations on peptide uptake, and this shows that the effects of such alterations on peptide and amino acid absorption are not the same. A fascinating observation, unexplained but of potential importance, is that in newborn animals peptide uptake is very rapid, occurring at many times the rate of amino acid uptake. As the animals grow older, peptide uptake is reduced so that it is only moderately faster than that of amino acids (21). Himukai et al. (8) have also shown that peptide uptake is more rapid in relation to amino acid uptake in very young animals than in adults.

Absorption of Biologically Active Peptides

Far too little is known about the mechanisms of absorption of biologically active peptides, in spite of the great interest of the subject to both independent investigators and pharmaceutical firms. In general, biologically active peptides are poorly absorbed. This is because many are too large for mediated uptake, or, if small enough, structurally unsuitable. For example, thyroliberin (thyrotropin releasing factor), the tripeptide pyroGlu-His-ProNH$_2$, has both terminal amino acid and carboxyl groups "blocked". Such absorption as does take place of such peptides, and there usually is absorption on a small scale, may be the result of diffusion through aqueous areas in the cell membrane. However, at least two biologically active oligopeptides *are* suitable for uptake by the mediated system(s) for absorption of dietary peptides and are very readily absorbed. These are carnosine (which is probably a neurotransmitter in the olfactory system and may promote wound healing) and cephalexin, an antibiotic. Some small cyclic peptides are lipid-soluble, and might be absorbed on a large scale by diffusion through membrane lipid. An example is the cyclic oligopeptide cyclochloritine, a fungal toxin. Large polypeptides such as insulin, which is known to be absorbed to some extent, might be absorbed on a small scale by the mechanisms responsible for absorption of whole proteins (see below). The possibility of small-scale absorption of biologically active peptides of dietary origin (17), which might exert hormonal or kinin-like effects, and possibly influence the central nervous system by enkephalin-like or neurotransmitter effects, is extremely exciting and demands further investigation. It has already been shown that neurologically active opioid peptides ("exorphins") may be derived from dietary proteins (27). An example of an effect which might be due to absorption of biologically active peptides is that in humans on a diet containing whole protein, the blood pressure is higher than when the protein component is replaced by free amino acids in a "chemically defined diet" (17).

Absorption of Peptides into the Portal Blood

For many years it has been generally believed that, with a few well-recognized exceptions such as carnosine and peptides of proline and hydroxyproline, and others mentioned above, only amino acids entered the portal blood. In a broad sense this may be true, but it is not satisfactorily proved, and recent work suggests that during absorption of a partial hydrolysate of casein, a proportion, maybe some 10%, may enter the blood in the form of small peptides (24). It has also been found that, in rats, there is some absorption of intact peptides after oral administration of heat-damaged protein, and certain proteins of poor nutritional value. Much more investigation is required in this area, especially with proteins of vegetable origin. Nothing is known about the mechanism by which readily absorbed hydrolysis-resistant peptides such as carnosine leave the absorptive cells. If, however, the process is analogous to that for amino acids, it will involve mediated transport.

General Comments

It would be a great mistake to suppose that active transmembrane transport of small peptides is an anomalous process, confined to the small intestine. It occurs in examples of all forms of life, including microorganisms, and in higher plants during the germination of seeds. In the mammalian body, active transport of peptides, or at least mediated transport, occurs in kidney, muscle, liver, and brain, to give but a few examples. Peptide transport may help to conserve metabolic energy, since it requires no more energy to transport a di-, tri-, or larger oligopeptide than a single amino acid. Some organisms, such as *E. coli* or germinating barley, can transport larger peptides than mammalian gut.

There appears to be a fundamental difference between the way the intestine handles small peptides and the way in which it handles disaccharides and oligosaccharides. With most peptides, there is some brush border hydrolysis followed by uptake of free amino acids by the absorptive cells, but this is accompanied by uptake of intact di- and tripeptides followed by intracellular hydrolysis. With oligo- and disaccharides, brush border hydrolysis precedes uptake of monosaccharides; while it has been suggested that hydrolysis and uptake of the products may be linked, there is no uptake of intact di- or oligosaccharides by the absorptive cells (22).

ABSORPTION OF AMINO ACIDS

When it was first shown in 1951 that L-amino acids were actively transported by the small intestine, and shortly afterwards two techniques (the everted sac and ring of everted small intestine) were developed which made *in vitro* studies easy, a burst of activity in the field followed, and this has by no means subsided. As the years went by, intense preoccupation with the details of amino acid absorption made it difficult to recruit workers to the new, equally attractive, and far more extensive field of peptide absorption.

Amino acids are transported into the absorptive cells by active, Na^+-dependent mechanisms, and leave them at the serosal poles of the cells (along with amino acids derived from intracellular hydrolysis of small peptides) by exit mechanisms also involving mediated transport. The importance of the specific exit mechanisms is illustrated by the disorder of lysinuric protein intolerance, in which lysine absorption is defective whether this amino acid is given in free or peptide form (20). It would appear that the disorder involves a defect in a specific mechanism by which lysine and related amino acids leave the absorptive cells. Many years ago it was suggested (10) that absorption of protein digestive products would be most severely affected if there were a defect, not in one of the uptake mechanisms, but in the *exit* of amino acids from the absorptive cells, which would block both major modes of absorption, that is, peptide uptake followed by intracellular hydrolysis and uptake of free amino acids. This suggestion seems to have been borne out by lysinuric protein intolerance, in which there is severe illness with diarrhea. In contrast, in cystinuria and Hartnup disease, in which only one mode of absorption is affected, obvious evidence of intestinal disturbance is unusual. The active uptake of amino acids, structural requirements, stereochemical specificity, kinetics of absorption and other topics are dealt with below.

Active Uptake of Amino Acids

The active transport of amino acids by the small intestine was first shown in 1951 by Wiseman, who demonstrated transmural transport against a concentration gradient. Active transport of dibasic amino acids was not shown until about 10 years later, by T. H. Wilson and his colleagues, using low concentrations. In recent years, evidence has accumulated suggesting that dicarboxylic amino acids, too, are actively transported. Active uptake of amino acids is greatly reduced or abolished by Na^+ replacement, anoxia, and metabolic inhibitors.

Structural Requirements for Active Uptake of Amino Acids

Amino acid uptake, like peptide uptake, requires free terminal amino and carboxyl groups, though a terminal imino agroup, as in proline or hydroxyproline, is tolerated. The systems prefer L-amino acids, but there is also active transport of several D-amino acids and, in fact, some D- and L-amino acids compete for transport. Probably the peptide uptake system(s) is more exacting in its stereochemically specific requirements than the systems for amino acid uptake.

The influence of the side-chains on amino acid uptake is very important, dividing amino acids into three major "transport groups", as well as influencing the kinetic characteristics of uptake of neutral amino acids. In man, a conventional classification of intestinal amino acid systems is as follows:

1. Systems for neutral amino acids:
   a. Favoring most neutral amino acids,
   b. Favoring proline, hydroxyproline, and glycine.
2. A system for dibasic amino acids (lysine, arginine, ornithine) and also cystine.
3. A system for dicarboxylic amino acids (glutamic, aspartic).

The evidence for these different uptake systems rests partly on the results of genetic disorders of amino acid transport in man, and partly on animal experiments, including experiments on competition for uptake between amino acids. Thus, in Hartnup disease, the ability to absorb from the intestine (or reabsorb in the kidney) most neutral amino acids is lost. The ability to absorb glycine is variably impaired, and the ability to absorb proline and hydroxyproline is retained, as is the ability to absorb dibasic and dicarboxylic amino acids. In iminoglycinuria, the ability to absorb proline, hydroxyproline, and glycine is impaired. In cystinuria, the ability to absorb lysine, arginine, ornithine, and cystine is lost. So far, no disorder of absorption of the dicarboxylic amino acids has been described. Within the system for neutral amino acids, the lipophilic properties of the side-chain have an important influence on the kinetic characteristics of the transport process. Amino acids with large, lipophilic side-chains, such as phenylalanine, methionine, or leucine, have a high apparent affinity for transport with a powerful inhibitory effect on the uptake of other neutral amino acids, and a relatively low maximal velocity of transport. Those with short side-chains such as glycine have a low apparent affinity and a relatively high maximal transport velocity. Owing to this relationship, it has been shown that in the series glycine, alanine, valine, and leucine, with increasingly lipophilic properties, at low and probably physiological concentrations, glycine is absorbed the least rapidly, and leucine the most rapidly. At high concentrations, the rate order is reversed.

Competition for Uptake Between Amino Acids

Not surprisingly, the amino acids within each transport group compete for uptake by the absorptive cells. The groups, however, do not have rigid boundaries, and an amino acid such as glycine, for example, may be taken up by both its "own" system (1b) and by system (1a). Consequently, its uptake may be inhibited in a competitive way by amino acids transported by system (1a). It has been estimated that appreciable quantities of basic amino acids are in fact taken up by the system "for" neutral amino acids. Some neutral amino acids inhibit uptake of basic amino acids. In addition, though this is not well known, some neutral amino acids, such as methionine, strongly inhibit the transport of the dicarboxylic amino acids, for reasons which are not yet properly understood. The subject of interactions for transport between amino acids is a confused one. "Cross-inhibition" of intestinal uptake between amino acids of different transport groups is not necessarily always competitive.

Kinetics of Amino Acid Uptake

Individual amino acids are absorbed at very different rates. It has been pointed out above, however, that the rate order among neutral amino acids, at least, may vary with concentration. When amino acids are perfused through the small intestine in man, a characteristic "stepladder" effect is seen (Fig. 5). This effect is partially or almost completely abolished when the perfusate consists largely of small peptides, as mentioned above. Studies of the relationship between rate and concentration often show (a) a saturable component, conforming approximately to Michaelis–Menten kinetics, and, often (at least *in vitro*), (b) a linear component, which may (but does not necessarily) represent diffusion. The same is true of small peptides. It is unlikely, however, that diffusion is of much importance in the absorption *in vitro* of physiological concentrations of amino acids, or of small peptides of dietary origin.

Site of Maximal Absorption of Amino Acids

It has already been pointed out that in man the site of maximal absorptive capacity for amino acids appears to be in the jejunum, whereas in two experimental animals the ileum is the site of maximal absorptive capacity. Little can be added to this beyond pointing out that the site of maximal absorptive capacity for a substrate may be, but need not necessarily be, the site at which most of that substrate is absorbed under physiological conditions.

Factors Affecting Absorption of Amino Acids

The factors affecting amino acid absorption include the presence or absence of sugars, dietary changes, various hormones, intestinal motility, and intestinal disease. They are too numerous for discussion here, especially as the area is very rich in conflicting results and the reader is referred to Wiseman (26), whose account, though some years old, is still the most comprehensive. Dietary and metabolic factors are discussed in Johnson (9).

General Comments

Like active transmembrane transport of small peptides, active transmembrane transport of amino acids has a very wide biological distribution. Though the details of the mechanisms of peptide transport and of amino acid transport, respectively, vary to some extent between one organ and another and between one species and another, it is important to note that in all known instances, amino acid and peptide transports are completely independent processes. In microorganisms, as in man, genetic error may lead to loss of one of the systems with retention of the other(s), and, in such cases, the duality of the normal processes for uptake of protein digestion products tends to permit survival. This has been referred to by D. S. Parsons as a physiological "fail-safe" mechanism.

ABSORPTION OF WHOLE PROTEINS

In newborn mammals, whole proteins, including immunoglobulins, are absorbed from the mother's milk on a massive scale by pinocytosis. This ceases in the first few weeks of life. However, there is little doubt that adult animals retain the ability to absorb whole proteins or very large protein fragments on a small scale, possibly partly by a residuum of the infantile uptake mechanism. In man, this ability is suggested by the occurrence of allergic reactions to dietary proteins. Absorption of whole proteins is unlikely to be of any nutritional importance in the adult mammal, since it accounts for only a small fraction, perhaps of the order of 1%, of total protein absorption.

CONCLUSION

It is clear that today we understand protein digestion and absorption far better than we did 15 years ago; our views have altered out of all recognition. There is no doubt whatsoever that mucosal peptide uptake is quantitatively important in protein absorption, and that the final stages of hydrolysis of protein digestion products occur, to a substantial extent, within the absorptive cells. The question of the extent of entry of peptides into the portal blood is still unresolved. This is remarkable after more than 100 years of investigation. If they do enter the blood on a significant scale, they may have important effects as yet unappreciated. Exactly how important peptide uptake is in relation to uptake of free amino acids we do not yet know, but it may well be the major mode of uptake of protein digestion products.

A recent reviewer (19), apparently finding modern views on peptide absorption unpalatable, and ignoring completely the occurrence and importance of peptide uptake in microorganisms and germinating plants, has asked rather plaintively whether it is really necessary, when considering absorption of protein digestion products, to revert to the views of the early years of the century. If one alters one obsolescent and slightly inappropriate word, "peptones" to "small peptides", there can be only one answer. Yes, it is.

ACKNOWLEDGMENTS

I am greatly indebted to the National Medical Research Fund, the Frank Odell Charity, Corporate Textiles Ltd., the Clouds Hill Breakers Club, and very many private donors for financial support.

REFERENCES

1. Adibi, S. A., and Phillips, E. (1968): Evidence for greater absorption of amino acid from peptide than from free form by human intestine. *Clin. Res.*, 16:446.
2. Barcroft, H., and Matthews, D. M. (1981): David Henry Smyth. *Biographical Memoirs of Fellows of the Royal Society*, 27:525–561.
3. Burston, D., Wapnir, R. A., Taylor, E., and Matthews, D. M. (1982): Uptake of L-valyl-L-valine and glycylsarcosine by hamster jejunum *in vitro. Clin. Sci.*, 62:612–626.
4. Cohnheim, O. (1901): Die Umwandlung des Eiweiss durch die Darmwand. *Z. Physiol. Chem.*, 33:451–465.
5. Craft, I. L., Geddes, D., Hyde, C. W., Wise, I. J., and Matthews, D. M. (1968): Absorption and malabsorption of glycine and glycine peptides in man. *Gut*, 9:425–437.
6. Fisher, R. B. (1954): *Protein Metabolism.* Methuen, London.

7. Ganapathy, V. and Leibach, F. H. (1982): Peptide transport in intestinal and renal brush border membrane vesicles. *Life Sci.,* 30:2137–2146.
8. Himukai, M., Konno, T., and Hoshi, T. (1980): Age-dependent change in intestinal absorption of dipeptides and their constituent amino acids in the guinea pig. *Pediatr. Res.,* 14:1272–1275.
9. Johnson, L. R. (editor) (1981): *Physiology of the Gastrointestinal Tract, Vol. 2.* Raven Press, New York.
10. Matthews, D. M. (1971): Protein absorption. *J. Clin. Pathol.,* 24 (Suppl.), 5:29–40.
11. Matthews, D. M. (1971): Experimental approach in chemical pathology. *Br. Med. J.,* 3:659–644.
12. Matthews, D. M. (1975): Intestinal absorption of peptides. *Physiol. Rev.,* 55:537–608.
13. Matthews, D. M. (1977): Memorial lecture: Protein absorption—Then and now. *Gastroenterology,* 73:1267–1279.
14. Matthews, D. M. (1978): Otto Cohnheim—The forgotten physiologist. *Br. Med. J.,* 2:618–619.
15. Matthews, D. M., and Adibi, S. A. (1976): Peptide absorption. *Gastroenterology,* 71:151–161.
16. Matthews, D. M., and Laster, L. (1965): The kinetics of intestinal active transport of five neutral amino acids. *Am. J. Physiol.,* 208:593–600.
17. Matthews, D. M., and Payne, J. W. (editors) (1975): *Peptide Transport in Protein Nutrition.* North Holland, Amsterdam.
18. Milne, M. D. (1972): In discussion following M. D. Milne: Peptides in genetic errors of amino acid transport. In: *Peptide Transport in Bacteria and Mammalian Gut (Ciba Foundation Symposium),* edited by K. Elliott and M. O'Connor, p. 104. Associated Scientific Publishers, Amsterdam.
19. Nutrition Reviews (1981): In what forms are digested proteins absorbed from the small intestine? *Nutr. Rev.,* 39:380–383.
20. Rajantie, J., Simell, O., and Perheentupa, J. (1980): Basolateral-membrane transport defect for lysine in lysinuric protein intolerance. *Lancet,* i:1219–1221.
21. Rubino, A., and Guandalini, S. (1977): Dipeptide transport in the intestinal mucosa of developing rabbit. In: *Peptide Transport and Hydrolysis, (Ciba Foundation Symposium),* edited by K. Elliot and M. O'Connor, pp. 61–71. Associated Scientific Publishers, Amsterdam.
22. Silk, D. B. A. (1981): Peptide transport. *Clin. Sci.,* 60:607–615.
23. Silk, D. B. A., Fairclough, P. D., Clark, M. L., Hegarty, J. E., Marrs, T. C., Addison, J. M., Burston, D., Clegg, K. M., and Matthews, D. M. (1981): Use of a peptide rather than free amino acid nitrogen source in chemically defined 'elemental' diets. *J.P.E.N.,* 4:548–553.
24. Sleisenger, M. H., Pelling, D., Burston, D., and Matthews, D. M. (1977): Amino acid concentrations in portal venous plasma during absorption from the small intestine of the guinea-pig of an amino acid mixture simulating casein and a partial enzymic hydrolysate of casein. *Clin. Sci. Mol. Med.,* 52:259–267.
25. Taylor, E., Burston, D., and Matthews, D. M. (1980): Influx of glycyl-sarcosine and L-lysyl-L-lysine into hamster jejunum *in vitro. Clin. Sci.,* 58:221–225.
26. Wiseman, G. (1964): *Absorption from the Intestine.* Academic Press, London, New York.
27. Zioudrou, D., and Klee, W. A. (1979): Possible roles of peptides derived from food proteins in brain function. *Nutrition and the Brain, Vol. 4,* edited by R. J. Wurtman and T. J. Wurtman, pp. 125–158. Raven Press, New York.

DISCUSSION

Dr. Perman: Many of the proteins in our diet are, in fact, sugar-containing proteins or glycoproteins. What do we know about the sequence of digestion of glycoproteins?

Dr. Matthews: This is, I'm afraid, slightly outside my area. I cannot help you on that.

Dr. Greene: With regard to the comparison in Fig. 4 between individual amino acids and a peptide mixture, was that mole per mole for the individual? or was that *in vivo* or *in vitro*? Could you explain that a little more in detail?

Dr. Matthews: The experiment was done by intestinal perfusion in human volunteers, measuring disappearance from the intestinal lumen over a period of 30 min.

Dr. Greene: Each of those was done separately—it was not a conglomerate of individual amino acids?

Dr. Matthews: It was a conglomerate—in this case, since the structure of lactalbumin is completely known, one merely made up a mixture corresponding to lactalbumin out of free amino acids for one set of experiments, and the other perfusate was made up from a partial hydrolysate of pure lactalbumin.

Dr. Kretchmer: I remember a couple of years ago that Tom Wilson, from Harvard, studied amino acid transport and showed that the transport of, I think, histidine in the intestine of the newborn was not oxygen-dependent, but was later on, in the adult. Is peptide transport oxygen-dependent?

Dr. Matthews: Peptide transport in adult gut is oxygen-dependent—I'm not sure that this question has been investigated in the newborn gut.

Dr. Kretchmer: Is it sodium dependent?

Dr. Matthews: We found it sodium dependent—there are some claims in the literature that, when transport is taking place down a concentration gradient, it is not sodium dependent.

Dr. Ribadeau Dumas: I didn't understand completely one of your slides—the one showing the relative absorption of lysine and dilysine. Was the total lysine content bound or unbound? And how do you explain the difference in absorption when you increase the amount of lysine?

Dr. Matthews: On the horizontal axis, it had the number of lysine residues or units per unit volume of solution peptide-bound or free. On the vertical axis, it had the rate of absorption expressed in terms of lysine residues or units. I can only explain differences in relative rates of absorption at different concentrations by saying that the kinetics of uptake of the amino acid and peptide are different. This is really no answer at all, but it is the only answer one can provide at the moment. K_t and V_{max} are different for lysine and lysyllysine.

Dr. Koldovský: If you get the intestine to absorb glycylglycine in a dipeptide, will it appear on the other side, in the bloodstream or whatever, as glycylglycine, or as glycine only, or in some given ratio?

Dr. Matthews: There may well be some definite relationship, but it has not been established. I can only tell you that, in man, it will be mainly in the form of glycine but with a small proportion of diglycine.

Dr. Salle: Do you think that the molecular weight of the peptides or dipeptides is important in transport? In other words, if you have a high molecular weight peptide, can it be transported through the cell?

Dr. Matthews: I think that di- and tripeptides are well absorbed by the peptide transport system, regardless of their molecular weight, but tetrapeptides and peptides with a larger number of residues are not. You could take a tetrapeptide, say tetraglycine, which would be poorly absorbed, and a tripeptide, such as trileucine, with an even higher molecular weight, which would be well absorbed.

CLINICAL ASPECTS OF GASTROINTESTINAL FUNCTION

Nutritional Adaptation of the Gastrointestinal Tract of the Newborn, edited by N. Kretchmer and A. Minkowski. Nestlé, Vevey/Raven Press, New York © 1983.

Noninvasive Techniques for the Evaluation of Gastrointestinal Function

Jay A. Perman

Department of Pediatrics, University of California at San Francisco, San Francisco, California 94143

The study of gastrointestinal function during infancy has been impeded by the invasiveness, impracticality, and imprecision of the conventional techniques of internal medicine transposed to newborn and young infants. Quantitative data on the intraluminal phase of digestion are usually obtained in adults from analyses of duodenal fluid, whereas mucosal functions are investigated with biopsies and intestinal perfusion techniques. However, the performance of biopsy and intubation procedures is more difficult in infants, and cannot be practiced in asymptomatic infants. Noninvasive techniques for the evaluation of gastrointestinal function are, therefore, appealing to clinicians and investigators dealing with infants.

This review will discuss well-established measurements using fluids obtained noninvasively: serum, urine, feces, and breath. Appropriate applications and limitations of the various methodologies will be considered, with particular emphasis on recently introduced techniques of breath analysis in the pediatric population. For purposes of discussion, techniques are organized according to the phase of digestion or absorption assessed by a particular method (Table 1).

INTRALUMINAL PHASE

Assessment of Pancreatic Function

Fat Digestion

Lipolysis is the process by which dietary fat or triglyceride is hydrolyzed by pancreatic lipase. Lipolysis results in the production of insoluble end-products in the form of long-chain fatty acids and β-monoglycerides. The quantitative fecal fat determination remains the most reliable measure of lipolysis. The infant should be maintained on a normal diet containing a minimum of 35% of total calories as fat for 2 days prior to the beginning of stool collections. Stools are collected for 72 hr in infants with diarrhea. Charcoal or carmine

TABLE 1. *Tests of digestion and absorption*

Function	Test
Intraluminal phase	
Pancreatic function	
Triglyceride → fatty acids, monoglycerides	Quantitative fecal fat Serum carotene ^{13}C-Lipid breath test
Carbohydrate → oligosaccharides, disaccharides	Breath H_2 test
Protein → peptides, amino acids	Fecal nitrogen
Micellar solubilization	Quantitative fecal fat ^{13}C-Lipid breath tests (multiple substrates)
Ileal dysfunction; bacterial overgrowth	^{13}C-Glycocholate breath test
Mucosal phase	
Nonspecific function	D-Xylose absorption or excretion
Specific functions	
Fat absorption	Quantitative fecal fat ^{13}C-Lipid breath tests
Disaccharides → monosaccharides	Fecal pH Fecal reducing substances Oral tolerance test Breath H_2 test
Peptides → amino acids	—

red markers administered at the beginning and end of a 72-hr balance period should be used in those without diarrhea, and all stools passed from the appearance of the first marker until the appearance of the second marker should be collected. A strict record of intake is to be maintained from which the dietary fat ingested during the 72-hr balance period can be calculated. Results are then expressed as a coefficient of absorption by the equation:

$$\frac{\text{Dietary fat} - \text{fecal fat}}{\text{Dietary fat}} \times 100 = \text{coefficient of absorption}$$

Normal values for infants are related to diet and age (11,26).

Measurement of serum carotene, a precursor of vitamin A, is useful as a screening test for efficiency of lipolysis in the older child and adult, but does not establish the extent of fat malabsorption (24). In early infancy, abnormally low serum carotene values may reflect limited dietary intake of carotene-containing foods, including carrots, squash, sweet potatoes, and green vegetables. Carotene measurements cannot estimate the adequacy of lipolysis in the infant whose diet consists entirely of breast milk or formulas.

Oral administration of carbon-labeled (^{14}C or ^{13}C) dietary fats, followed by collection and measurement of labeled carbon dioxide excreted in breath, permits assessment of fat absorption without 72-hr stool collection. Appropriate enrichment of labeled CO_2 in breath following administration of labeled lipid indicates normal digestion, absorption, and oxidation of fat. Since ^{14}C represents a small but finite radiation burden to the child, Watkins et al. have validated the use of ^{13}C-labeled lipids in breath tests (30). ^{13}C is a nonradioactive naturally occurring stable isotope representing approximately 1.1% of all carbon atoms, and is differentiated from ^{12}C by its mass using a mass spectrometer. Administration of the labeled long-chain triglyceride ^{13}C-triolein has recently been shown to establish the presence of steatorrhea in children ages 3 months to 17 years with lipolytic defects (28) (Fig. 1). The ^{13}C-triolein breath test does not, however, differentiate lipolytic from other intraluminal phase (micellar solubilization) or mucosal abnormalities. Subsequent administration of ^{13}C-palmitic acid and measurement of expired $^{13}CO_2$ in breath appears to discriminate lipolytic function from micellar phase and mucosal function, since palmitic acid is a free fatty acid which does not require lipolysis for digestion but depends on micellar solubilization and normal mucosal function for absorption (Fig. 1).

It is important to note that the usefulness of ^{13}C-lipid breath tests has not yet been established in small, immature infants or in populations with extensive malnutrition. Both groups may have altered rates of CO_2 production at rest, potentially affecting the results of ^{13}C breath tests. In addition, substrates are generally expensive and facilities for the analysis of $^{13}CO_2$ are not widespread. With greater use, the price per gram of substrate should decrease and com-

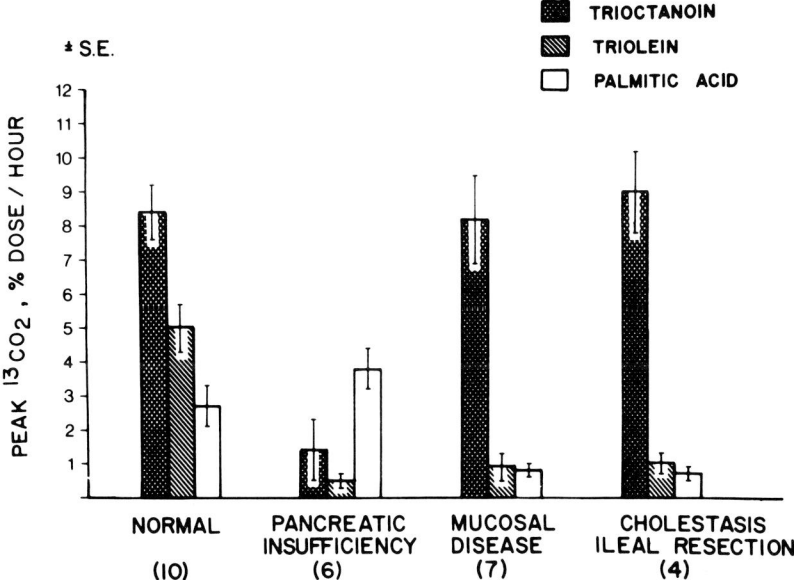

FIG. 1. Peak excretion rate for each substrate in normal individuals and patients with fat malabsorption. Depicted according to substrate and diagnosis. N = number of patients in each group. (From Watkins et al., ref. 28, with permission. Copyright American Gastroenterological Society, 1982.)

mercial services for isotopic measurements on breath should expand. It is, therefore, anticipated that these procedures will become both cost effective and accessible for general use.

Carbohydrate Digestion

Unlike fat, hydrolysis of starch and glucose polymers by measurement of starch content in stools does not accurately assess adequacy of intraluminal carbohydrate digestion. Starch balance cannot be determined in a fashion analogous to fat balance because bacterial fermentation in the colon significantly modifies starch escaping small bowel absorption. Performance of starch balance requires measurement of lactic acid, glucose, dextrins, and starch in 3-day collections of feces while simultaneously quantifying the starch content in the diet (10). The practicality of this method is limited.

The same fermentation processes which modify starch escaping small bowel absorption result in gaseous products which can be measured noninvasively, providing an index of starch digestion and absorption. Endogenous H_2 production is exclusively due to fermentation of luminal substrate by intestinal bacteria. H_2 elaborated by bacterial processes is not metabolized in man, and is excreted in the lungs in proportion to its production in the intestine (16). Breath H_2 measurement has been established as a sensitive indicator of carbohydrate malabsorption, and incomplete digestion or absorption of starches and flours may be detected using this methodology (2). In a preliminary report, Mackie et al. (17) have utilized H_2 measurements to demonstrate that 15% to 50% of a starch load is malabsorbed in individuals with pancreatic insufficiency secondary to chronic pancreatitis. Breath H_2 tests for detection of disaccharide and monosaccharide malabsorption will be discussed below.

Protein Digestion

Accurate noninvasive measures of protein digestion are currently not available. Fecal nitrogen determinations are affected by the large contribution of endogenous sources of nitrogen to the intraluminal nitrogen content, and by bacterial catabolism of nitrogen in the colon (12,13). Controversy exists regarding whether quantitative fecal nitrogen determinations are linearly related to the amount of dietary nitrogen ingested and malabsorbed (8,23). However, 72-hr collections of feces followed by nitrogen determination are sufficient to distinguish children with pancreatic insufficiency from normal controls and patients with celiac disease. Recent studies using experimental animals (7) and *in vitro* fecal incubation studies (20) suggest that breath H_2 measurements following ingestion of proteins, or carbohydrate-containing proteins (glycoproteins), may be useful in quantifying protein absorption. These techniques have not been validated at present.

Assessment of Micellar Solubilization

The products of lipolysis, fatty acids, and monoglycerides, must gain aqueous solubility for absorption across the intestinal mucosa. Bile acids cluster in complexes called "micelles" which are capable of bringing fatty acids and monoglycerides into solution. Duodenal concentrations of bile acids inadequate for the formation of micelles may occur in infants with cholestatic liver disease, small bowel bacterial overgrowth syndromes associated with deconjugation of bile acids, and in ileal disease or resection which interrupts the enterohepatic circulation.

Assessment of micellar solubilization may be performed by quantitative fecal fat determination. Whereas neither this test nor the triolein breath test will alone discriminate between abnormalities of lipolysis and micelle formation, the ^{13}C-palmitic acid breath test should, because palmitic acid requires micellar solubilization only. A labeled carbon breath test using trioctanoin, a medium-chain triglyceride, would also be expected to achieve this discrimination, since absorption of trioctanoin does not require micellar solubilization, but digestion of this substrate is enhanced by lipolysis (Fig. 1). Ileal dysfunction or bacterial overgrowth causing defective micellar solubilization may also be detected by a breath test using ^{13}C-glycocholic acid. In this test, glycocholic acid is labeled on the carboxyl carbon atom of the glycine moiety. The glycine is liberated when the amide bond linking the glycine to the bile acid is hydrolyzed by intestinal bacteria present in the colon or, in the case of small bowel bacterial overgrowth, in the upper small intestine. Subsequently, the liberated glycine is metabolized by the bacteria or within the body, resulting in elaboration of labeled CO_2 in expired air. In individuals with ileal resection or disease, large amounts of bile acid are exposed to colonic bacteria and deconjugated, resulting in a measurable increase in the excretion of $^{13}CO_2$. An identical process occurs in the upper small bowel in the case of small bowel bacterial overgrowth. ^{13}C-Glycocholate breath tests have recently been validated for the detection of both ileal dysfunction and bacterial overgrowth in infants (29).

MUCOSAL PHASE

Nonspecific Mucosal Function

The functional integrity of the jejunum may be assessed by measurement of D-xylose absorption or excretion. D-Xylose is a 5-carbon monosaccharide absorbed chiefly by passive transport in the proximal small intestine. Serum samples for xylose determination are obtained at 30-min intervals for 2 hr following administration of a xylose test dose of 0.5 g/kg (maximum 5 g). The values obtained are compared with a blank or fasting xylose concentration. Some investigators have advocated the use of a single determination at 1 hr following administration of xylose, but the accuracy of this approach is controversial (6,9). In children old enough to void on command, all urine is collected for 5 hr following the administration of xylose and the quantity of xylose in the urine is determined. Normal values based on age are available (25).

Xylose absorption is not a measure of carbohydrate absorption, since uptake of xylose is independent of intestinal mucosal disaccharidases, pancreatic exocrine secretions, and bile salts. Intraluminal bacterial overgrowth may modify the results of the test. Xylose absorption is affected by delayed gastric emptying, and excretion may be impaired in patients with abnormal intravascular volumes or renal disease.

Specific Mucosal Functions

Uptake of fatty acids and monoglycerides may be assessed by quantitative fecal fat determination. A xylose excretion test may then be used to distinguish fat malabsorption due to mucosal disease from that due to intraluminal phase defects. Alternatively, serial ^{13}C-labeled breath tests will discriminate abnormalities in absorption of fat from abnormalities in lipolysis (Fig. 1).

Hydrolysis of Disaccharides and Uptake of Monosaccharides

Tests for Carbohydrates in Feces

Sugars escaping small bowel absorption enter the colon where a portion is fermented by bacteria to short-chain fatty acids. This process may be detected by measuring the fecal pH. A value of 5.5 or less is indicative of carbohydrate malabsorption (1). Unfermented sugar passes into the feces, and may be detected by the Clinitest method for reducing sugars (14). Measurements of fecal pH and reducing substances are useful screening tests for sugar malabsorption, but are not quantitative.

Disaccharide and Monosaccharide Absorption Tests

Oral tolerance tests in which a dietary carbohydrate such as lactose, sucrose, or glucose is administered to test a specific disaccharidase or transport function, require repeated determinations of serum glucose, and can be distorted by variations in gastric emptying and intermediary glucose metabolism. These uncontrolled variables lead to difficulties in interpretation of oral tolerance tests (15,18). A fundamental limitation of oral sugar tolerance tests is that, in contrast with fat absorption tests, *un*absorbed sugar cannot be measured by these means. Oral tolerance tests for the identification of lactase and sucrase deficiency should therefore be interpreted with caution.

Lactose and Sucrose Breath H_2 Tests

Simplified H_2 collection, storage, and measurement techniques have been developed for detection of childhood lactose and sucrose malabsorption (4,19). Samples of expired air are collected by nasal prong (19) from fasting patients before and at 30-min intervals for 3 hr after administration of 20% lactose or sucrose solution (2 g/kg; maximum 50 g). A rise in expired air H_2 concentration indicates malabsorption of the substrate (Fig. 2). The amount of nutrient carbohydrate escaping absorption can be estimated by measuring H_2 produced after sequential administration of equivalent amounts of nonabsorbable (lactulose) and potentially absorbable carbohydrate (5). This procedure is based on the demonstration that H_2 increases linearly with increasing amounts of lactulose, and that equivalent amounts of H_2 are produced from different carbohydrate substrates by fecal flora from individual patients (5,21).

Criteria for interpretation of breath H_2 tests have largely been established on the basis of studies in older children and adults with primary disaccharidase deficiencies. Comparisons of mucosal histology and enzyme activity with breath H_2 excretion indicate that increases in expired air H_2 concentrations in children with isolated lactase deficiency are of greater magnitude and occur more rapidly after an oral lactose load when compared with children with lactase insufficiency secondary to mucosal injury (4). These differences in magnitude and time course of the H_2 response among primarily and secondarily deficient individuals may simply be attributable to the amount of carbohydrate escaping small bowel absorption. In early infancy, however, additional factors may affect the relationship between absorptive capacity for a given sugar, and H_2 production and excretion. The colonic contents of normal neonates and of infants with carbohydrate malabsorption are generally acidic (3). Using an *in vitro* fecal incubation system, studies in our laboratory have established that H_2 production within human colonic ecosystems is inhibited at acid pH (21). Acidification of colonic contents by repeated administration of nonabsorbable carbohydrate confirmed the effect of acid pH on H_2 production *in vivo* (Fig. 3). Thus, the presence of acid luminal contents at the time a test carbohydrate is administered may affect resultant H_2 production.

Similarly, the H_2 signal in certain infants may be blunted by low mesenteric blood flow. H_2 excretion is dependent on transfer of H_2 into the portal circulation. Premature newborns may have decreased mesenteric perfusion secondary to left-to-right cardiac shunts, hypoplastic left heart, polycythemia, and placement of umbilical catheters. The effect of intestinal ischemia on H_2 excretion was examined in adult and newborn dogs by insufflating ileal segments with H_2, modifying mesenteric perfusion by hemorrhage or occlusion, and monitoring of H_2 excretion in breath (22). Breath H_2 measurements were shown to decrease in ischemia and rise upon relief of ischemia (Fig. 4), suggesting that altered intestinal perfusion may affect the H_2 signal.

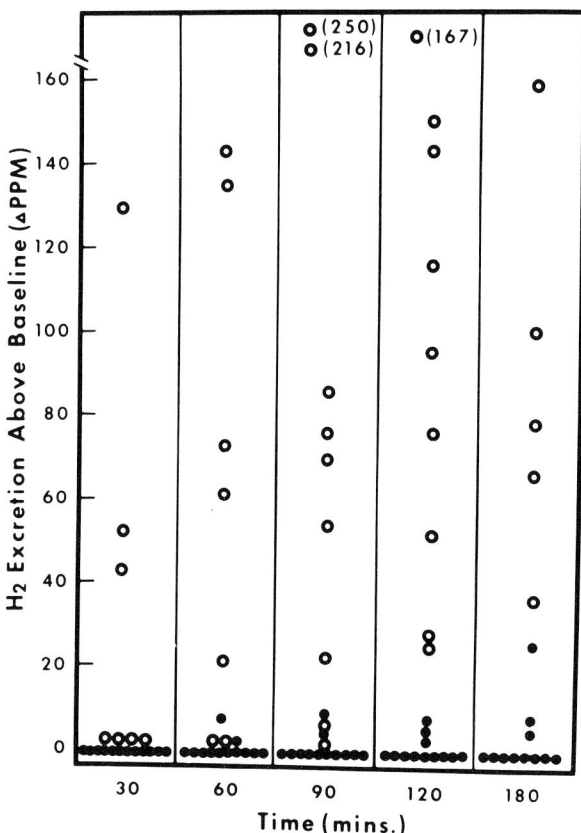
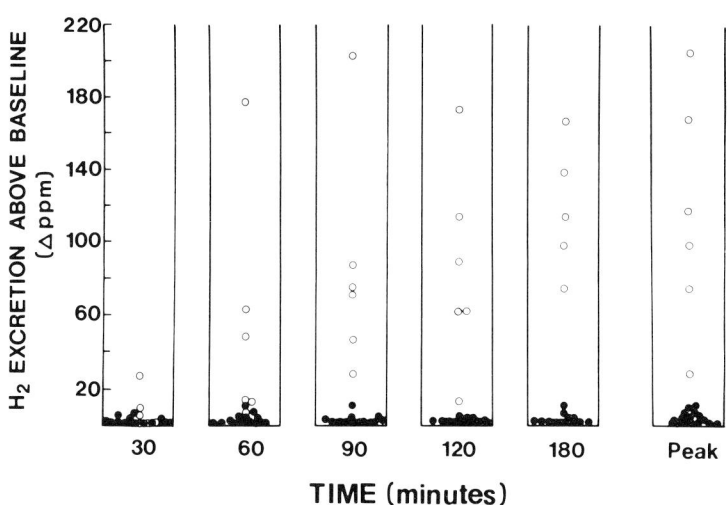

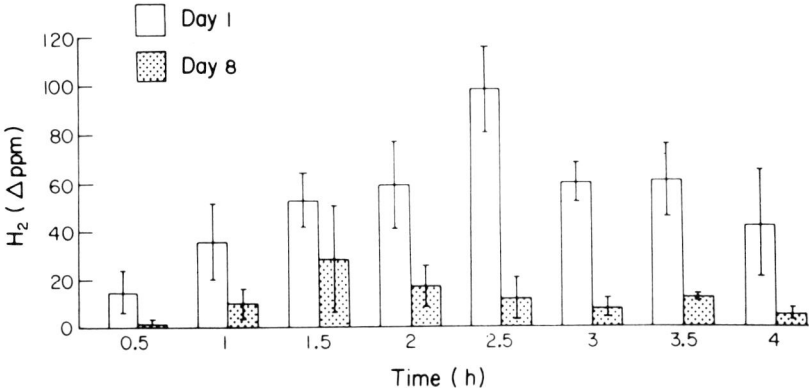

FIG. 3. Breath H_2 responses to lactulose test doses on day 1 and on day 8, and after the lactulose maintenance period. Samples of expired air were obtained at half-hour intervals following administration of lactulose 0.3 g/kg. The average change in H_2 concentration in parts per million above base-line (fasting) levels (Δppm) for 5 subjects is represented by the *bars* (mean ± SEM). (From Perman et al., ref. 21, with permission. Copyright American Society for Clinical Investigation, 1981.)

These variables should be considered when interpreting breath H_2 measurements in infants, since they potentially affect the relationship between the absorptive capacity for a given carbohydrate and H_2 production/excretion. Recognition of these variables may ultimately add to the utility of breath H_2 measurements for evaluation of gastrointestinal function.

Peptide and Amino Acid Absorption

Noninvasive tests for specific assessment of peptide hydrolysis, and peptide and amino acid absorption are currently unavailable. Conversely, transmucosal protein loss from the circulation can be detected by measurement of random fecal alpha-1-antitrypsin concentration in stool (27).

CONCLUSIONS

In summary, gastrointestinal function in infancy may be assessed by a variety of noninvasive techniques. Many of the methods are adequate only for

---

FIG. 2. Top: Hydrogen excretion in parts per million above base line (Δppm) in lactase-normal children (*closed circles*) and isolated lactase-insufficient (*open circles*) children following ingestion of 20% aqueous lactose solution (2 g/kg, maximum 50 g). In 4 lactase-insufficient children no 180-min sample was obtained; in 2 children, no 30- or 60-min samples were obtained. (From Barr et al., ref. 4, with permission. Copyright American Academy of Pediatrics, 1981.) **Bottom:** Time course of breath hydrogen excretion following a 2 g/kg (maximum 50 g) sucrose load. *Closed circles,* sucrose-tolerant patients; *open circles,* intolerant patients. Peak value is the highest hydrogen determination obtained from each patient. A sample was not obtained from 1 sucrose-intolerant patient at 180 min. (From Perman et al., ref. 19, with permission.)

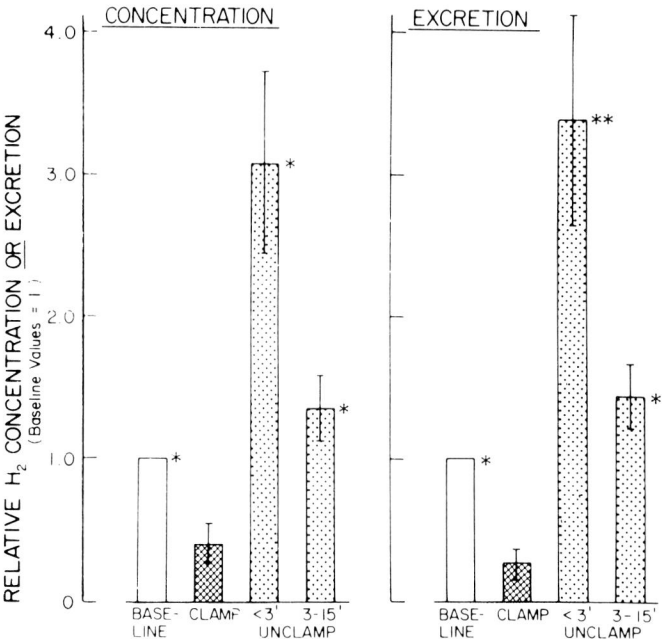

FIG. 4. Effect of local mesenteric vascular clamping on breath H_2 concentration (*left panel*, 4 dogs) and breath H_2 excretion [*right panel*, 3 dogs (expired air volume was not measured in 1 dog)]. Excretion was calculated from the product of H_2 concentration and total volume of gas excreted per timed collection. Bars ± SD represent average multiples of base-line H_2 (*open bars*) during the 10-min period of occlusion (*cross-hatched bars*) and the periods after relief of occlusion (*stippled bars*). Values obtained during the clamp period were compared with values from baseline and postocclusion periods by the paired *t*-test (* $p < 0.025$; ** $p < 0.05$). (From Perman et al., ref. 22, with permission.)

screening purposes, whereas others, such as fecal fat determinations, yield quantitative information. Breath tests are particularly attractive because they are accurate and painless, and permit the study of digestive and metabolic processes otherwise not readily accessible to investigation. Important questions regarding sensitivity and specificity of breath tests in infants remain to be resolved, but the promise of these simple procedures is considerable.

ACKNOWLEDGMENTS

The studies performed in the author's laboratory were supported by a research grant (HD 12449) and Research Career Development Award HD 00297 from the National Institute of Child Health and Human Development.

REFERENCES

1. Ament, M. E. (1972): Malabsorption syndromes in infancy and childhood. *J. Pediatr.*, 81:685–697.

2. Anderson, I. H., Levine, A. S., and Levitt, M. D. (1981): Incomplete absorption of the carbohydrate in all-purpose wheat flour. *N. Engl. J. Med.*, 304:891–892.
3. Barbero, G. J., Runge, G., Fischer, D., Crawford, M. N., Torres, F. E., and Gyorgy, P. (1952): Investigations on the bacterial flora, pH, and sugar content in the intestinal tract of infants. *J. Pediatr.*, 40:152–163.
4. Barr, R. G., Watkins, J. B., and Perman, J. A. (1981): Mucosal function and breath hydrogen excretion: Comparative studies in the clinical evaluation of children with non-specific abdominal complaints. *Pediatrics*, 68:526–533.
5. Bond, J. H., Jr., and Levitt, M. D. (1972): Use of pulmonary hydrogen (H_2) measurements to quantitate carbohydrate malabsorption. *J. Clin. Invest.*, 51:1219–1225.
6. Butt, J.-P, Morin, C. L., Roy, C. C., Weber, A., and Bonin, A. (1978): One-hour blood xylose test: A reliable index of small bowel function. *J. Pediatr.*, 92:729–733.
7. Carter, E. A., Bloch, K. J., Cohen, S., Isselbacher, K. J., and Walker, W. A. (1981): Use of hydrogen gas (H_2) analyses to assess intestinal absorption. *Gastroenterology*, 81:1091–1097.
8. Cheng, A., Gomez, A., Bergen, J., Lee, T., Monckeberg, F., and Chichester, C. (1978): Comparative nitrogen balance study between young and aged adults using three levels of protein intake from a combination of wheat–soy–milk mixture. *Am. J. Clin. Nutr.*, 31:12–22.
9. Christie, D. L. (1978): Use of the one-hour blood xylose test as an indicator of small bowel mucosal disease. *J. Pediatr.*, 92:725–728.
10. DeVizia, B., Ciccimarra, F., DeCicco, N., and Auricchio, S. (1975): Digestibility of starches in infants and children. *J. Pediatr.*, 86:50–55.
11. Fomon, S. J., Ziegler, E. E., Thomas, L. N., Jensen, R. L., and Filer, Jr., L. J. (1970): Excretion of fat by normal full-term infants fed various milks and formulas. *Am. J. Clin. Nutr.*, 23:1299–1313.
12. Freeman, H. J., and Kim, Y.-S. (1978): Digestion and absorption of protein. *Annu. Rev. Med.*, 29:99–116.
13. Gibson, I., Sladen, G., and Dawson, A. (1976): Protein absorption and ammonia production: The effect of dietary protein and removal of the colon. *Br. J. Nutr.*, 35:61–65.
14. Kerry, K. R., and Anderson, C. M. (1964): A ward test for sugar in feces. *Lancet*, i:981–982.
15. Krasilnikoff, P. A., Gudmand-Hoyer, E., and Moltke, H. H. (1975): Diagnostic value of disaccharide tolerance tests in children. *Acta Pediatr. Scand.*, 64:693–698.
16. Levitt, M. D. (1969): Production and excretion of hydrogen gas in man. *N. Engl. J. Med.*, 281:122–127.
17. Mackie, R. D., Levine, A. S., and Levitt, M. D. (1981): Malabsorption of starch in pancreatic insufficiency. *Gastroenterology*, 80:1220.
18. Paige, D. M., Mellits, E. D., Chiu, F.-Y, Davis, L., Bayless, T. M., and Cordano, A. (1978): Blood glucose rise after lactose tolerance testing in infants. *Am. J. Clin. Nutr.*, 31:222–225.
19. Perman, J. A., Barr, R. G., and Watkins, J. B. (1978): Sucrose malabsorption in children: Noninvasive diagnosis by interval breath hydrogen determination. *J. Pediatr.*, 93:17–22.
20. Perman, J. A., and Modler, S. (1982): Glycoproteins as substrates for production of hydrogen and methane by colonic bacterial flora. *Gastroenterology*, 83:388–393.
21. Perman, J. A., Modler, S., and Olson, A. C. (1981): Role of pH in production of hydrogen from carbohydrates by colonic bacterial flora: Studies *in vivo* and *in vitro*. *J. Clin. Invest.*, 67:643–650.
22. Perman, J. A., Waters, L. A., Harrison, M. R., Yee, E. S., and Heldt, G. P. (1981): Breath hydrogen reflects canine intestinal ischemia. *Pediatr. Res.*, 15:1229–1233.
23. Reifenstein, E., Albright, F., and Wells, S. (1945): The accumulation, interpretation and presentation of data pertaining to metabolic balances. *J. Endocrinology*, 5:367–395.
24. Roy, C. C., Silverman, A., and Cozzetto, F. J. (1975): *Pediatric Clinical Gastroenterology.* C. V. Mosby, St. Louis, p. 696.
25. Santiago, P. J., Santini, R., Jr., and Maldonado, N. (1971): The xylose excretion test in normal children and in pediatric patients with tropical sprue. *Pediatrics*, 48:59–63.
26. Schmerling, D. H., Forrer, J. C. W., and Prader, A. (1970): Fecal fat and nitrogen in healthy children and in children with malabsorption or maldigestion. *Pediatrics*, 46:690–695.
27. Thomas, D. W., Sinatra, F. R., and Merritt, R. J. (1981): Random fecal alpha-1-antitrypsin concentration in children with gastrointestinal disease. *Gastroenterology*, 80:776–782.
28. Watkins, J. B., Klein, P. D., Schoeller, D. A., Kirschner, B. S., Park, R. and Perman, J. A. (1982): Diagnosis and differentiation of fat malabsorption in children using ^{13}C-labeled lipids: Trioctanoin, triotein and palmitic acid breath tests. *Gastroenterology*, 82:911–917.

29. Watkins, J. B., Park, R., Perman, J. A., Schoeller, D. A., and Klein, P. D. (1980): Ileal dysfunction vs. bacterial overgrowth: Detection by ^{13}C glycocholate breath test and fecal combustion. *Pediatr. Res.,* 14:512.
30. Watkins, J. B., Schoeller, D. A., Klein, P. D., Newcomer, A. D., and Hofmann, A. F. (1977): ^{13}C-Trioctanoin—A nonradioactive breath test to detect fat malabsorption. *J. Lab. Clin. Med.,* 90:422–430.

DISCUSSION

Dr. Aurrichio: Do you have any experience on the breath test in patients with cystic fibrosis? What kind of relationship is there between the increase in the breath content of hydrogen and the bacterial overgrowth?

Dr. Perman: Approximately 50% of our patients with cystic fibrosis have elevated basal hydrogen excretion. There are a number of interpretations of the elevated basal hydrogen excretion in cystic fibrosis, all of which need to be explored. One is the fact that perhaps glycoproteins, which are substrates for hydrogen production, are increased in the lumen of patients with cystic fibrosis. There are other possible interpretations. It is conceivable that a portion of the elevated basal hydrogen excretion even in fasting patients with cystic fibrosis may be due to malabsorption of carbohydrates. All our patients who had cystic fibrosis and elevated basal hydrogen excretions had been on antibiotics, and it is conceivable that what we are seeing is a change in the flora due to the antibiotics.

With regard to bacterial overgrowth, we don't have a close correlation between the number of organisms, for example, in the upper small bowel and basal hydrogen excretion, but in each situation where we have aspirated duodenal contents and documented overgrowth, an elevated basal hydrogen was found.

Nutritional Adaptation of the Gastrointestinal Tract of the Newborn, edited by N. Kretchmer and A. Minkowski. Nestlé, Vevey/Raven Press, New York © 1983.

Necrotizing Enterocolitis

John Barnard, Harry Greene, and Robert Cotton

Department of Pediatrics, Division of Pediatric Gastroenterology/Nutrition, Nutrition Center, Vanderbilt School of Medicine, Nashville, Tennessee 37232

Neonatal necrotizing enterocolitis (NEC) is a well-described and extensively investigated affection of the high-risk newborn. It is a cosmopolitan disease, the clinical course of which ranges from modest abdominal distention and gastrointestinal dysfunction to a fulminant course of sepsis, disseminated intravascular coagulation, cardiovascular collapse, and death. The etiology remains largely unknown, but almost certainly is multifactorial with important contributions from infectious, immunologic, and structural origins. The purpose of this review is to highlight some of the current concepts regarding pathogenesis, clinical features, and management of NEC.

Genersich has been credited with the first case description (30). In 1891, he reported a fatal illness in a 2-day-old premature infant with vomiting and abdominal distention. Autopsy revealed inflammation and perforation of the distal ileum. During the first half of this century, numerous reports of abdominal catastrophies resembling NEC appeared in the literature. Various terminology was used, including malignant enteritis, neonatal appendicitis, ulcerative enterocolitis, and neonatal gut infarction. In 1965, the first American series was described by Mizrahi et al. (64). Since then, the literature has been inundated with clinical experience and investigation of pathogenic factors.

The recent surge of interest in NEC is not only the result of better recognition of the disease, but also there appears to be an increasing incidence in the United States and Canada. The increased incidence appears to stem from the larger number of very-low-birth-weight infants coupled with more sophisticated treatment which allows salvage of smaller, and apparently, more vulnerable infants. The incidence varies widely, some centers reporting only rare, isolated cases (16,88), while others report an incidence of 4% to 5% of all neonatal admissions (29,76,101). Yearly incidence within a single nursery may vary considerably as the result of the occasional epidemic nature of NEC. Though term infants may be affected (72), low-birth-weight neonates are at highest risk. Figure 1 illustrates the relationship between birth weight and incidence of disease in 51 neonates from the Vanderbilt nursery. This distribution is typical of that experience in the literature. No racial or gender differences in incidence have been described.

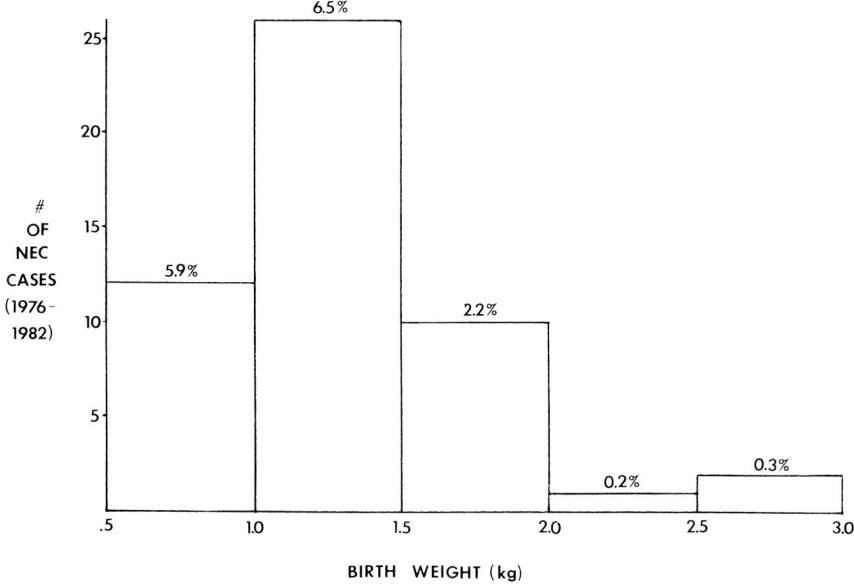

FIG. 1. Relationship between birth weight and NEC. The percent figure represents the percent of all neonatal intensive care unit admissions for each weight category who developed NEC. Data were collected over a 6-year period.

Mortality rates also vary from center to center. During the past 17 years, reported mortality rates range from 15% to 80% (29,72,76,80,101). With advances in physiologic support of critically ill neonates, survival rates have significantly improved. Schullinger reviewed 25 years of experience and found a dramatic increase in survival, from 17% prior to 1972, to 68% in 1980 (80).

SIGNS AND SYMPTOMS

The age of onset of NEC is extremely variable (49,101). Figure 2 shows the postnatal age of onset in 51 infants at Vanderbilt University Hospital. Note that 8 patients were diagnosed after 1 month of age and 1 infant was afflicted on the 63rd day. Two cases occurred within the first 24 hr of life. The mean age at diagnosis was 16 days, the median 11.5 (49). In a review of 123 patients, Kliegman noted the mean age at diagnosis was 12 days and the median was 7 days. Little is known about the determinants of age at presentation. Yu found an inverse relationship between birth weight and age of onset (101). deLemos found that the administration of parenteral antibiotics delayed the onset of the disease (21). Infants who had received no antibiotics were diagnosed at 8.9 days, whereas those previously receiving antibiotics first manifested signs and symptoms at 19.9 days of age. The onset of disease as late as

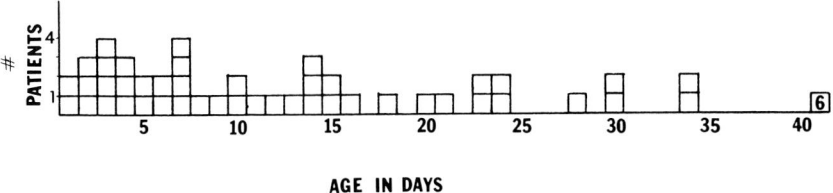

FIG. 2. Postnatal age of infants at the time of diagnosis. Note that 6 patients were diagnosed beyond 40 days of age.

the second or third month suggests that perinatal problems and complications are not necessary precursors of NEC.

Table 1 lists the usual signs and symptoms (7,49,85,101). None are considered absolute for diagnosis; many are quite nonspecific. According to Hodson (42), the most common signs are temperature instability 57%, lethargy 33%, and apnea 29%, none of which are distinctive enough to establish the diagnosis. An abdominal radiography may show considerable disease in the face of minimal or no clinical signs or symptoms (73).

It is clear that NEC may assume a broad spectrum of clinical severity. Some infants have little in the way of signs and symptoms, isolated colonic pneumatosis, and a benign course (59). Others have fulminant disease characterized by extensive gangrene, early perforation, cardiovascular collapse, and death within hours of onset of disease (55). Determinants of the severity are as yet ill defined.

LABORATORY EVALUATION

Laboratory investigations are nondiagnostic. However, some data may be important prognostically and serial determinations of coagulation function, platelet counts, hematocrits, acid–base balance, and electrolytes are crucial to aggressive, conscientious medical support. Thrombocytopenia is a frequent

TABLE 1. *Signs and symptoms of NEC*

Abdominal distention	68–100%
Bloody stools	55–89%
Apnea/bradycardia	34–94%
Vomiting	13–89%
Diarrhea	15–50%
Abdominal tendernesss	26–36%
Hypothermia	5–89%
Hypotension	14%
Abdominal wall erythema	4%
Abdominal mass	2%

Data from refs. 7, 49, 85, and 101.

occurrence but was not first reported in association with NEC until 1969 (99). Hutter reviewed 40 cases of NEC and found clinical bleeding and platelet counts < 50,000 in 12 infants (44). Curiously, disseminated intravascular coagulation (DIC) was documented in only 6 infants. He hypothesized that platelet microthrombi or local intestinal consumption might account for thrombocytopenia in the absence of DIC. Nadir platelet counts did not differ in survivors and those who died. In survivors, the platelet count returned to normal in 1 to 31 days (median = 7 days).

Leukopenia is sometimes present. In Hutter's series, 14 of 38 had white counts less than 1,500 and this group had a significantly increased mortality (44).

DIC occurs in 10% to 50% of patients and may be fulminant. Roback (76) found an 85% mortality rate in association with DIC. In Frantz's (29) series, 26 of 51 infants developed DIC and all required surgical intervention.

A metabolic acidosis, often refractory to alkali therapy, is not infrequent. Hyponatremia may be profound and is a manifestation of massive fluid shifts and "3rd spacing" of fluid into the edematous bowel wall and the peritoneal space.

RADIOGRAPHIC EVALUATION

In addition to careful serial physical examinations, radiographic assessment of the abdomen is critical to diagnosis and evaluation of progression of the disease. X-ray abnormalities may be subtle and nonspecific early in the course, but as disease progresses, they may be diagnostic. Early signs of gastrointestinal dysfunction include diffuse gaseous distention, often with air fluid levels and separation of adjacent bowel loops (8,75).

The hallmark of roentgenographic diagnosis is demonstration of pneumatosis intestinalis on the plain abdominal film. It is present in 90% to 100% of cases (8,85) and typically is first seen in the ileocecal area. In widespread disease, though, intramural air may be demonstrated anywhere from the stomach to the rectum. Two patterns of pneumatosis are described (8). Linear pneumatosis is appreciated as a curvilinear intramural radiolucency and probably represents subserosal gas. Cystic pneumatosis is less easily appreciated and assumes a foamy or bubbly pattern which can be confused with fecal material. The cystic pattern probably represents submucosal gas collection. Curiously, pneumatosis intestinalis may rapidly appear and disappear. The extent of pneumatosis is not usually considered a reflection of disease severity, though this point is subject to controversy (8,29,73,74). One must be mindful that pneumatosis may be present in other clinical situations such as intestinal gangrene secondary to vascular occlusion, Hirschsprung's disease with enterocolitis, obstruction at the site of bowel atresia, pyloric stenosis, and meconium ileus. In addition, it is possible that premature infants requiring mechanical ventilation with high airway pressure may have extension of mediastinal air direction into the abdomen resembling pneumatosis.

Any clinical circumstance resulting in pneumatosis intestinalis may cause hepatic portal venous or lymphatic gas. It appears as fine arborizing channels in the hepatic area and is best demonstrated on a lateral supine view of the abdomen. Formerly, this radiographic sign was considered particularly ominous prognostically (89,99); it is demonstrable in 30% of cases and is no longer believed to be of grave consequence (49,88). Portal venous gas may also be seen for several hours after umbilical vein catheterization (8).

Ascites is represented by bulging of the flanks, a diffuse, ground glass appearance, separation of adjacent bowel loops, and a central position of floating bowel. Leonidas noted that these signs often developed coincident with clinical deterioration and suggested that they were an indication of progressive peritonitis (60). Ascites is present in 10% to 20% of cases (101).

Free peritoneal air may be minuscule and escape radiographic detection, or may be massive as demonstrated by "the football sign" with stitching represented by the falciform ligament. A pneumoperitoneum in association with the proper clinical setting is a sign of perforation and indicates need for prompt surgical intervention. Curiously, 50% to 60% of patients with documented perforation at laparotomy have no detectable free peritoneal air (8,73).

While evaluating serial abdominal films during the course of disease, one should be particularly mindful of a persistently dilated bowel loop. Wayne noted this pattern in 10/30 neonates requiring surgery, and the anatomic location of necrotic bowel frequently corresponded to the position of dilation (9).

Although abdominal roentgenograms are crucial adjuncts to the diagnosis and assessment of infants with NEC, dramatic interobserver variability in the radiographic diagnosis has been reported. Mata asked six pediatric radiologists and four neonatologists to review 17 unlabeled abdominal X-rays of neonates with clinical NEC. Full agreement was reached only on one film (62).

PATHOLOGY

At laparotomy or autopsy, the areas most frequently involved are the distal ileum, cecum, and right colon. Occasionally, extensive disease is found with necrosis extending from the stomach to rectum. Grossly, the affected segments are dilated. Serosal surfaces are dull gray, hemorrhagic, or necrotic. Intramural gas collections and areas of perforation may be apparent. The diseased bowel is quite friable when manipulated. The intestinal wall and mesentery may be edematous and purulent peritonitis may be observed.

Microscopic sections initially show vascular congestion, hemorrhages into the lamina propria, and sloughing of the surface epithelium forming superficial ulcerations. A pseudomembrane consisting of inflammatory cells, fibrin, and cellular debris may be apparent. Mucosal or submucosal necrosis progresses to transmural involvement with an intact serosa acting as the only barrier to impending perforation. Gaseous collections are found in the submucosa and subserosa. Large vessel thrombosis is unusual although platelet–fibrin microthrombi are noted in intramural arterioles (9,79,89).

MANAGEMENT

Professionals involved in the care of high-risk neonates must maintain a constant index of suspicion for signs and symptoms of NEC. If the diagnosis is made, prompt institution of medical measures is indicated and preparations for laparotomy should be made if the initial evaluation reveals a reason for surgical intervention. Surgical consultation should be obtained on any suspect case, with frequent clinical reassessment and review of laboratory and roentgenographic data conducted by both medical and surgical teams.

Cultures should be obtained from blood, stool, cerebrospinal fluid, urine, and peritoneal fluid. Parenteral ampicillin and an aminoglycoside, such as gentamicin, should be started; adaptations should be made as determined by routine surveillance cultures and sensitivities. The efficacy of enteral aminoglycosides is controversial. Bell (3) used traditional medical management techniques and, additionally, topical gavage antibiotics given at 4-hr intervals. With this regimen, none of 14 cases progressed to perforation. This same investigator later studied fecal microflora in 22 patients with NEC (4). Each infant received topical gentamicin in addition to intravenous antibiotic therapy. Cultures obtained during therapy showed significantly fewer gram-negative aerobes when compared with pretreatment cultures. This effect was attributed to topical gentamicin. In a recent randomized controlled study, Hansen found that enteral administration of gentamicin did not influence morbidity or mortality (36). He did, however, demonstrate significantly increased peak serum gentamicin concentrations in study patients, some of which were greater than potentially ototoxic levels.

Initial management often must be directed toward restoring the intravascular volume and cardiac output. Patients with NEC may lose 30% to 50% or more of their circulating volume into the affected mesentery and bowel. In addition, clinical findings of endotoxic shock often occur, a feature which is not unexpected in view of the common involvement of gram-negative organisms. These conditions may demand massive volume replacement with colloids, including blood. When an increasing central venous pressure is observed without improvement in systemic perfusion, improvement in myocardial performance should be sought with an ionotropic agent such as dopamine or digoxin. The aggressive and rapid management of shock is of paramount importance in order to minimize the possibility of additional ischemic necrosis of the bowel.

Other important therapeutic maneuvers include gastric decompression by nasogastric suction, removal of umbilical vessel catheters, withholding oral feedings, and introducing central or peripheral hyperalimentation. Support of altered cardiodynamics and electrolyte balance is adjusted as dictated by frequent determinations of electrolyte and acid–base parameters and with attention to vital signs, systemic blood pressure, central venous pressure, and urine flow. Platelet and coagulation abnormalities should be followed closely and prompt intervention made when appropriate.

As medical management has become more refined and physiologic support of critically ill prematures more sophisticated, early surgical intervention is no longer indicated. Much debate has centered around establishing accurate criteria for operative therapy. Laparotomy in a fragile premature infant without surgically remedial disease, such as for gangrene or perforation, is laden with unacceptable hazard. Similarly, a delay in operative intervention can be fatal, as the mortality rate in infants with gangrene and perforation is double those with gangrene alone (54). Kosloske has recently evaluated 10 criteria for operation based on previous recommendations by several authors (54). Of these, gangrene was best predicted by the presence of a pneumoperitoneum, a persistently dilated intestinal loop on serial radiographs, erythema or cellulitis of the abdominal wall, and a "positive" paracentesis. Invalid indications included clinical deterioration, persistent tenderness of the abdominal wall, profuse lower gastrointestinal hemorrhage, a gasless abdomen with ascites, and severe thrombocytopenia. Though some investigators have strongly supported thrombocytopenia and clinical deterioration as a reliable indicator of gangrene (68), in our study, clinical deterioration and severe thrombocytopenia were relatively frequent in patients without gangrene.

A promising technique for diagnosis of early gangrene is paracentesis, with lavage if necessary (52). A brown color of peritoneal fluid obtained by direct aspiration or lavage is highly suggestive of gangrene, whereas a yellow or pink color is found in cases without gangrene. The technique is successful even if abdominal roentgenograms fail to show ascites.

Utilizing correct medical therapy and prompt operative intervention when indicated, mortality rates for medically and surgically managed babies may be as low as 15% to 30% (7,54). The surgical procedure most commonly performed is segmental resection of the devitalized bowel with proximal diversion and a distal mucous fistula.

Independent of the well-described neurodevelopmental sequellae in low-birth-weight infants, neonates surviving NEC may experience a multiplicity of complications. First, there is a 20% incidence of intestinal stricture 1 to 2 months after the acute illness (6,56,74,80). The majority are colonic and are characterized histologically by fibrous tissue, edema, and granulation tissue. It is recommended that all infants recovering from NEC undergo a contrast barium enema prior to reestablishing intestinal continuity or if symptoms of intestinal obstruction develop.

Second, resection of long lengths of small bowel may result in a severe malabsorption syndrome. Schullinger found postoperative malabsorption in 8% of patients (80). Third, lymphoid polyposis, transient lactose malabsorption, and intraabdominal abcesses have been described (53,74). Finally, perhaps the most far-reaching morbidity of NEC is the occurrence of iatrogenic malnutrition in infants who are kept NPO (nothing per os) or who are inadequately fed for the first few days or weeks of life because of respect for this potentially devastating disease.

PATHOGENESIS OF NEC

Early reports of NEC were laden with speculation about pathogenesis and causal associations were frequently made from descriptive studies without controls. In an effort to more accurately delineate the neonate at risk, controlled studies have been conducted in order to identify perinatal complications and problems unique to the infant who will develop disease (17,29,50,78,87,101). Table 2 demonstrates the persistence of considerable confusion surrounding predisposing phenomena and factors of etiologic importance. No one perinatal complication or management technique is consistently implicated. In fact, Stoll determined that affected infants were quite similar to controls and identified no risk factors (87). Kliegman's study, the most recent and perhaps the most appropriately controlled, failed to delineate any important risk factor. He therefore concluded that perinatal problems which precede NEC are indeed equally common to all high-risk infants (50). These findings are perhaps the most powerful testimony to the multifactorial etiology of NEC.

IMPORTANT FACTORS IN PATHOGENESIS

Enteric Feedings

The observation that most neonates have been fed prior to the diagnosis has been an issue of intense interest and speculation. Controlled studies comparing feeding management techniques in infants with and without NEC fail to consistently support feeding as an important precursor, though controversy certainly persists. There are multiple ways by which feeding might contribute to the pathogenesis or progression of disease: (a) direct mucosal injury by hypertonic feedings, (b) the absence of an immunologically protective effect in formula-fed infants, (c) the alteration of intestinal microflora, (d) structural immaturity of the premature intestine, and (e) the effect of early or large-volume feedings on an alimentary tract compromised by adverse perinatal events. Immunologic and infectious considerations are discussed later.

Both animal studies and clinical data have implicated hypertonic feedings in production of mucosal injury. Hypertonic solutions applied to the intestine produce functional and microscopic damage to the epithelial surface (45).

TABLE 2. *Purported risk factors for NEC (summary of seven controlled studies)*

RISK FACTOR FOR NEC	REFERENCE						
	78	101	51	87	29	76	17
APGAR 1		S					S
APGAR 5	S						S
UMBILICAL ARTERIAL CATH					S		S
UMBILICAL VENOUS CATH					S		S
EXCHANGE TRANSFUSION		S					
NO RDS			S				
ENTERIC FEEDING		■			S	S	
PROM	S	S				■	
PDA	S			■		■	
HYPEROSMOLAR FEEDS	S	S			■		
RECURRENT APNEA		S					
PLACENTAL ABRUPTION			S				
SHOCK		S			■		
GAVAGE FEEDING	S			■			
HYPERALIMENTATION	S						
10% DEXTROSE	S						
MARRIED MOTHERS	■		■				
MATERNAL ANTIBIOTICS	S						
MATERNAL ANESTHESIA	S						
NO GENTAMICIN	S						

KEY

S — Parameter significantly more common in patients with NEC

☐ — Parameter not significant

■ — Parameter not investigated

deLemos produced an enterocolitis closely resembling NEC when he fed goats a dialyzed, hypertonic goat's milk formula (22). In a very small prospective study, Book noted an 87% incidence of NEC in infants < 1,200 g who were fed an elemental formula containing 650 mosm/liter (10). In contrast, only 25% of neonates fed standard cow's milk formula (359 mosm/liter) developed the disease. Willis described a group of premature infants with an increased incidence of disease presumably because a high-osmolality calcium lactate solution (>1,700 mosm/liter) was added to the standard formula (98). Osmolalities of preterm cow's milk formulas have been determined by freezing point depression (69): 20 cal./oz. formula yields 252 to 319 mosm/liter. $D_{10}W$ (10% dextrose in water) and formulas containing >20 cal./oz. yield >400 mosm/liter and some powdered formulas may be even more hypertonic. Hypertonic enteric feedings are best used with caution.

Debate surrounds the importance of early institution and rapid volume advancement of feedings in a premature neonate with a structurally and functionally immature alimentary system (66). An increased incidence of NEC has been temporally associated with a change to more aggressive feeding policies, and clusters of cases have "disappeared" with the institution of a more conservative feeding schedule (12,26,31). Eyal et al. performed a 2-year study of the influence of feeding practices on the incidence of the disease (26). During the first year, neonates were fed expressed breast milk on days 2 to 5 of life and were advanced at increments of 10 to 20 ml/kg/day. In the second year, infants were first fed at 2 to 3 weeks of age. The incidence of NEC was 18% and 3% in the first and second study years, respectively. Brown felt that NEC was virtually eliminated in his nursery coincident with the institution of an extremely cautious feeding protocol which fostered late initiation of enteral feedings, slow advancement of feedings, and prompt discontinuance of feedings when untoward signs suggesting hypoxia, hypoperfusion, or gastrointestinal dysfunction developed (16). Book, however, has published a small prospective study comparing fast and slow feeding rates designed to attain complete enteral alimentation at 7 and 14 days, respectively. No difference in the incidence of NEC was found (12). The controversy involving early feedings and optimal feeding rates remains quite unsettled.

Infection

By virtue of its clinical presentation, occasional epidemic nature, and association with laboratory evidence of systemic infection, NEC is considered a primary infectious disease by some authors. Since a wide variety of organisms have been isolated from stool, peritoneal, and blood cultures, a single etiologic agent seems unlikely. Table 3 lists the bacteria most commonly isolated from blood and stool specimens. Blood cultures are positive in 18% to 60% of cases and usually correlate well with the isolates from stool and peritoneal fluid (7,4,46,49,76,85,100); these bacteria are common enteric organisms, even in healthy subjects. Therefore, the existence of a superimposed predisposition, such as hypoxic injury, immunologic immaturity, or the administration of hypertonic feedings must be important in the pathogenesis. Additionally, altered virulence of the organisms, the size of bacterial inoculum, or the multiple complex interactions between the "normal flora" and potential pathogens may contribute to NEC (61). Bell and co-workers showed that Enterobacteriaceae such as *Escherichia coli* and *Klebsiella* were recovered with greater frequency from stools of infants with NEC when compared with controls without the disease (2). In a later study, Bell demonstrated a changing incidence of NEC

TABLE 3. *Organisms commonly isolated from blood and stool cultures in infants with NEC*

Organism	Stool (%)	Blood (%)
Escherichia coli	31–50	20–85
Klebsiella	19–57	6–40
Enterobacter	46	1–6
Citrobacter	3	1
Pseudomonas	8–40	6–30
Staphylococcus epidermidis	30–54	30
Clostridia	3	2–20
Enterococcus	5–12	4–6

Data from refs. 4, 7, 46, 49, 76, 85, and 101.

in his nursery and noted an association with the changing prevalence of *E. coli* and *Klebsiella* (5). Frantz, too, found that stool cultures obtained at the time of diagnosis were statistically more likely to grow *Klebsiella* than similarly timed cultures from controls (29). Stanley reported a striking decrease in the incidence of NEC concurrent with the emergence of *Serratia* as the predominant nursery stool flora. These observations (83) suggest that as yet ill-defined microbial characteristics and interrelationships are important pathogenetic factors.

NEC can be an epidemic disease with clustering as shown in Fig. 3. Efforts aimed at identification of epidemic pathogens are variably successful. Virnig performed careful bacteriologic and viral studies during an outbreak (92). Blood, cerebrospinal fluid, and urine samples were incubated for bacterial and fungal growth. Blood and stool specimens were submitted for viral isolation. No transmissible agent was found consistently, even from 5 cases clustered in a 3-week period. Incubator position within the nursery and nursing assignments were not suggestive. All individuals having contact with the infants were screened for infectious disease and none was found. The author concluded

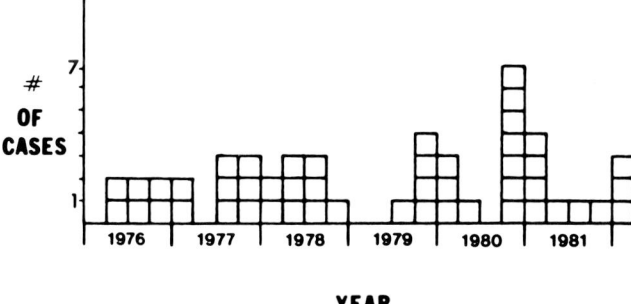

FIG. 3. Distribution of cases with respect to time; each *square* represents a 3-month interval and clustering of cases is apparent.

that organisms associated with NEC were normal enteric microflora which were invasive because of altered host defense. Book reported a temporal cluster during which the incidence increased from 0.3% to 3.6% of all admissions (13). Ten cases occurred during a 2½-week period and in only two of four nursery rooms. Interestingly, several cases of gastrointestinal illness occurred in nursing personnel during this interval. Despite a diligent search for bacterial or viral causation, none was identified. Aggressive infectious disease control measures were implemented, including case isolation, strict handwashing, gowns and gloves, and a cohort nursing system. The incidence of disease promptly decreased to 0.7%. Because of the suggestion of a transmissible agent in this epidemic, the author called for more sophisticated methods of search for an infectious etiology.

Instances of epidemic NEC associated with specific pathogens have been well documented. Outbreaks caused by *Clostridium butyricum* (43), *Salmonella* (84), *E. coli* (27,100), and *Klebsiella* type 26 (40) have recently been described.

Clostridial organisms are gas-forming anaerobes with a propensity to infect ischemic, devitalized tissue. The isolation of several clostridial species and toxins from infants with NEC, as well as identification of clostridial-mediated NEC-like illnesses in other mammals, has stimulated a recent interest in this organism and its role in neonatal NEC. Conflicting data have emerged. Fulminant and rapidly fatal NEC has been associated with blood and peritoneal fluid culture positivity for clostridia (55). An unusual outbreak in term infants has been described in England (43), where 9 of 12 infants were blood-culture positive for *C. butyricum*. Kliegman reviewed 12 cases presumably secondary to *C. perfringens* (47) and Cashore cultured clostridia from confirmed and suspect cases more frequently than in infants without disease (18). Pedersen likened NEC to gas gangrene of the bowel (70). On the other hand, clostridia are ubiquitous organisms and enteric colonization with these bacteria is usual in the first week of life (57,63). Shurentz cultured *C. difficile* from a nurse's hand, the nursery floor, and in respiratory therapy equipment. Both *C. difficile* and its toxin were found with regularity in infants with and without NEC (82). Donta detected *C. difficile* toxin in 55% of all infants in the intensive care nursery (24), while Chang found no toxin in 18 infants with NEC (19). These observations suggest that the exact relationship between clostridial organisms and their toxins and the pathophysiology of NEC remains quite obscure.

Immunologic Considerations

A normal child has a multiplicity of host defense mechanisms, both immunologic and nonimmunologic, which assist to protect against gastrointestinal mucosal invasion and also to moderate microbial colonization of intraluminal surfaces. The subject has recently been reviewed and is vastly complex (61,93). Presently, only a superficial understanding of the premature mucosal immune system exists. We are even more ignorant about the functional and structural integrity of the system in the face of profound prematurity, severe cardiopulmonary distress, and malnutrition. The role of altered host defense in the pathogenesis of NEC is similarly obscure. After local gastrointestinal defense mechanisms have been violated, undoubtedly an immature systemic immune system can contribute to the progression of fulminant disease. The development and relative immaturity of the premature's systemic immune system is the subject of several recent reviews and will not be further considered here (34,86). Since the majority of premature mucosal immunity is acquired from breast milk, this discussion centers on breast milk and some of the theoretical, experimental, and clinical considerations in the pathogenesis of NEC.

Human breast milk offers a number of immunologic advantages over cow's milk formula. Of these, the most widely investigated is secretory immunoglobulin A. In term infants SIgA is not demonstrable in intestinal fluids until 1 week of age and reaches "adult" values at 1 month postnatal age (81). It functions in several ways, the most significant of which appears to be inhibition of bacterial adherence to epithelial surfaces, which influences invasion and governs luminal colonization (97). Additionally, other antigenic materials such as toxins may be prevented from binding to the intestinal surface (94). Thus, during the first days of life, a time when microbial colonization occurs, the non-breast-fed premature is deficient in what may well be the "backbone" of mucosal immunity. An interesting "homing" mechanism has been described in humans and experimental animals whereby SIgA-producing plasma cells in the maternal gut are antigenically stimulated and migrate to the breast where specific antibodies are secreted into colostrum (94). In this way a breast-feeding infant may receive some passive protection against bacteria he is most likely to harbor, that is, his mother's. In summary, then, a distressed premature, who receives either no enteral feedings or cow's milk feeding, is without the potential protection of SIgA. Also, with the advent of regionalization of neonatal intensive care, infants fed pooled breast milk may not have specific and optimal SIgA function protective against maternally acquired flora.

Another component of breast milk which may have particular relevance to NEC is the *Lactobacillus bifidus* "growth factor". Breast-fed infants harbor a predominance of enteric lactobacilli and fewer gram-negative organisms such as *E. coli* (63,96). This effect is present as early as 48 hr postnatally and potentiates growth of nonpathogenic organisms which have not been regarded as important agents in NEC.

The presence of other factors in breast milk, such as cell-mediated mucosal immune responses, intraluminal immunoglobulins (IgG), and viable breast milk cells, such as neutrophils, lymphocytes, and macrophages, is of interest but, as yet, is not well studied in the premature infant.

There are a limited number of experimental observations on the importance of breast milk in NEC. Most popular is Barlow's work with newborn rats with experimental enterocolitis (1). Using an hypoxic insult, she consistently produced a disease similar to NEC in rats fed an artificially prepared formula. All breast-fed, asphyxiated rats were protected from disease, even if orally contaminated with a *Klebsiella* inoculum. Additionally, asphyxiated animals fed dam's breast milk for the first 24 hr and then switched to artificial formula were protected. Barlow concluded that breast milk induced a protective passive enteric immunity in the rat newborn and that it may similarly protect the premature infant. In a related study, the same investigators demonstrated that frozen milk was not protective until viable cells were added (71).

NEC has repeatedly been documented in neonates fed exclusively human milk. Moriarty described 15 cases (65). Kliegman reviewed 109 cases of NEC and showed that the incidence in infants fed only refrigerated human milk was comparable to that in infants fed with commercial formula (51). Possible explanations for development of the disease in the face of significant theoretical advantages offered by breast milk included the absence of an intact "homing" mechanism, the use of pooled, banked milk, contamination of milk and, perhaps most importantly, the adverse effects of storage on the viability and functional integrity of the cellular components.

Hypoxic/Ischemic Considerations

Since the earliest reports of NEC, investigators have noted that the disease frequently is associated with perinatal asphyxia, umbilical vessel manipulation, cold stress, and hypoxia. Interest in gastrointestinal ischemia as a contributor to NEC was further stimulated by documentation of the arterial constrictor response in diving animals (15). This "survival reflex" involves arterial constriction in vascular beds of muscle, skin, kidney, liver, and gastrointestinal tract in an attempt to preserve cardiac and cerebral blood flow during prolonged diving. Premature neonates may respond to repeated stresses in a similar fashion resulting in intermittent ischemia to the gastrointestinal tract.

Several animal studies have demonstrated structural violation of mucosal surfaces following severe hypoxia. Under experimental hypoxic conditions, a clinical syndrome resembling NEC can be produced in laboratory animals. Harrison studied histologic and ultrastructural changes in the gastrointestinal tract of puppies exposed to hypoxia and hypovolemia for 1- to 2-hr periods (38). Alterations were most common in the ileum and proximal colon and consisted of vascular microthrombosis, swollen or "blistered" endothelial cells, disruption of tight junctions, swelling and rupture of mitochondria, and perivascular edema. All these observations were made with electron microscopy. With the exception of vascular congestion, light microscopy was normal. Touloukian designed an experimental model whereby mucosal perfusion and histology were evaluated in asphyxiated and resuscitated neonatal piglets (91). Perfusion of all portions of the gut, with the exception of the esophagus, was dramatically decreased. The most impressive reduction occurred in the stomach, distal ileum, and colon—common sites of necrosis and perforation in

NEC. Histologic evidence of vascular congestion and hemorrhage was most common in the ileum and colon. Barlow induced gastrointestinal catastrophies in newborn rats by exposing them to a 3- to 5-min hypoxic insult and then formula feedings (1). The fatal illness closely resembled fulminant NEC.

Speculation about the role of umbilical vessel manipulation in the production of mucosal ischemia has been widespread. Distinct arterial thrombi have been found in 95% of infants with umbilical artery catheters (67). Lehmiller implicated umbilical artery catheters in the formation of mesenteric thromboemboli found in postmortem NEC specimens (58). Hillman quantified plasticizer levels in tissues of neonates with indwelling umbilical catheters (41). The mean levels in gastrointestinal tissues from three infants with NEC were significantly higher than those in infants without disease. Each of these studies identified a potential hazard of umbilical vessel catheterization. With particular reference to the alimentary tract, there are numerous reports of ischemic gastrointestinal lesions after umbilical venous exchange transfusion (37). Touloukian measured portal venous pressure in newborn piglets during exchange transfusion through the portal venous system (90). A significant increase in portal pressure was recorded during the injection phase of the exchange, and the author hypothesized that dramatic alterations in mucosal vascular pressures produced ischemia secondary to vascular congestion and hemorrhage. As noted in the above section on controlled studies of NEC, no clinical data consistently implicate utilization of umbilical vessel catheters in the pathogenesis.

Low-flow states such as exist with left-to-right shunting through a patent ductus arteriosus (39) or polycythemic hyperviscosity syndrome (35,39) are potential contributors to mucosal ischemia. Hakanson (35) found a significantly increased incidence of NEC in small-for-gestational-age infants with hyperviscosity. A propensity for NEC has been reported following cardiac catheterization for evaluation of congenital heart disease, implying that hemodynamic disturbances, severe cyanosis, or angiographic contrast hypertonicity can contribute to alimentary mucosal ischemia and possibly NEC (20,23).

PREVENTION

Definitive recommendations on prevention of NEC await further elucidation of etiologic mechanisms. Several studies have addressed prevention by prophylactic administration of an enteral aminoglycoside antibiotic. Two of four similarly designed trials have supported gentamicin or kanamycin enteral prophylaxis in low-birth-weight infants (25,32). The remaining two studies concluded that no protection was afforded, as controls and study infants both developed NEC at similar rates (14,77). It is agreed that enteric bacterial colonization rate is reduced, but antibiotic-resistant gram-negative organisms have emerged during such therapy. Currently, it would seem that this type of prophylaxis is not helpful and may, indeed, be deleterious.

In an attempt to identify early mucosal damage and secondary decreased capacity for carbohydrate absorption, Book et al. screened for reducing substances in stool specimens from formula-fed infants at risk of NEC. Seventy-one percent of infants who developed NEC had 3 to 4^+ reducing substances from 1 to 4 days prior to clinical manifestations of disease. The presence of stool-reducing substances may signal the need for altered management and close scrutiny for signs and symptoms of NEC. A more sensitive and specific indicator for early disease or a predisposition to disease is lacking.

Some investigators have suggested that delay of enteral feedings and institution of slowly progressive feeding regimens help prevent NEC (16). Well-designed prospective controlled studies are presently not available.

ACKNOWLEDGMENTS

The authors express their appreciation to Debora Carroll for typing and aid in preparation of this manuscript. Research supported in part by NIH grant AM26657 and funds from Bristol Meyers Company.

REFERENCES

1. Barlow, B., Santulli, T. V., Heird, W. C., Pitt, J., Blanc, W. A., and Schullinger, J. N. (1974): An experimental study of acute neonatal enterocolitis—The importance of breast milk. *J. Pediatr. Surg.,* 9:587–595.
2. Bell, J. H., Feigin, R. D., Ternberg, J. L., and Brotherton, T. (1978): Evaluation of intestinal microflora in necrotizing enterocolitis. *J. Pediatr.,* 92:589–592.
3. Bell, J. H., Kosloske, A. M., Benton, C., and Martin, L. W. (1973): Neonatal necrotizing enterocolitis: Prevention of perforation. *J. Pediatr. Surg.,* 8:601–605.
4. Bell, J. H., Shackelford, P. G., Feigin, R. D., Ternberg, J. L., and Brotherton, T. (1979): Alterations in gastrointestinal microflora during antimicrobial therapy for necrotizing enterocolitis. *Pediatrics,* 63:425–428.
5. Bell, J. H., Shackelford, P., Feigin, R. D., Ternberg, J. C., and Brotherton, T. (1979): Epidemiologic and bacteriologic evaluation of neonatal necrotizing enterocolitis. *J. Pediatr. Surg.,* 14:1–4.
6. Bell, M. J., Ternberg, J. L., Askin, F. B., McAlister, W., and Shackelford, G. (1976): Intestinal stricture in necrotizing enterocolitis. *J. Pediatr. Surg.,* 11:319–327.
7. Bell, M. J., Ternberg, J. L., Feigin, R. D., Keating, J. P., Marshall, R., Barton, L., and Brotherton, T. (1978): Neonatal necrotizing enterocolitis: Therapeutic decisions based on clinical staging. *Ann. Surg.,* 187:1–7.
8. Bell, R. S., Graham, C. B., and Stevenson, J. K. (1971): Roentgenologic and clinical manifestations of neonatal necrotizing enterocolitis. *Am. J. Roent. Rad. Ther. Nuc. Med.,* 112:123–134.
9. Benirschke, K. (1975): In: *Necrotizing Enterocolitis in the Newborn Infant.* Report of the 68th Ross Conference on Pediatric Research, p. 29.
10. Book, L. S., Herbst, J. J., Atherton, S. O., and Jung, A. L. (1975): Necrotizing enterocolitis in low-birth-weight infants fed an elemental formula. *J. Pediatr.,* 87:602–605.
11. Book, L. S., Herbst, J. J., and Jung, A. L. (1976): Carbohydrate malabsorption in necrotizing enterocolitis. *Pediatrics,* 57:201–204.
12. Book, L. S., Herbst, J. J., and Jung, A. L. (1976): Comparison of fast and slow feeding rate schedules to the development of necrotizing enterocolitis. *J. Pediatr.,* 89:463–465.
13. Book, L. S., Overall, J. C., Herbst, J. J., Britt, M. R., Epstein, B., and Jung, A. L. (1977): Clustering of necrotizing enterocolitis: Interruption by infection-control measures. *N. Engl. J. Med.,* 297:984–986.

14. Boyle, R., Nelson, J. S., Stonestreet, B. S., Peter, G., and Oh, W. (1978): Alterations in stool flora resulting from oral kanamycin prophylaxis of necrotizing enterocolitis. *J. Pediatr.*, 93:857–861.
15. Bron, K. M., Murdaugh, H. V., Millen, J. E., Lenthall, R., Raskin, P., and Robin, E. D. (1966): Arterial constrictor response in a diving mammal. *Science*, 152:540–543.
16. Brown, E., and Sweet, A. (1978): Preventing necrotizing enterocolitis in neonates. *J.A.M.A.*, 240:2452–2454.
17. Bunton, G. L., Durbin, G. M., McIntosh, N., Shaw, D. G., Taghizadeh, A., Reynolds, E. O., Rivers, R. P., and Urman, G. (1977): Necrotizing enterocolitis: Controlled study of three years experience in a neonatal intensive care unit. *Arch. Dis. Child.*, 52:772–777.
18. Cashore, W. J., Peter, G., Lauermann, M., Stonestreet, B., and Oh, W. (1981): Clostridia colonization and clostridial toxin in neonatal necrotizing enterocolitis. *J. Pediatr.*, 98:308–311.
19. Chang, T., and Areson, P. (1978): Neonatal necrotizing enterocolitis: Absence of enteric bacterial toxins. *N. Engl. J. Med.*, 299:424.
20. Cooke, R. W., Meradji, M., and De Villenevue, V. H. (1980): Necrotizing enterocolitis after cardiac catheterization in infants. *Arch. Dis. Child.*, 55:66–68.
21. deLemos, R. A., Null, D. A., and Franklin, L. C. (1976): The effect of previously administered antibiotics on the time of onset and clinical course of necrotizing enterocolitis. *Pediatr. Res.*, 10:422.
22. deLemos, R. A., Roger, J. H., and McLaughlin, G. W. (1974): Experimental production of necrotizing enterocolitis in newborn goats. *Pediatr. Res.*, 8:380.
23. Dickinson, D. F., Galloway, R. W., Wilkinson, J. L., and Arnold, R. (1982): Necrotizing enterocolitis after neonatal cardiac catheterization. *Arch. Dis. Child.*, 57:431–433.
24. Donta, S. T., and Myers, M. G. (1982): *Clostridium difficile* toxin in asymptomatic neonates. *J. Pediatr.*, 100:431–435.
25. Egan, E. A., Mantilla, G., Nelson, R. M., and Eitzman, D. V. (1976): A prospective controlled trial of oral kanamycin in the prevention of neonatal necrotizing enterocolitis. *J. Pediatr.*, 89:467–471.
26. Eyal, F., Sagi, E., and Avital, A. (1982): Necrotizing enterocolitis in the very-low-birth-weight infant: Expressed breast milk feeding compared with parenteral feeding. *Arch. Dis. Child.*, 57:274–276.
27. Farmer, K., and Hassell, I. B. (1973): An epidemic of *E. coli* type 055:k59(BS) in a neonatal unit. *N. Z. Med. J.*, 77:372–375.
28. Franklin, R. H., Schofestall, R. O., and Amoury, R. A. (1979): Neonatal necrotizing enterocolitis: Five year experience at Children's Mercy Hospital. *Am. Surg.*, 45:636–642.
29. Frantz, I. D., L'Heureux, P., Engel, R. R., and Hunt, C. E. (1975): Necrotizing enterocolitis. *J. Pediatr.*, 56:259–263.
30. Genersich, A. (1891): Bauchfellentzundung beim, neugebornen in folge von perforation des ileums. *Arch. Anat. Pathol.*, 126:485.
31. Goldman, H. I. (1980): Feeding and necrotizing enterocolitis. *Am. J. Dis. Child.*, 134:553–555.
32. Grylack, L. J., and Scanlon, J. W. (1978): Oral gentamicin therapy in the prevention of neonatal necrotizing enterocolitis: A controlled double-blind trial. *Am. J. Dis. Child.*, 132:1192–1194.
33. Gunn, T., and Outerbridge, E. (1977): Polycythemia as a cause of necrotizing enterocolitis. *Can. Med. Assoc. J.*, 117:438.
34. Gutoff, S. P. (1974): Neonatal immunity. *J. Pediatr.*, 85:149–154.
35. Hakanson, D. O., and Oh, W. (1977): Necrotizing enterocolitis and hyperviscosity in the newborn infant. *J. Pediatr.*, 90:458–461.
36. Hansen, T. N., Ritter, D. A., Speer, M. E., Kenny, J. D., and Rudolph, A. J. (1980): A randomized, controlled study of oral gentamicin in the treatment of neonatal necrotizing enterocolitis. *J. Pediatr.*, 97:836–839.
37. Hardy, J. D., Savage, T. R., and Shirodaria, C. (1972): Intestinal perforation following exchange transfusion. *Am. J. Dis. Child.*, 124:136–140.
38. Harrison, M. V., Connell, R. S., Campbell, J. R., and Webb, M. C. (1975): Microcirculatory changes in the gastrointestinal tract of the hypoxic puppy: An electron microscope study. *J. Pediatr. Surg.*, 10:599–608.

39. Heath, R. E., and Bowen, F. W. (1976): Necrotizing enterocolitis and the patent ductus arteriosus. *Pediatr. Res.,* 10:424.
40. Hill, H. R., Hunt, C. E., and Matsen, J. M. (1974): Nosocomial colonization with *Klebsiella* type 26, in a neonatal intensive care unit associated with an outbreak of sepsis, meningitis and necrotizing enterocolitis. *J. Pediatr.,* 85:415–419.
41. Hillman, L. S., Goodwin, S. L., and Sherman, W. R. (1975): Identification and measurement of plastilizer in neonatal tissues after umbilical catheters and blood products. *N. Engl. J. Med.,* 292:381–386.
42. Hodson, W. A. (1975): In: *Necrotizing Enterocolitis in the Newborn Infant.* Report of the 68th Ross Conference on Pediatric Research, p. 19.
43. Howard, F. M., Flynn, D. M., Bradley, J. M., Noone, P., and Szawatkowski, J. (1977): Outbreak of necrotizing enterocolitis caused by *Clostridium butyricum. Lancet,* ii:1099–1102.
44. Hutter, J. J., Hathaway, W. E., and Wayne, E. R. (1976): Hematologic abnormalities in severe neonatal necrotizing enterocolitis. *J. Pediatr.,* 88:1026–1031.
45. Kameda, H., Abei, T. et al. (1968): Functional and histologic injury to intestinal mucosa produced by hypertonicity. *Am. J. Physiol.,* 214:1090–1097.
46. Kliegman, R. M. (1979): Necrotizing enterocolitis: Implications for an infectious disease. *Pediatr. Clin. North Am.,* 26:327–344.
47. Kliegman, R. M., Fanaroff, A. A., Izant, R., and Speck, W. T. (1979): Clostridia as pathogens in neonatal necrotizing enterocolitis. 95:287–289.
48. Kliegman, R. M., and Fanaroff, A. A. (1981): Neonatal necrotizing enterocolitis: A nine year experience, II. Outcome assessment. *Am. J. Dis. Child.,* 135:608–611.
49. Kliegman, R. M., and Fanaroff, A. A. (1981): Neonatal necrotizing enterocolitis: A nine year experience: Epidemiology and uncommon observations. *Am. J. Dis. Child.,* 135:603–607.
50. Kliegman, R. M., Hack, M., Jones, P., and Fanaroff, A. A. (1982): Epidemiologic study of necrotizing enterocolitis among low birth weight infants: Absence of identifiable risk factors. *J. Pediatr.,* 100:440–445.
51. Kliegman, R. M., Pittard, W. B., and Fanaroff, A. A. (1979): Necrotizing enterocolitis in neonates fed human milk. *J. Pediatr.,* 95:450–453.
52. Kosloske, A. M., and Lilly, J. R. (1978): Paracentesis and lavage for diagnosis of intestinal gangrene in neonatal necrotizing enterocolitis. *J. Pediatr. Surg.,* 13:315–320.
53. Kosloske, A. M., and Martin, L. W. (1973): Surgical complications of neonatal necrotizing enterocolitis. *Arch. Surg.,* 107:223–228.
54. Kosloske, A. M., Papile, L., and Burstein, J. (1980): Indications for operation in acute necrotizing enterocolitis of the neonate. *Surgery,* 87:502–508.
55. Kosloske, A. M., Ulrich, J. A., and Hoffman, H. (1978): Fulminant necrotizing enterocolitis associated with Clostridia. *Lancet,* 2:1014–1016.
56. Krasna, I. H., Becker, J. M., Schneider, K. M., and Beck, A. R. (1970): Colonic stenosis following necrotizing enterocolitis of the newborn. *J. Pediatr. Surg.,* 5:200–206.
57. Laverdiere, M., Robert, A., Chicoine, R., Salet, D., and Rosenfeld, R. (1978): Clostridia in necrotizing enterocolitis. *Lancet,* 2:377.
58. Lehmiller, D. H., and Kanto, W. F. (1978): Relationships of mesenteric thrombolmolism, oral feeding and necrotizing enterocolitis. *J. Pediatr.,* 92:96–100.
59. Leonidas, J. C., and Hall, R. T. (1976): Neonatal pneumatosis coli: A mild form of neonatal necrotizing enterocolitis. *J. Pediatr.,* 89:456–459.
60. Leonidas, J. C., Krasna, I. H., Fox, H. A., and Broder, M. S. (1973): Peritoneal fluid in N.E.C.: A radiologic sign of clinical deterioration. *J. Pediatr.,* 82:672–675.
61. Mackowiak, P. A. (1982): The normal microbial flora. *N. Engl. J. Med.,* 307:83–93.
62. Mata, A. G., and Rosengart, R. M. (1980): Interobserver variability in the radiographic diagnosis of necrotizing enterocolitis. *Pediatrics,* 66:68–71.
63. Mata, L. J., and Urrutia, J. J. (1971): Intestinal colonization of breast-fed children in a rural area of low socioeconomic level. *Ann. N. Y. Acad. Sci.,* 176:93.
64. Mizrahi, A., Barlow, O., Berdon, W., Blanc, W., and Silverman, W. (1965): Necrotizing enterocolitis in premature infants. *J. Pediatr.,* 66:697–706.
65. Moriartey, R. R., Finer, N. N., Cox, S. F., Phillips, H. J., Theman, A., Stewart, A. R., and Ulan, O. A. (1979): Necrotizing enterocolitis and human milk. *J. Pediatr.,* 94:295–296.
66. Moxey, P. C., and Trier, J. S. (1975): Structural features of the mucosa of human fetal small intestine. *Gastroenterology,* 68:1002, A-145.

67. Neal, W. A., Reynolds, J. W., Jarvis, C. W., and Williams, J. H. (1972): Umbilical artery catheterization: Demonstration of arterial thrombosis by aortography. *Pediatrics,* 50:6–12.
68. O'Neill, J. A., Stahlman, M. T., and Meng, H. C. (1975): Necrotizing enterocolitis in the newborn: Operative indications. *Ann. Surg.,* 182:274–279.
69. Paxson, C. L., Adcock, E. W., and Morriss, F. H. (1976): Infant formula osmolality: A consideration in necrotizing enterocolitis. *Clin. Res.,* 24:1962.
70. Pedersen, P. V., Hansen, F. H., Halveg, A. B., and Christiansen, E. D. (1976): Necrotizing enterocolitis of the newborn—Is it gas-gangrene of the bowel? *Lancet,* ii:715–716.
71. Pitt, J., Barlow, B., Heird, W. C., and Santulli, T. V. (1974): Macrophages and the protective action of breast milk in NEC. *Pediatr. Res.,* 8:384.
72. Polin, R. A., Pollack, P. F., Barlow, B., Wigger, H. J., Slovis, T. L., Santulli, T. V., and Heird, W. C. (1976): Necrotizing enterocolitis in term infants. *J. Pediatr.,* 89:460–462.
73. Rabinowitz, J. G., and Siegle, R. L. (1976): Changing clinical and roentgenographic patterns of necrotizing enterocolitis. *Am. J. Roent.,* 126:560–566.
74. Rabinowitz, J. G., Wolf, B. S., Feller, M. R., and Klasna, I. (1968): Colonic changes following necrotizing enterocolitis of the newborn. *Am. J. Roent.,* 103:359–364.
75. Reid, W. D., and Shannon, M. P. (1973): Necrotizing enterocolitis—A medical approach to treatment. *Can. Med. Assoc. J.,* 108:573–576.
76. Roback, S., Foker, J., Frantz, I., Hunt, C., Engel, R., and Leonard, A. (1974): Necrotizing enterocolitis: An emerging entity in the regional infant intensive care facility. *Arch. Surg.,* 109:314–319.
77. Rowley, M. P., and Dahlenburg, G. W. (1978): Gentamicin in prophylaxis of neonatal necrotizing enterocolitis. *Lancet,* i:532.
78. Ryder, R. W., Sheldon, J. D., Guinan, M. E., and the Committee on Necrotizing Enterocolitis (1980): Necrotizing enterocolitis: A prospective multicenter investigation. *Am. J. Epidemiol.,* 112:113–123.
79. Santulli, T. V., Schullinger, J. N., Heird, W. C., Gongaware, R. D., Wigger, J., Barlow, B., Blanc, W. A., and Berdon, W. E. (1975): Acute necrotizing enterocolitis in infancy: A review of sixty-four cases. *Pediatrics,* 55:376–387.
80. Schullinger, J. N., Mollitt, D. L., Vinocur, C. D., Santulli, T. V., and Driscoll, J. M. (1981): Neonatal necrotizing enterocolitis: Survival, management and complications: A 25 year study. *Am. J. Dis. Child.,* 135:612–614.
81. Selner, J. C., Merrill, D. A., and Claman, H. N. (1968): Salivary immunoglobulin and albumin: Development during the newborn period. 72:685–689.
82. Sherertz, R. J., and Sarubbi, F. A. (1982): The prevalence of *Clostridium difficile* and toxin in a nursery population: A comparison between patients with necrotizing enterocolitis and an asymptomatic group. *J. Pediatr.,* 100:435–440.
83. Stanley, M. D., Null, D. M., and deLemos, R. A. (1977): Relationship between intestinal colonization with specific bacteria and the development of NEC. *Pediatr. Res.,* 11:543 (abstr.).
84. Stein, H., Beck, J., Solomon, A., and Schmaman, A. (1972): Gastroenteritis with necrotizing enterocolitis in premature babies. *Br. Med. J.,* 2:616–619.
85. Stevenson, D. K., Graham, C. B., and Stevenson, J. R. (1980): Neonatal necrotizing enterocolitis: 100 new cases, In: *Year Book of Pediatrics,* pp. 319–340. Year Book, Chicago.
86. Stiehm, E. R. (1975): Fetal defense mechanisms. *Am. J. Dis. Child.,* 129:439–443.
87. Stoll, B. J., Kanto, W. B., Jr., Glass, R. I., Nahmias, A. J., and Brann, A. W., Jr. (1980): Epidemiology of necrotizing enterocolitis: A case control study. *J. Pediatr.,* 96:447–451.
88. Torma, J., deLemos, R., Rogers, J., and Deserens, H. (1973): Necrotizing enterocolitis in infants, analysis of forty-five consecutive cases. *Am. J. Surg.,* 126:758–761.
89. Touloukian, R. J., Berdon, W. E., Amoury, R. A., and Santulli, T. V. (1967): Surgical experience with necrotizing enterocolitis in the infant. *J. Pediatr. Surg.,* 2:389–401.
90. Touloukian, R. J., Kadar, A., and Spencer, R. P. (1973): The gastrointestinal complications of umbilical venous exchange transfusion: A clinical and experimental study. *Pediatrics,* 51:36–42.
91. Touloukian, R. J., Posch, J. N., and Spencer, R. (1972): The pathogenesis of ischemic gastroenterocolitis of the neonate: Selective gut mucosal ischemia in asphyxiated neonatal piglets. *J. Pediatr. Surg.,* 7:194–205.

92. Virnig, N. L., and Reynolds, J. W. (1974): Epidemiologic aspects of neonatal necrotizing enterocolitis. *Am. J. Dis. Child.,* 128:186–190.
93. Walker, W. A. (1976): Host defense mechanisms in the gastrointestinal tract. *Pediatrics,* 57:901–916.
94. Walker, W. A., and Wu, A. L. (1976): The immunologic control mechanism for toxigenic diarrhea. *Pediatr. Res.,* 10:361.
95. Wayne, E. R., Burrington, J. D., and Hutter, J. (1975): Neonatal necrotizing enterocolitis: Evolution of new principles in management. *Arch. Surg.,* 110:476–480.
96. Wilkinson, B., Marks, K. H., Gamsu, H. R., and Cunliffe, A. C. (1976): Stool bacteria in low birth weight infants: Changes with milk formula. *Pediatr. Res.,* 10:361.
97. Williams, R. C., and Gibbons, R. J. (1972): Inhibition of bacterial adherence by secretory immunoglobulin A: A mechanism of antigen disposal. *Science,* 177:697–699.
98. Willis, D. M., Chabot, J., Radde, I. C., and Chance, G. W. (1977): Unsuspected hyperosmolality of oral solutions contributing to necrotizing enterocolitis in very-low-birth-weight infants. *Pediatrics,* 60:535–538.
99. Wilson, S. E., and Woolley, M. M. (1969): Primary necrotizing enterocolitis in infants. *Arch. Surg.,* 99:563–566.
100. Yeager, A. S., McNabb, M. B., Sullivan, D. W., Johnson, J. D., and Sunshine, P. (1977): Cluster of cases of necrotizing enterocolitis associated with *E. coli* 085. *Pediatr. Res.,* 11:545.
101. Yu, V., Tudehope, D., and Gill, G. (1977): Neonatal necrotizing enterocolitis: I. Clinical aspects. *Med. J. Aust.,* 1:685–688.

DISCUSSION

Dr. Räihä: I don't agree with you entirely about necrotizing enterocolitis as being very common. I say this because between 1970 and 1980, when I worked in a large neonatal unit in Helsinki, I saw very few cases. There were about 20,000 deliveries per year in this unit and about 1,000 infants were hospitalized each year. We went through the records of 7 years looking for the incidence of necrotizing enterocolitis. Every infant that died was autopsied and every small premature infant had an X-ray of the abdomen; we looked very carefully for necrotizing enterocolitis. In all this material concerning about 7,000 infants we found five cases of necrotizing enterocolitis, and three of these five were full-term infants that contracted this condition after exchange transfusions. If we take the lowest percentage you gave, which is 1%, we should have seen 70 cases.

Dr. Zetterström: My experience is much the same as that of Dr. Räihä. In the Stockholm area, the incidence of necrotizing enterocolitis is much lower than 1% of all babies born. Do you have any figures about the incidence in the United States and Canada, for instance, that can demonstrate that there are any differences in different centers? That is my first question. My second question refers to the fluid given to the babies. On the basis of studies made by Bill Owen and co-workers, it is thought that one of the reasons for the development of necrotizing enterocolitis may be a high fluid intake.

Dr. Greene: I don't know why our incidence of necrotizing enterocolitis is 1% to 2%, but those are the statistics and I cannot argue with them. I don't believe that we are doing anything different from any other center in the United States. Of those patients that developed necrotizing enterocolitis, 30% were fed nothing but their own mother's milk during the time that they developed necrotizing enterocolitis. Regarding fluid intake, our babies are kept relatively dry during the first week of life.

Dr. Guesry: When you were listing the possible etiologies of necrotizing enterocolitis, you didn't mention the possibility of viral infection.

Dr. Greene: That was clearly an oversight on my part. I think that it is equally a possibility.

Dr. Sunshine: I think there is some confusion about the basic etiological premises that Dr. Greene pointed out. Although viruses have been suggested, it is difficult to imagine that a viral organism could lead to gas production, and that is the hallmark of the disease. Therefore, it has to be bacterial overgrowth. I am convinced that the reason why people see more or less of this disease depends upon what type of organism is colonizing their particular nursery, and those institutions that have a high incidence often have an increased colonization of invasive bacteria which tend to be resistant to the usual antibiotics. Perhaps the low incidence that you are seeing, Dr. Räihä, may be due to the fact that you are not using many antibiotics and that you do not have the development of resistant organisms.

Dr. Räihä: This is probably a very important issue and I would like to ask Dr. Greene whether another reason for the difference of frequencies in different areas could have something to do with bacterial colonization, for instance, maternal and vaginal colonization, in different parts of the world? And secondly, since it may also have something to do with the frequency of intrauterine hypoxia, could the obstetricians do something about decreasing the frequency?

Dr. Greene: My guess is that it is not only the type of organism, be it invasive or not, but also the quantity of the organism that is important.

Dr. Metcoff: There are clearly striking differences between centers; we have heard of two important centers where the difference of incidence is remarkable. I would imagine that an epidemiological assessment of what is done differently in each of these nurseries might prove to be quite useful. A plan could be developed both prospectively and retrospectively to attempt to define the differences.

Dr. Ransome-Kuti: Up until about 2 years ago in Lagos, this condition was very common in our newborn unit and the children were being fed with formula milk. Then it was decided to change to pooled expressed breast milk which was collected every morning from the mothers and fed to the babies fresh; since then the condition has become very rare in our newborn nursery.

Dr. Samarra: In Paris, as in Nashville, there is necrotizing enterocolitis among high-risk newborns. The rate in the intensive care unit of Port Royal is 1.2%, but 2 years ago there was an outbreak of 28 cases among low-risk newborns over an 18-month period. No cases had been reported from other maternity hospitals and no case has been reported after December 1979. No single bacteria, no toxin, no drug could be incriminated. A virus was found in half the cases where electron microscopy of the stool had been carried out, but the prevalence of positive results was the same among nonaffected newborns. Do you have any data about viral infections responsible for necrotizing enterocolitis?

Dr. Greene: We have been looking for rotavirus and we have not found it in our nursery in association with necrotizing enterocolitis. As far as any other viral infection is concerned, we have not been able to detect any either, but I think that our ability to look for them is something that could be improved.

Dr. Zetterström: In your group of patients, how many had been fed fresh mother's milk before they got enterocolitis?

Dr. Greene: Thirty percent of the infants who had developed necrotizing enterocolitis were consuming their own mother's milk at the time of development.

Dr. Zetterström: Was this milk treated and pasteurized or completely fresh?

Dr. Greene: The mothers brought the milk in after it had been refrigerated for 24 hr. It was not pasteurized.

Dr. Räihä: As far as we are concerned, we only have one diet for the infants and this is untreated breast milk. A premature infant, especially one weighing less than 1,500 g, will get the mother's own milk supplemented with nonpasteurized, fresh-pooled breast milk, or if this is not available, pasteurized, frozen, pooled milk. One difference between our routine and the routine that I have seen in the United States is that we increase the volume intakes very slowly.

I would like to ask Dr. Sunshine and Dr. Rigo whether they are really giving complete total parenteral nutrition, because in our experience, and from what I have seen in the Swedish units over the past 2 years, we never use total parenteral nutrition unless it is a case of surgical complication of the gut, like atresia. We always use parenteral nutrition in combination with enteral nutrition. I have not seen a case in which we have used total parenteral nutrition in many years. This may also have some bearing on the incidence of necrotizing enterocolitis.

Dr. Salle: We use a combination of supplemental parenteral nutrition and oral nutrition and we increase the amount of milk very slowly. We use human milk only in premature infants; we use the mother's own milk if she agrees to give her milk to feed the baby, otherwise we use bank milk, but this milk is pasteurized and frozen. The rate of necrotizing enterocolitis in my department is less than 1%—0.3% over the last 5 years.

Dr. Perman: I think we should be careful in ascribing any difference in the incidence of necrotizing enterocolitis in infants on breast milk solely to the protective effects of breast milk. It is very clear that there are major differences in the establishment of enteric microflora, at least significant qualitative differences between infants that are breast fed and infants who are formula fed, and although this has not been investigated in the neonate, there are probably significant differences in the infant that is fed total parenteral nutrition versus the infant that is fed parenterally and enterally with regard to the flora as well.

Dr. Sunshine: A study was carried out in the United States involving 13 institutions looking at whether or not there was any protective effect if human milk was used in the nursery, which compared fresh human milk, processed human milk that had been pasteurized, pooled human milk, formulae, etc. Dr. Ryder published the results in the *American Journal of Epidemiology*. This study showed that there was no difference in the incidence of necrotizing enterocolitis among the 13 institutions. The only thing that was evident was that the severity of the disease was much less and the babies did not require surgery as frequently if they were fed whole fresh human milk that had not been processed.

INFANT NUTRITION

Some Pathophysiologic Changes in Experimental Intrauterine Malnutrition

A. Minkowski and C. Chanez

Centre de Recherches Biologiques du Développement Foetal et Neonatal (INSERM U. 29), Université René Descartes, Hôpital Port-Royal, F-75014 Paris, France

The two major causes (48) of intrauterine human growth retardation (IUGR) (63), which has become a major concern to neonatalogists (3,4), are a reduction in the blood flow to the fetus and maternal malnutrition. The physiological and biological changes observed in both human and animal species include a delay or arrest in cell multiplication, which may spare some organs while affecting others. Experimentation on intrauterine retarded growth has been conducted on rats (48,67), guinea pigs (46), lambs, monkeys, and pigs; IUGR has been induced either by maternal proteinocaloric deprivation or by vascular ligature or microemboli caused by plastic microspheres during gestation (Fig. 1). The following consequences have been observed in the animal and occasionally also in the human being (48):

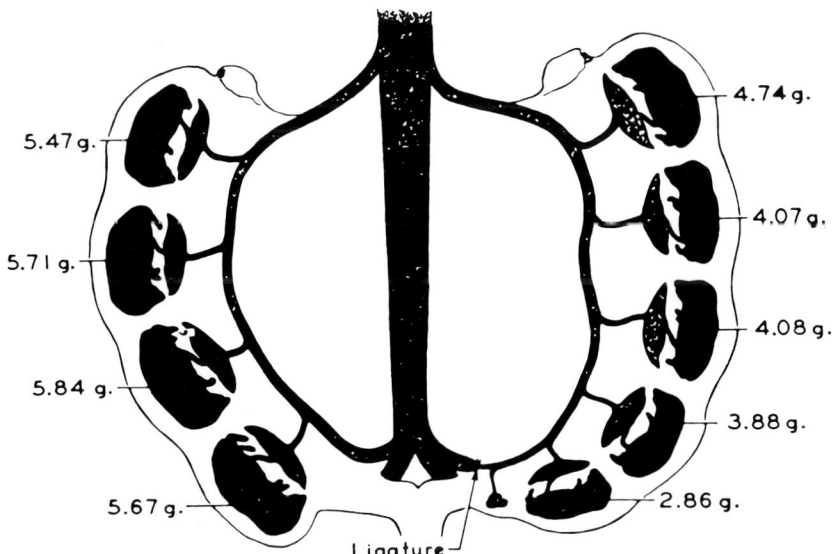

FIG. 1. Schematic diagram of the experimental model. The fetal weights are taken from one experiment. (Modified from Wigglesworth, ref. 63.)

1. Relative preservation of the brain volume and weight versus excessive reduction of the liver (19,39,43,48)
2. Hypoglycemia (17,20,49)
3. Reduction in cell number (DNA) in the liver and preservation of cell size (18)
4. No catch-up growth when the total body weight reduction exceeds 30% (in rats) (51,61)
5. Specific pathological involvement of the cerebellum
6. Alteration of brown fat
7. Hypoproteinemia and alterations of the plasma aminogram
8. Premature appearance of the surfactant
9. Early opening of the eyes

Experimentally produced IUGR is now commonly induced by: (a) reducing the blood supply to the uterus (ligature of the uterine artery), or (b) total or selective deprivation of nutrients in the gestant animal. Sheep have been used for the experimental production of IUGR either by ligaturing one umbilical artery or by producing microemboli by injecting small plastic spheres into the uterine artery. This procedure also provides a means of measuring uterine blood flow and its distribution. Rhesus monkeys have been used to produce IUGR at 100 days gestation by ligaturing the fetal umbilical vessels leading to the secondary placental disk. The multiple pregnancy of the pig sometimes results in "runts" that weigh about 50% of the normal weight. Widdowson and Adams have used such material for their studies.

In general, most of the factors producing IUGR are environmental, either vascular or nutritional (63). The role of hormones is rather obscure; genetic factors are certainly to be taken into consideration, and it is well known that weight and body length of the offspring are dependent on maternal weight and size.

THE GENERAL PROBLEM OF ORGAN REDUCTION

If we accept a certain reduction in body weight (below the 10th percentile or 2 SD in the human, below 30% in rats, etc.) as indicative of IUGR, we can describe a general "large brain, small liver" syndrome, which is encountered in various species. This pattern is observed *in all animals* (48) whether IUGR is spontaneous or provoked, or of vascular or nutritional origin. In the human being, the brain is usually relatively large although it may sometimes be reduced; in contrast, the liver is more reduced than the rest of the body. In addition to the liver, the thymus and the lungs are also very reduced in size. In the rat, spleen and liver are reduced. In the monkey the spleen is markedly affected, whereas the piglet is the only animal in which the heart is also reduced (Fig. 2).

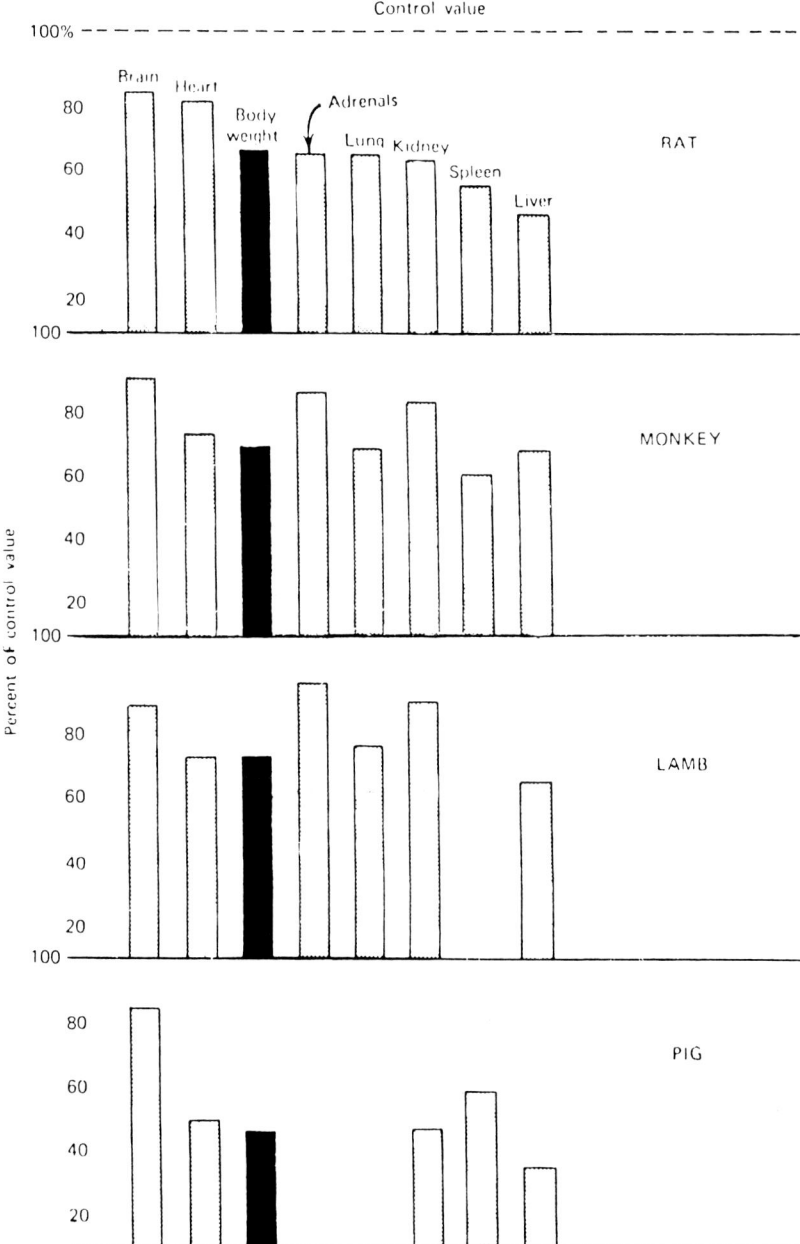

FIG. 2. Mean body and organ weight of IUGR rats, monkeys, lambs, and pigs, plotted as percentages of the control values.

The protein/DNA ratio and total RNA are unaffected in the liver of animals with IUGR which is related to the preservation of cell function (11). Liver glycogen is also markedly decreased in the rat. Glycogen content per unit wet weight of liver is not modified, but the total content is diminished because the liver is reduced in size.

The Reduction of Blood Flow to the Organs

The reduction of blood flow to the organs is one of the main mechanisms involved in the production of IUGR. Vascular lesions in the human being were mentioned by Gruenwald. Ligature of the uterine artery (rat, monkey, etc.) and nonradioactive-microsphere emboli obviously raise the problem of hemodynamic factors.

Some Peculiarities in Brain Involvement (8–10)

Winick (64) has shown that there are differences in the decrease of cell multiplication in various parts of the brain in intrauterine malnutrition. Whereas the cerebral cortex is hardly decreased in IUGR, the cerebellum (6,7,21,55) is markedly affected (it is the organ where cell multiplication is most rapid during fetal life). These differences have been studied by different methods and it has been shown (48,61) that oxygen uptake is the same in the cerebrum of IUGR rats and controls. On the other hand in our group, Privat (*unpublished data*) has shown, by using tissue cultures of IUGR rat brains, that there is a sharp decrease in the growth pattern of the cerebellum.

Another important point made by Winick (65,68) is that whereas prenatal or postnatal malnutrition in the pregnant mother produces very little decrease (15%) in the multiplication of the cells of the cerebrum in the offspring, the combination of both produces an enormous decrease in DNA.

Glucose Metabolism (17,45,48,49)

IUGR individuals can be very hypoglycemic. In the human, Sabata and Stembera have described a decrease in the glucose supply from the mother to the fetus and the absence of an arterial–venous difference in glucose, indicative of an absence of glucose utilization by the fetus; both features are abolished by a continuous infusion of glucose to the mother for short periods during labor. Lactate and pyruvate are high in the umbilical arterial blood of IUGR, a sign of chronic fetal distress. Melichar has studied hypoglycemia in IUGR newborns and has shown that intravenous administration of glucose is followed by a higher blood glucose level than in controls.

We have studied (19,20,59) enzymatic activities and their relation to blood glucose levels and hepatic glycogen content in the rat. The IUGR rat fetus has a very low plasma glucose level. After birth, the level does not rise as in the control, but remains low until the 10th day. In contrast, the lactate level is quite normal, except at day 3, when IUGR animals have significantly higher levels than do control. In spite of a normal glycogen concentration, as expressed per gram of wet tissue, the total glycogen stores of the liver are decreased by the reduction of the liver size. The IUGR newborn rat has only 60 mg of glycogen per gram body weight, which is only half that of the control. Glycogen is normally mobilized within 24 hr and becomes similar soon afterwards in both groups. It thus appears that the hypotrophic liver is enzymically well equipped for the synthesis of glycogen.

Glucose-6-phosphatase activity in fetal liver is extremely low. It increases just after birth in both IUGR rats and controls. The activity of fructose-1,6-diphosphatase is also very low in fetal liver and rises soon after birth, the increase being slower in the IUGR newborn; 48 hr after birth it is significantly lower than in controls ($p < 0.01$). Normal levels are reached 3 days later. At 10 days of age a significant difference in lactate dehydrogenase activity is found, the IUGR having a higher level of activity than the control animals. No modifications in the pattern of glucose-6-phosphate dehydrogenase have been found in hypotrophic liver. Asparte aminotransferase, which is involved in the conversion of amino acid to carbohydrates, has the same activity in both IUGR and controls.

Lipids, Free Fatty Acids, Glycerol, and Brown Fat (12,13,23–25,37,44)

The three main functions of lipids are to act as insulation, energy stores, and structural components of certain membranes. At birth the first two functions predominate. The newborn rat is deprived of lipid stores, mainly white adipose tissue. One can follow the utilization of stores by studying the levels of free fatty acids and glycerol in the plasma. During development, the level in IUGR rats and controls is the same. In the IUGR rabbit (caused by hyponutrition of the pregnant mother during last period of gestation) the fatty acid level in the fetus is unmodified.

In the human, Sabata and Sternbera have shown that in umbilical artery samples, the levels of esterified and free fatty acids are higher in the IUGR newborn than in the control. The same observation has been made for free fatty acids in the serum of the hypoglycemic IUGR newborn. This could be interpreted as a mobilization of fat reserves in the absence of sufficient carbohydrate stores (the decreased rate of glucose supply from the mother to the fetus; the small liver with a reduced total amount of available glycogen). Within 12 hr after birth, blood ketone bodies rise due to an increased breakdown of fatty acids in the IUGR newborn.

In IUGR rats, total body lipids decrease until the age of 10 days. This is associated with an increase in water content. The livers of IUGR rats contain more total lipids 48 hr after birth than do the livers of controls. This tendency to develop fatty liver has also been found in newborn rabbits born from malnourished mothers. A decrease in hepatic hydroxybutyrate dehydrogenase has been found in spontaneous IUGR rabbits. This could be a consequence of an impaired catabolism of fatty acids. Lipogenesis from glucose is unaffected in the liver of IUGR rats (the activities of glucose-6-phosphate dehydrogenase and ATP citrate lyase are identical with those in controls). The percentage of fatty acids is identical in both IUGR and controls. The composition of brain lipids is unchanged in IUGR.

Interscapular brown fat in the IUGR rat is reduced from 12 hr before birth until 5 days after (60). Until that date the percentage of water is higher and triglyceride levels lower in IUGR. The activities of glucose-6-phosphate dehydrogenase and glycerokinase in brown fat tissue are lower. The incorporation of labeled glucose into brown fat lipids is very much reduced in IUGR. This indicates a marked reduction in the metabolism of brown fat.

Long-Lasting Effects of Intrauterine Malnutrition on Neurotransmitter Metabolism in the Brain of Developing Rats (16)

A number of studies have shown that malnutrition during the perinatal period may result in long-term alterations of the central nervous system (CNS) (31–34,52). Studies on neurotransmitter metabolism (1,2,53,54,57,58) in the CNS of undernourished developing rats have been conducted using food-deprived gestating or lactating mothers. However, the biochemical alterations observed may result not only from food deprivation of the fetus or newborn animal, but also from secondary changes in the food-deprived maternal organism. This led us to reinvestigate the effects of undernutrition on the metabolism of monoaminergic neurotransmitters in the CNS of developing rats using the uterine vessel ligature model (Fig. 3).

Although the blood supply was restricted for the last 5 days of gestation only, marked alterations in the levels of serotonin (5-HT) (35,36) dopamine (DA) and norepinephrine (NE) were noted in the offspring for at least the first 2 postnatal weeks. The high concentrations of tryptophan and 5-hydroxyindoleacetic acid (5-HIAA) (26) detected in the brain of IUGR rats strongly suggest that the turnover of 5-HT is accelerated in IUGR as compared with control rats.

MATERIALS AND METHODS (see also ref. 16)

Female rats of the Sherman strain were used. IUGR of the fetus was obtained according to Wigglesworth's method (63). On the 17th day of gestation, the artery and vein of one uterine horn were ligatured after laparotomy under

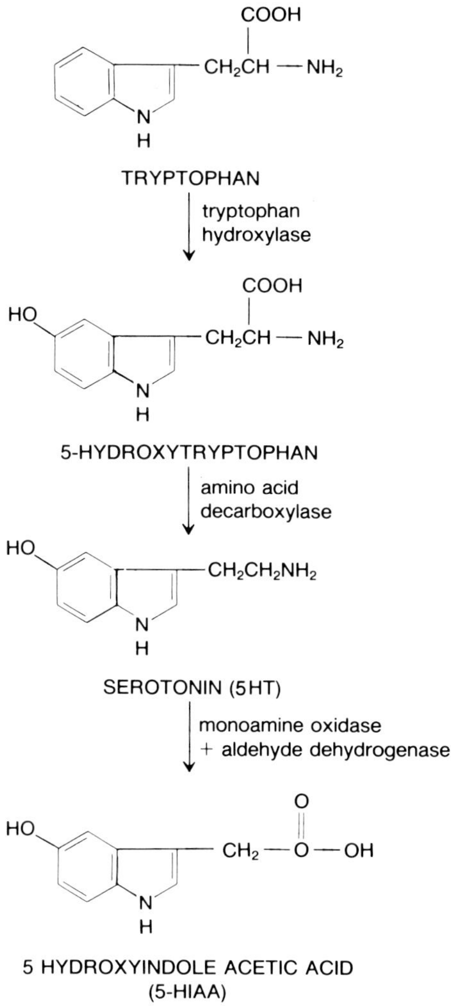

FIG. 3. Metabolic pathway for 5-HT synthesis and degradation.

light ether anesthesia; the opposite horn was left as a control. The fetus next to the ligature died and was partially resorbed.

In many cases, there was a gradient in fetal size between the upper and lower end of the experimental horn. No postoperative problems occurred, and about 58% of the operated mothers gave birth to IUGR rats. Eighty-seven percent of the IUGR offspring were viable and exhibited no malformation. At birth, an animal was considered as being IUGR when the body weight was reduced by at least 40% compared with controls. During development the IUGR rats never reached the weight of control rats, whatever the rearing conditions. All organs presented an important reduction, particularly the liver and the brown adipose tissue. The brain weight was reduced by about 10% (up to 20%). At weaning, the average weight reduction of the organs was approximately 30%.

Throughout the study, all mother rats were fed a normal diet *ad libitum* and were housed in separate cages with 6 to 8 pups. Lactation was normal and weaning was established at 22 days. Both male and female offspring were used at random and killed at 1, 8, 15, or 22 days (between 10 a.m. and 12 a.m.). Blood was collected from trunk vessels, and serum was obtained by centrifugation at 3,000 $\times$ g for 30 min at 6°C.

All values were expressed as milligrams of amine, amino acid, or acid per gram of fresh tissue or per milliliter of serum. They were corrected for recoveries calculated with internal standards. In all cases these recoveries were at least equal to 75%.

Statistical calculations were performed according to Snedecor and Cochran (56). When the p value was higher than 0.05 (Student's t-test), the difference was considered to be nonsignificant.

RESULTS

Whole Body, Brainstem, and Forebrain Weight Gain in Developing Controls and IUGR Rats

Although body weight was reduced by about 40% at birth in IUGR compared with control rats, differences in brain weights were rather small (Table 1). The reduction affected primarily the forebrain mass (-20%); the brainstem weight of IUGR rats did not differ from controls. The differences noted at birth were still present at the end of the third postnatal week. The precursors of 5-HT have been estimated in blood and forebrain of IUGR and controls (see Figs. 4 and 5).

Ontogenic Changes in 5-HT, DA, and NE Levels in the Brainstem and the Forebrain of Control and IUGR Rats

5-HT levels increased markedly for the first 2 postnatal weeks and then leveled off in the brainstem; they slightly decreased in the forebrain during the following week (Fig. 6). Although this developmental pattern was similar in both groups of rats, absolute 5-HT levels were generally higher in the IUGR animals. This was particularly striking in the brainstem since the concentration

TABLE 1. Body and brain growth of control and IUGR rats during the first 3 postnatal weeks

Age	Body wt (g)	Forebrain wt (mg)	Brain stem wt (mg)
1 Day			
Control	7.21 ± 0.09 (40)	174.19 ± 1.58 (47)	47.11 ± 1.20 (17)
IUGR	4.46 ± 0.12 (40)^a	139.51 ± 1.95 (41)^a	46.88 ± 0.77 (18)
8 Days			
Control	19.20 ± 0.10 (30)	616.55 ± 6.69 (20)	94.00 ± 4.19 (14)
IUGR	10.90 ± 0.24 (29)^a	519.89 ± 6.81 (19)^a	87.06 ± 2.53 (16)
15 Days			
Control	34.27 ± 0.08 (30)	857.97 ± 10.87 (37)	124.15 ± 3.0 (13)
IUGR	23.61 ± 0.36 (30)^a	746.65 ± 9.22 (40)^a	123.86 ± 2.52 (15)
22 days			
Control	54.39 ± 0.87 (30)	1022.42 ± 8.78 (40)	155.92 ± 2.69 (25)
IUGR	36.85 ± 0.51 (30)^a	905.74 ± 9.65 (43)^a	151.88 ± 2.20 (36)

IUGR rats were selected at birth as those exhibiting a reduction in body weight at least equal to 40% as compared with control animals in the same litter. For the whole lactating period until weaning (28th postnatal day), IUGR and control developing rats were fed by mothers maintained under the same environmental conditions.

Each value is the mean ± SEM of N individual determinations at each age (N expressed in parentheses).

^{a} $p \leq 0.001$, when compared with values from pair-aged control rats.

of the indoleamine in this region was significantly higher in IUGR than in control rats at all ages examined.

Little difference between control and IUGR rats was noted in the levels of the two other monoamine neurotransmitters, NE and DA (Table 2). NE levels were generally higher in IUGR than in control rats; the difference, however, was not statistically significant except in the forebrain at day 1. As already noted for 5-HT, the ontogenetic evolution of the concentration of DA followed the same pattern in the forebrain of controls and IUGR rats. DA levels were significantly higher in IUGR animals, except on day 8.

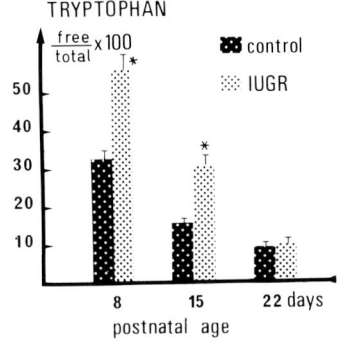

FIG. 4. Percentage of serum free tryptophan in IUGR rats (white bars) and control rats (black bars) at various ages after birth.

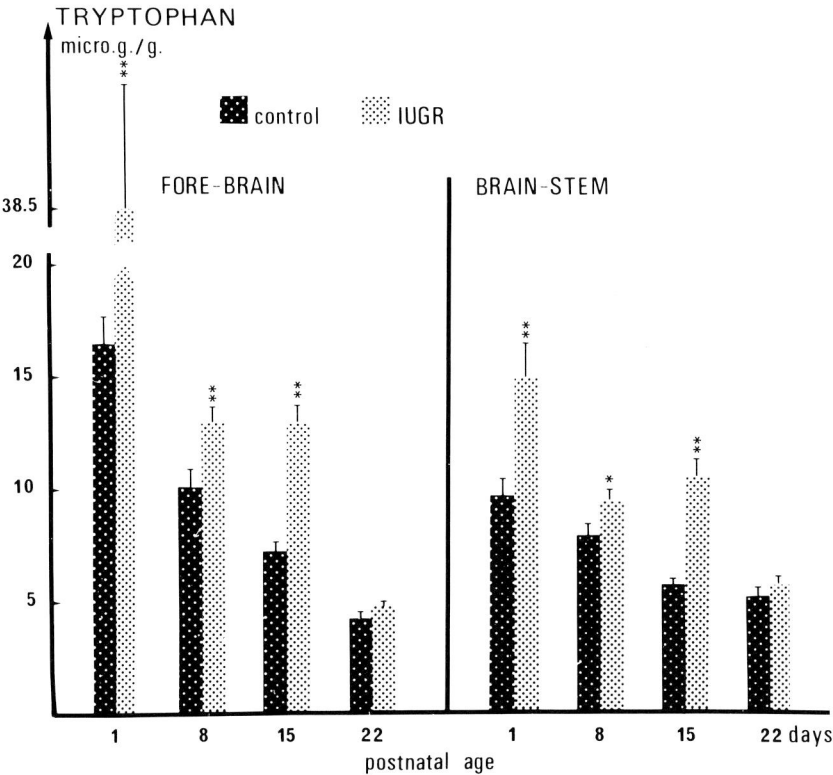

FIG. 5. Tryptophan levels in the forebrain and the brainstem of IUGR (*white bars*) and control rats (*black bars*). The results are given at various ages after birth and are expressed in mg/g of wet tissues. Each bar represents the mean based on 20–30 samples. The asterisks denote statistically significant differences between IUGR and control animals (Student's *t*-test). ** At least $p < 0.01$; * at least $p < 0.05$.

Ontogenetic Changes in Tryptophan and 5-HIAA Levels in the Brainstem and the Forebrain of Controls and IUGR Rats (14,15,27,28,30,38,40,41,47)

Since an increase in 5-HT levels can result from either a reduction or an acceleration (42) of the turnover of this neurotransmitter, it was of interest to measure the concentration of 5-HIAA in tissues to explain the differences between controls and IUGR rats. The ontogenetic evolution of 5-HIAA levels were markedly different in the brainstem and the forebrain in both groups of rats. Thus, at birth, the concentration of the 5-HT metabolite in the brainstem was already as high as in weaning rats and only discrete changes were noted during the first 3 postnatal weeks. In contrast, the concentration of 5-HIAA gradually increased in the forebrain during the same period and reached, on the 22nd postnatal day, a level twice as high as that found at birth. Although

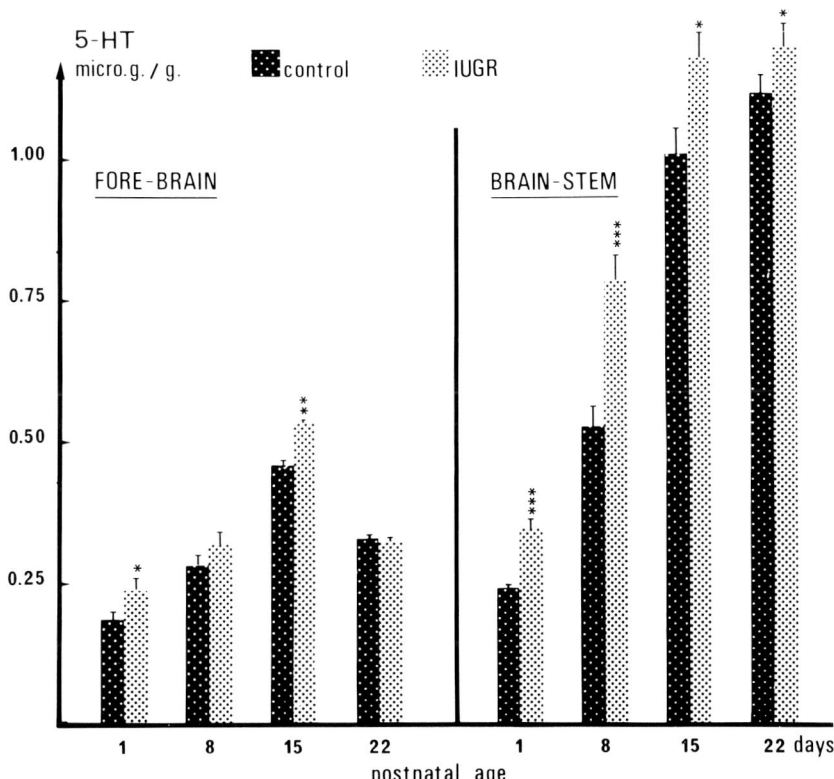

FIG. 6. 5-HT levels in the forebrain and the brainstem of IUGR (*white bars*) and control rats (*black bars*). The results are given at various ages after birth and are expressed in mg/g of wet tissues. Each bar represents the mean based on 20–30 samples. The asterisks denote statistically significant differences between IUGR and control animals (Student's *t*-test). ** $p < 0.01$; * $p < 0.05$.

these evolution patterns were very similar in controls and IUGR rats, absolute levels were markedly higher in hypotrophic animals.

A comparison of data indicates that the ratio of 5-HIAA to 5-HT levels is more elevated during the early period of life. Except at 8 days of age, this ratio is higher (10% to 36%) in IUGR than in control rats.

Under many circumstances, parallel fluctuations in the respective levels of 5-HIAA and tryptophan have been observed in the CNS leading to the proposal that an acceleration of 5-HT turnover may be due to an increased availability of the precursor amino acid in the tissues. In the present case, IUGR-induced increases in 5-HIAA levels were associated with significant elevations in the concentration of tryptophan in the brainstem and in the forebrain. Before tryptophan level fell to the adult value, that is, on the 22nd postnatal day, it

TABLE 2. NE and DA levels in the brain of IUGR and control rats at various postnatal ages

Age	NE Forebrain		NE Brainstem		DA Forebrain	
1 Day						
Control	0.127 0.009	(N = 18)	0.300 0.010	(N = 13)	0.232 0.010	(N = 18)
IUGR	0.158^a 0.016^a	(N = 19)	0.326 0.029	(N = 18)	0.282^b 0.013^b	(N = 18)
8 Days						
Control	0.131 0.005	(N = 19)	0.315 0.021	(N = 18)	0.339 0.012	(N = 16)
IUGR	0.146 0.008	(N = 18)	0.362 0.015	(N = 18)	0.348 0.007	(N = 18)
14 Days						
Control	0.151 0.008	(N = 12)	0.420 0.018	(N = 16)	0.421 0.014	(N = 14)
IUGR	0.154 0.008	(N = 15)	0.472 0.025	(N = 14)	0.470^b 0.015^b	(N = 14)
22 Days						
Control	0.191 0.008	(N = 14)	0.555 0.021	(N = 14)	0.491 0.012	(N = 13)
IUGR	0.187 0.012	(N = 14)	0.559 0.029	(N = 14)	0.564^a 0.022^a	(N = 14)

Each value, expressed as micrograms of NE or DA per gram of fresh tissue, is the mean of N separate determinations. The SEM is indicated underneath.
^{a} $p \leq 0.05$ when compared with respective control values.
^{b} $p \leq 0.01$ when compared with respective control values.

remained significantly higher in tissues of hypotrophic compared with control growing animals (Fig. 7).

Ontogenetic Changes in the Concentration of Tryptophan and Tyrosine in the Serum of Control and IUGR Rats

In both control and IUGR rats, the concentration of free tryptophan progressively decreased as a function of age to reach adult values at weaning. These changes were mainly due to the progressive increase in the capacity of serum proteins to bind tryptophan since the concentration of total tryptophan and of tyrosine did not follow the same evolution pattern. A reduction in their concentration was noted only at weaning.

Except at 22 days of age, marked differences were detected between control and IUGR rats. Both the absolute concentration and the relative proportion of free tryptophan in serum were significantly higher in hypotrophic than in control animals. These changes in peripheral free tryptophan were closely related to those previously observed in brain. Such a relationship between tissue and serum free levels of tryptophan is particularly obvious when comparing values in 8- and 15-day-old animals in both groups (Table 3).

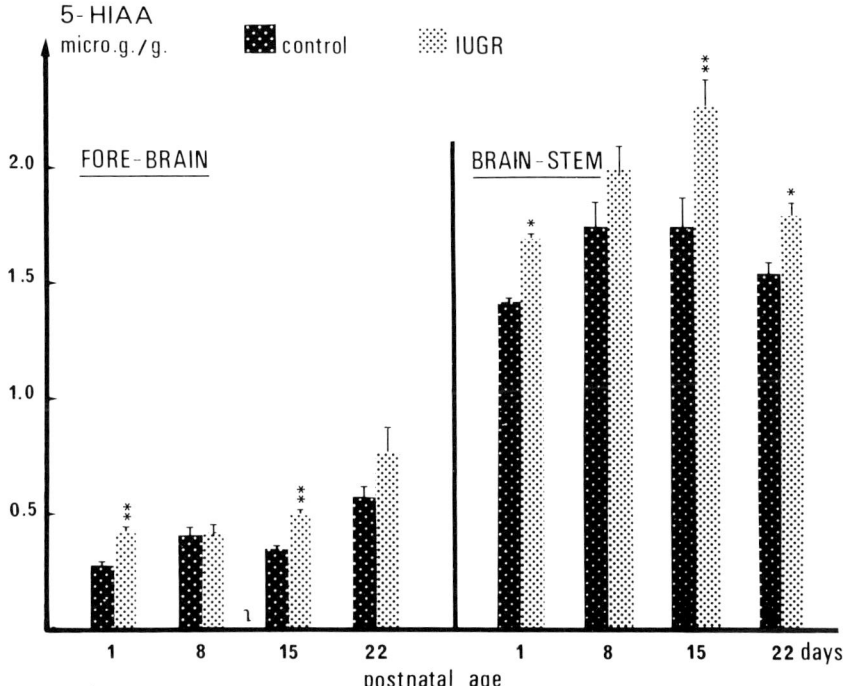

FIG. 7. 5-HIAA concentration levels in the forebrain and brainstem of IUGR (*white bars*) and control rats (*black bars*). The results are given at various ages after birth and are expressed in mg/g of wet tissues. Each bar represents the mean based on 20–30 samples. The asterisks denote statistically significant differences between IUGR and control animals (Student's *t*-test). ** $p < 0.01$; * $p < 0.05$.

The reduction in tryptophan levels occurring in tissues of 15-day-old compared with 8-day-old control rats only paralleled that found in the concentration of free amino acids in serum, since that of total tryptophan remained constant for the period considered. In IUGR rats, tryptophan levels in tissue and concentrations of free tryptophan in serum were not significantly different in 8- and 15-day-old rats.

DISCUSSION

A restriction of the maternal blood flow during the last 5 days of pregnancy markedly affects the growth of the offspring. In spite of a normal lactation for the first 3 postnatal weeks, body weight is still more than 30% lower in IUGR compared with control rats. The brain growth is apparently comparatively less affected since a slight reduction (10% to 20%) is noted only for the forebrain mass in IUGR animals.

TABLE 3. *Tryptophan and tyrosine concentrations in the serum of control and IUGR rats*

Age	N	Total tryptophan	Free tryptophan	Tyrosine
8 Days				
Control	(15)	29.59 ± 3.41	9.60 ± 1.62	56.69 ± 2.88
IUGR	(11)	25.42 ± 2.62	13.14 ± 0.72[a]	52.06 ± 3.25
15 Days				
Control	(12)	27.85 ± 1.48	3.65 ± 0.28	61.08 ± 2.15
IUGR	(8)	31.57 ± 2.73	9.82 ± 1.19[a]	65.96 ± 3.95
22 Days				
Control	(12)	22.46 ± 2.67	1.94 ± 0.23	25.93 ± 2.45
IUGR	(19)	21.07 ± 1.50	1.93 ± 0.30	21.55 ± 1.39

Control and IUGR rats were killed on the 8th, 15th, or 22nd postnatal day and blood was collected from trunk vessels. Whole and free tryptophan and tyrosine levels were measured in the serum as described in Materials and Methods. Each value (in μg/ml) is the mean ± SEM of N individual determinations.

[a] $p \leq 0.05$ when compared with respective control values.

During that time, changes in monoamines—particularly 5-HT, its percursor, and its metabolite—are detected in the CNS of IUGR animals. The increased levels of 5-HT, 5-HIAA, and tryptophan in IUGR rats are real since the most striking differences between IUGR and control animals are observed in the brainstem, that is, a region with the same weight in both groups of rats. Therefore, the simultaneous increases in tryptophan, 5-HT, and 5-HIAA levels very likely reflect an acceleration of 5-HT turnover in the CNS of IUGR rats. However, this acceleration may not necessarily represent an overall increase in 5-HT-dependent synaptic activity.

Two factors could be responsible for the changes in 5-HT turnover in the developing rat. Indeed, the restriction of the maternal blood flow not only results in undernutrition but also in partial hypoxia of the fetus. Although the latter can produce a marked increase in the turnover of 5-HT in the immature rat brain, it is not likely to be responsible for the long-term alterations presently observed, since no significant changes in brain tryptophan, 5-HT, and 5-HIAA levels are detected 24 days after resuscitation. Several authors have already mentioned that undernutrition can increase tryptophan, 5-HT, and 5-HIAA levels in the CNS of developing rats. Furthermore, in contrast to hypoxia, undernutrition exerts long-lasting effects since significant increases in 5-HT turnover are observed in several brain areas at 20 days after birth. The present results indicate that undernutrition for a short period (i.e., the last 5 days) during gestation induces a long-lasting acceleration of 5-HT turnover in the CNS of growing rats.

As already observed in adult as well as in normal developing rats, a close relationship exists between the concentration of circulating free tryptophan and the level of this amino acid in the brain tissue of IUGR rats. We have confirmed that the evolutionary pattern of tissue tryptophan parallels that of the free form of the amino acid in the serum of developing animals. Although other factors, notably the level of neutral amino acids in serum, may be involved in the transport of tryptophan to brain, the present findings strongly suggest that the increased accumulation of tryptophan in brain tissues of IUGR rats is due to a higher concentration of peripheral free tryptophan. Previous studies have shown that several factors are responsible for the high level of serum free tryptophan in newborn animals. The concentration of unesterified fatty acids, which competes with tryptophan for its specific binding site onto serum albumin, is elevated during the lactation period. In addition, the concentration of the binding protein, serum albumin, is rather low in young as compared with adult rats. Accordingly, the higher level of serum free tryptophan in IUGR rats might result from changes in the concentration of unesterified fatty acids and/or serum albumin. However, neither of these two parameters is different in developing control and IUGR rats. Bourgoin et al. (15) have reported that a particular form of serum albumin with less capacity to bind tryptophan is present in the serum of normal developing rats during the early postnatal period. Since a pronounced retardation in liver maturation occurs in IUGR rats, a delay in the synthesis of the adult form of serum albumin with maximal capacity to bind tryptophan might well be responsible for the relative lack of tryptophan binding in hypotrophic animals. However, further experiments are required to establish this point.

On the basis of experiments using drugs, particularly 5-HT, which reduce the brain concentration of monoamines during development, several authors have proposed that these molecules may exert a trophic effect on brain maturation. One may thus speculate that the increased 5-HT turnover in IUGR rats could correspond to a faster maturation of the CNS in those animals, and thus represent a compensatory mechanism for retarded brain growth. Although such speculation has to be looked at with great caution, one may recall that IUGR animals open their eyes 1.5 days before controls do. A similar precocity in eye opening is obtained by daily administration of 5-HT during the early postnatal period. In this respect, IUGR rats differ markedly from offspring of mothers subjected to a low-protein diet during lactation where a delay of 2 days in eye opening is observed. This further illustrates the point that protein restriction in the mother may produce effects different from those observed in undernutrition of the offspring.

Although informative with regard to the level of neurological maturation of animals, data on the time of eye opening are, however, not precise enough to reveal alterations in the functional status of the brain of IUGR rats. In this respect the increased levels of DA and NE might be due to a more rapid differentiation of the storage capacities of the catecholaminergic neuron in developing IUGR rats. However, further studies with more appropriate neuronal markers are necessary to characterize the temporal changes in brain maturation in hypotrophic animals.

REFERENCES

1. Adlard, B. P. F., and Dobbing, J. (1971): Vulnerability of developing brain. III. Development of four enzymes in the brains of normal and undernourished rats. *Brain Res.,* 28:97–107.
2. Adlard, B. P. F., Dobbing, J., and Smart, J. L. (1974): Adult brain nerve-ending content and acetylcholinesterase activity in rats growth retarded for different periods in early life. *Biochem. Soc. Trans.,* 2:124–127.
3. Altman, J., Das, G. D., and Sudarshan, K. (1970): The influence of nutrition on neural and behavioral development. I. Critical review of some data on the growth of the body and the brain following dietary deprivation during gestation and lactation. *Dev. Psychobiol.,* 3:281–301.
4. Andrews, B. F. (1970): Symposium on the small for date infant. *The Pediatric Clinics of North America, Vol. 17,* No. 1. W. B. Saunders, Philadelphia.
5. Bakke, J. L., Lawrence, J. L., Robinson, S. A., Bennett, J., and Browers, C. (1978): Late endocrine effects of L-DOPA, 5-HTP and 6 OH-DOPA administrated to neonatal rats. *Neuroendocrinology,* 25:291–302.
6. Barnes, D., and Altman, J. (1973): Effects of different schedules of early undernutrition on the preweaning growth of the rat cerebellum. *Exp. Neurol.,* 38:406–419.
7. Barnes, D., and Altman, J. (1973): Effect of two levels of gestational–lactational undernutrition on the postweaning growth of the rat cerebellum. *Exp. Neurol.,* 38:420–428.
8. Bass, J. H., Netsky, M. G., and Young, E. (1970): Effect of neonatal malnutrition on developing cerebrum. I. Microchemical and histologic study of cellular differentiation in the rat. *Arch. Neurol.,* 23:289–302.
9. Bass, N. H., Netsky, M. G., and Young, E. (1970): Effect of neonatal malnutrition on developing cerebrum. III. Micro-chemical and histologic study of myelin formation in the rat. *Arch. Neurol.,* 23:303–313.
10. Benton, J. W., Moser, H. W., Dodge, P. R., and Carr, S. (1966): Modification of the schedule of myelination in the rat by early nutritional deprivation. *Pediatrics,* 38:801–807.
11. Boivin, A., Vendrely, R., and Vendrely, C. (1948): L'acide desoxyribonucléique du noyau cellulaire dépositaire des caractères héréditaires: Arguments analytiques. *C.R. Acad. Sci. Paris,* 226:1051–1053.
12. Borgman, R. F., Bursey, R. G., and Caffrey, B. C. (1975): Influence of dietary fat upon rats during gestation and lactation. *Am. J. Vet. Res.,* 36:795–798.
13. Borgman, R. F., Bursey, R. G., and Caffrey, B. C. (1975): Influence of maternal dietary fat upon rat pups. *Am. J. Vet. Res.,* 36:799–805.
14. Bourgoin, S., Faivre-Bauman, A., Benda, P., Glowinski, J., and Hamon, M. (1974): Plasma tryptophan and 5-HT metabolism in the CNS of the newborn rat. *J. Neurochem.,* 23:319–327.
15. Bourgoin, S., Faivre-Bauman, A., Hery, F., Ternaux, J. P., and Hamon, M. (1977): Characteristics of tryptophan binding in the serum of the newborn rat. *Biol. Neonate,* 31:141–154.
16. Chanez, C., Priam, M., Flexor, M. A., Hamon, M., Bourgoin, S., Kordon, C., and Minkowski, A. (1981): Long lasting effects of intrauterine growth retardation on 5-HT metabolism in the brain of developing rats. *Brain Res.,* 207:397–408.
17. Chanez, C., Roux, J. M., and Tordet-Caridroit, C. (1969): Glycémie, glycogène et glucose-6-phosphatase dans le foie à la période périnatale chez le rat dysmature. *C.R. Soc. Biol.,* 163:2272–2274.
18. Chanez, C., Tordet-Caridroit, C., and Roux, J. M. (1971): Studies on experimental hypotrophy in the rat. II. Development of some liver enzymes of gluconeogenesis. *Biol. Neonate,* 18:56–65.
19. Chanez-Bel, C. (1972): Retard de croissance intra-uterin chez le rat. Recherches allométriques et métaboliques. Thèse de Doct. es. Sci. Univ. Paris VI.
20. Chanez-Bel, C., and Tordet-Caridroit, C. (1972): Glucose—Acides gras libres et glycérol du plasma. *Arch. Franc. Ped.,* 29:593–601.
21. Chase, H. P., Lindsley, W. F. B., and O'Brien, D. (1968): Undernutrition and cerebellar development. *Nature (Lond.),* 221:554–555.
22. Clos, J., Rebiere, A., and Legrand, J. (1973): Differential effects of hypothyroidism and undernutrition on the development of glia in the rat cerebellum. *Brain Res.,* 63:445–449.
23. Cogneville, A. M. (1973): Etude de quelques aspects du métabolisme lipidique du tissu adipeux brun interscapulaire du rat hypotrophique au cours du developpement. Thèse Doct. 3e Cycle. Paris Sud Orsay.

24. Cogneville, A. M., Civodino, N., and Tordet-Caridroit, C. (1975): Lipid composition of brown adipose tissue as related to nutrition during the neonatal period in hypotrophic rat. *J. Nutr.*, 105:982–988.
25. Cogneville, A. M., and Tordet-Caridroit, C. (1974): Developmental patterns of glycerokinase and cytochrome-*c*-oxidase in the brown adipose tissue of hypotrophic rats. *Biomedicine*, 21:323–326.
26. Curzon, G., and Green, A. R. (1970): Rapid method for the determination of 5-hydroxytryptamine and 5-hydroxyindole acetic acid in small regions of rat brain. *Br. J. Pharmacol.*, 39:653–655.
27. Curzon, G., and Knott, P. J. (1974): Effects on plasma and brain tryptophan in the rat of drugs and hormones that influence the concentration of unesterified fatty acid in plasma. *Br. J. Pharmacol.*, 50:197–204.
28. Denckla, W. D., and Dewey, H. H. (1967): The determination of tryptophan in plasma, liver and urine. *J. Lab. Clin. Med.*, 69:160–169.
29. Dobbing, J. (1978): Effects of experimental undernutrition on development of the nervous system. In: *Malnutrition, Learning and Behavior*, edited by N. S. Scrimshaw and J. Gordon. M.I.T. Press, Cambridge, Mass.
30. Dobbing, J., and Smart, J. L. (1974): Vulnerability of developing brain and behavior. *Br. Med. Bull.*, 30:164–168.
31. Dobbing, J., Hopewell, J. W., and Lynch, A. (1971): Vulnerability of developing brain. VII. Permanent deficit of neurons in cerebral and cerebellar cortex following early mild undernutrition. *Exp. Neurol.*, 32:439–477.
32. Dobbing, J., and Sands, J. (1971): Vulnerability of developmental brain. IX. The effects of nutritional growth retardation on the timing of the brain growth spurt. *Biol. Neonate*, 19:363–378.
33. Dobbing, J., and Smart, J. L. (1973): Early undernutrition brain development and behaviour. In: *Ethology and Development: Clinics in Developmental Medicine, Vol. 47*, edited by S. A. Barnett, pp. 16–36. Heinemann Medical Books, London.
34. Dobbing, J., and Widdowson, E. (1965): The effect of undernutrition and subsequent rehabilitation of myelination of rat brain as measured by its composition. *Brain*, 88:357–366.
35. Fernstrom, J. D., and Hirsch, M. J. (1975): Rapid repletion of brain serotonin in malnourished corn-fed rats following L-tryptophan injection. *Life Sci.*, 17:455–464.
36. Fernstrom, J. D., and Wurtman, R. J. (1972): Brain serotonin content: Physiological regulation by plasma neutral amino acids. *Science*, 178:414–416.
37. Fishman, M. A., Prensky, A. L., and Dodge, P. R. (1969): Low content of cerebral lipids in infants suffering from malnutrition. *Nature (Lond.)*, 221:552–553.
38. Gessa, G. L., and Tagliamonte, A. (1974): Serum free tryptophan: Control of brain concentrations of tryptophan and of synthesis of 5-hydroxytryptamine. In: *Aromatic Amino Acids in the Brain. Ciba Foundation Symposium 22*, edited by G. E. W. Wolstenholme and D. W. Fitzsimons, pp. 207–216. Elsevier, Excerpta Medica, Amsterdam.
39. Guthrie, H. A., and Brown, M. L. (1968): Effect of severe undernutrition in early life on growth, brain size, and composition in adult rats. *J. Nutr.*, 94:419–426.
40. Hamon, M., Bourgoin, S., and Glowinski, J. (1973): Feed-back regulation of 5-HT synthesis in rat striatal slices. *J. Neurochem.*, 20:1727–1745.
41. Hamon, M., Bourgoin, S., Morot-Gaudry, Y., Hery, F., and Glowinski, J. (1974): Role of active transport of tryptophan in the control of 5-HT biosynthesis. In: *Serotonin—New Vistas, Vol. 11*, edited by E. Costa, G. L. Gessa, and M. Sandler, pp. 153–162. Raven Press, New York.
42. Hamon, M., and Glowinski, J. (1974): Regulation of serotonin synthesis. *Life Sci.*, 15:1533–1548.
43. Hatai, S. (1907): Effects of partial starvation followed by a return to normal diet on the growth of the body and central nervous system of albino rats. *Am. J. Physiol.*, 18:309.
44. Howard, E., and Granoff, D. M. (1968): Effect of neonatal food restriction in mice on brain growth. DNA and cholesterol and on adult delayed response learning. *J. Nutr.*, 95:111–121.
45. Kollee, L. A. A. (1980): Neonatal hypoglycemia in intrauterine growth retarded rats. Thesis Drukkerig Vitgenerij, H. Gianotten, B. V. Tilburg.
46. Lafeber, H. N. (1981): Experimental intra-uterine growth retardation in guinea-pig. Thesis—Zeemanstraat 27 2912 BK Nieuwekerk a/j Ijsse.
47. Miller, M., Leahy, J. P., Stern, W. C., Morgane, P. J., and Resnick, O. (1977): Tryptophan

availability: Relation to elevated brain serotonin in developmentally protein malnourished rats. *Exp. Neurol.,* 57:142–157.
48. Minkowski, A., Roux, J. M., and Tordet-Caridroit, C. (1974): Pathophysiologic changes in intra-uterine malnutrition. In: *Nutrition and Fetal Development,* edited by M. Winick, pp. 45–77. Wiley and Sons, N.Y.
49. Nitzan, M., and Groffman, H. (1971): Glucose metabolism in experimental intra-uterine growth retardation, *in vitro* studies with liver and brain slices. *Biol. Neonate,* 17:420–426.
50. Roux, J. M., Chanez-Bel, C., Degremont, C., Gaben-Cogneville, A. M., Fulchignoni-Lataud, M. C., Swierczewski, E., Tordet-Caridroit, C., and Minkowski, A. (1979): Effect of intrauterine growth retardation on cellular proliferation and differentiation in developing rat. *Ann. Biol. Anim. Bioch. Biophys.,* 19:135–150.
51. Roux, J. M., Tordet-Caridroit, C., and Chanez, C. (1970): Studies on experimental hypotrophy in the rat. I. Chemical composition of the total body and some organs in the rat foetus. *Biol. Neonate,* 15:342–347.
52. Shoemaker, W. J., and Bloom, F. E. (1977): Effect of undernutrition on brain morphology. *Nutrition and the Brain, Vol. 2,* edited by R. J. Wurtman and J. J. Wurtman. Raven Press, New York.
53. Shoemaker, W. J., and Wurtman, R. J. (1971): Perinatal undernutrition: Accumulation of catecholamines in rat brain. *Science,* 171:1017–1019.
54. Shoemaker, W. J., and Wurtman, R. J. (1973): Effect of perinatal undernutrition on the metabolism of catecholamines in the rat brain. *J. Nutr.,* 103:1537–1547.
55. Sima, A., and Persson, L. (1975): The effect of pre- and postnatal undernutrition on the development of the rat cerebellar cortex. I. Morphological observations. *Neurobiology,* 5:23–24.
56. Snedecor, G. W., and Cochran, W. G. (1967): *Statistical Methods.* Iowa State Univerity Press, Ames, Iowa.
57. Sobotka, T. J., Cook, M. P., and Brodie, R. F. (1974): Neonatal malnutrition. Neurochemical, hormonal and behaviour manifestations. *Brain Res.,* 65:443–457.
58. Stern, W. C., Miller, M., Forbes, W. B., Morgane, P. J., and Resnick, O. (1975): Ontogeny of levels of biogenic amines in various parts of the brain and in peripheral tissue in normal and protein malnourished rats. *Exp. Neurol.,* 49:314–326.
59. Tordet-Caridroit, C. (1971): Evolution périnatale de l'aspartate-amino-transférase hépatique chez le rat ayant subi un ralentissement de croissance intra-utérine. *Ann. Biol. Anim. Bioch. Biophys.,* 11:389–397.
60. Tordet-Caridroit, C., and Cogneville, A. M. (1973): Developmental changes in intra-uterine growth retardation of rat interscapular brown adipose tissue. In: *The Regulation of the Adipose Tissue Mass,* edited by J. Vague and J. Boyer, pp. 18–22. Excerpta Medica, Amsterdam.
61. Tordet-Caridroit, C., Roux, J. M., and Chanez, C. (1969): Etude du developpement postnatal du rat né dysmature. *C.R. Soc. Biol.,* 163:1321–1322.
62. Von Euler, J. S., and Lishajko, F. (1961): Improved technique for fluorometric estimation of catecholamines. *Acta Physiol. Scand.,* 51:348–355.
63. Wigglesworth, J. S. (1964): Experimental growth retardation in the foetal rat. *J. Pathol. Bact.,* 88:1–13.
64. Winick, M. (1969): Malnutrition and brain development. *J. Pediatr.,* 74:667–679.
65. Winick, M. (1974): *Nutrition and Fetal Development, Vol. 2.* Wiley and Sons, N.Y.
66. Winick, M. (1977): Early malnutrition. Brain structure and function. *Prev. Med.,* 6:358–360.
67. Winick, M., and Noble, A. (1965): Quantitative changes in DNA, RNA, and protein during prenatal and postnatal growth in the rat. *Dev. Biol.,* 12:451.
68. Winick, M., and Noble, A. (1966): Cellular response in rats during malnutrition at various ages. *J. Nutr.,* 89:300–306.

DISCUSSION

Dr. Semenza: Do you have any data on the degree of respiratory control of the brown fat during development, and particularly when you say that the animals are very sensitive to cold, because obviously the physiological function of brown fat is supposed to be that.

Dr. Minkowski: I think you are right. It has not been looked at for the moment, but it should.

Dr. Rey: Dr. Minkowski, you used a special model to produce small-for-date rats or animals. Did you study the carcass composition of these animals at birth, because it seems to me that the main difference between small-for-dates infants and normal babies is a low content of fat in the organism. It seems also that the number of adipocytes is related to gestational age and that the size of the cells depends on the rate of growth. I wonder if with this special model you don't produce alterations of the body composition that are different in your experimental animals from what they are in humans.

Dr. Minkowski: I will try to reply to your question concerning fats. As you know, the rat does not deposit fat in intrauterine life. There are species that do this, for example, the human, guinea pig, and bat. Lafeber has studied it in guinea pigs because this animal deposits large amounts of fats, and as you would rightly suppose, the deposit of fat in the carcass is very much diminished in IUGR animals. The epidermal growth factor has been described by Dr. Stanley Cohen in the United States and, at the moment, its study requires a sophisticated radioimmunoassay. The interesting thing is that epidermal growth factor is activated by a certain number of compounds like hydroxytryptophane and thyroxine.

Dr. Greene: We have just finished a study which will be published in *Endocrinology* in which we gave pharmacological doses of epidermal growth factor to rats that were 12 days postdelivery, and we were able to demonstrate that at least calcium transport in an *in vivo* perfusion is converted from an almost passive process to an active one. In other words, we moved the development of the gastrointestinal tract as far as calcium transport was concerned backwards by a factor of 5 days, and this would tend to coincide with another observation we made, i.e., that those animals that were small, those that were in the horn of the uterus, tended to have a more rapid onset of calcium transport from the passive to the active phase. So it may be that your observations with epidermal growth factor, as far as the eyes opening is concerned, may, in fact, have some relevance as far as rapid onset of the maturation of the gastrointestinal tract of rats anyway is concerned.

Dr. Jacquot: Just a comment concerning the glucogen and the apparent lack of activity of the enzymes of the gluconeogenic pathway. I believe it has been clearly demonstrated in the rat that glucagon does not show the gluconeogenetic effects you might expect if the newborn is deprived of fatty acids. Since these small newborns do not get access to milk, they are in competition with the others, they don't suckle normally, they have a rather low content of free fatty acids in their blood, and glucagon cannot induce a gluconeogenetic pathway. As far as rats and guinea pigs are concerned, they are just as different as a newborn infant is from an adolescent. A newborn rat has nothing to do with a newborn guinea pig.

Dr. Minkowski: This is quite obvious. Nevertheless, comparative physiology does not deal necessarily with animals of some degree of maturity.

Fetal Growth Retardation Caused by Maternal Dietary Amino Acid Imbalance

*Jack Metcoff, **T. Cole, **P. Lunn, and **S. Salem

*University of Oklahoma Health Sciences Center, Oklahoma City, Oklahoma, 73190; and **MRC-Dunn Nutritional Laboratories, Cambridge, United Kingdom

This chapter presents some preliminary experimental data which indicate that maternal dietary amino acid imbalance affects fetal growth. As background, among approximately 1,164 mother–baby pairs studied at midpregnancy, we found that mothers who later had small babies had a pattern or "profile" of amino acids and nutrient levels in their plasma which differed from mothers who later had large babies (1,3) (Fig. 1). At midpregnancy, mothers having smaller babies had rather higher levels of plasma amino acids, with more positive deviations relative to the standard score means for the entire group. In contrast, mothers who later had large babies had standardized values for most of the amino acid values which were below the mean. This seemed rather paradoxical. We interpreted the observation to mean that mothers with a well-growing fetus had better deposition and utilization of amino acids in their own tissues and better placental transport and fetal uptakes of the amino acids; therefore, they had lower plasma amino acid levels. Since these values were obtained at midpregnancy, before the fetal growth rate had peaked and before significant expansion of body fluid volumes is usually observed, it was not likely that the differences between the two groups of mothers resulted from significant differences in volume expansion. Further, the pattern for the amino acids was not uniform; some, like methionine and isoleucine, deviated below the mean, while some nonessentials like serine, glycine, and alanine were above the mean at midpregnancy in mothers who delivered small babies 18 to 20 weeks later. This suggested an amino acid imbalance. At about that time, Tews, in Harper's laboratory, where amino acid imbalances had been studied for many years, showed that small neutral and large neutral amino acids competed with threonine for uptake into brain slices *in vitro*, and *in vivo* (5). With reduced amounts of threonine in the diet, the transport of amino acids into, and of protein synthesis by, the brain slices was markedly reduced in experimental animals (rats). She later showed that a diet limited in threonine, but containing an excess of small and large neutral amino acids, would lead to postnatal growth retardation in rats (6). Based on the work of Harper's group, we hypothesized that a similar diet during pregnancy might

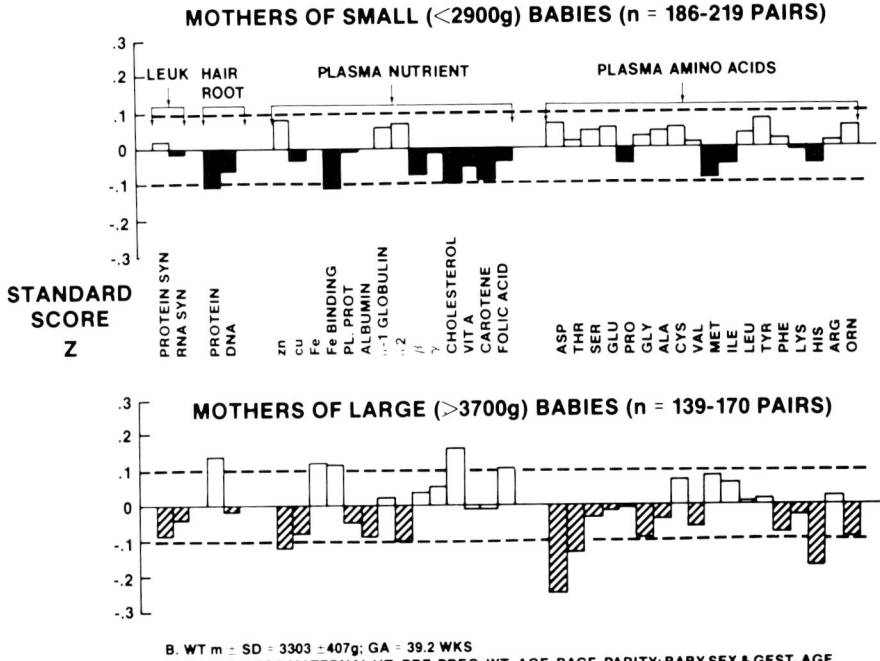

FIG. 1. Standard score values for nutrient variables measured in the mother at midpregnancy are illustrated. The first two bars refer to maternal leukocyte measures, the second two refer to protein and DNA levels in hair roots, respectively. The remaining bars refer to plasma nutrient measures. The pattern for the amino acids in mothers who later had small babies is almost opposite that for mothers who later had large babies. For the former, most of the amino acid levels show positive deviations from the group mean, whereas for the latter, most of the deviations are negative. (From Metcoff, ref. 1, with permission.)

cause fetal growth retardation as a consequence of maternal amino acid imbalance.

METHODS

Three diets were prepared: control, basal, and experimental. The basal diet contained 6% casein and was supplemented with 4.5 g of small neutral and 4.5 g large neutral amino acids per 100-g diet (Table 1). Methionine also was added (0.2%) to all diets. The essential difference between the basal and the experimental diets was the elimination of a threonine supplement from the latter. The control diet contained 20% casein, but otherwise was similar to the basal diet. All diets were equicaloric and contained about 4 cal./g of diet. The basal and experimental diets, with the added amino acids, had a protein equivalence of 15%, but the experimental diet was imbalanced with respect to threonine. Virgin female, infection-free, hooded rats (220–240 g) were kept indi-

TABLE 1. *Composition of control, basal, and experimental diets*[a]

Component	Diets (g/100 g)[b]		
	Control	Basal	Experimental
Casein	20	6	6
Added amino acids			
Small neutrals[c]	4.5	4.5	4.5
Large neutrals[d]	4.5	4.5	4.5
Threonine	0.4	0.4	—
Protein equivalent	30.1	15.0	15.0
Calories (cal./g)	4.03	4.03	4.03

[a] See ref. 3 for a detailed description of the diet.
[b] Usual salt, vitamin, fats, and CHO.
[c] Serine, glycine, alanine.
[d] Isoleucine, leucine, valine, phenylalanine, tyrosine, tryptophan, histidine.

vidually caged, bred, and, when vaginal plugs were detected, were started on the basal diet. After three days the experimental or control diets were substituted for the basal in alternate rats. Animals and food intake were weighed daily. After a 20–24 hr fast, the fetuses were delivered by cesarean section, generally on day 21 of pregnancy, but occasionally on day 20 or 22. The dams then were sacrificed as blood was drawn from the abdominal aorta. The details of the diet and management of the experiment were previously published (2). The tissue protein content was determined by an automated procedure. Plasma amino acid levels were obtained with a Technicon analyzer.

RESULTS AND DISCUSSION

Dams getting the control diet had about an 8% net increase (total body weight—conceptus weight) in their body weight during the course of pregnancy, but the basal group had no net increase. Dams getting the experimental, threonine-limited diet had a net weight loss of about 12% (Fig. 2) (2).

The grams of diet intake required to produce a 1 g weight gain in the mother—called the "converting efficiency" of the diet—is illustrated in Table 2. With the performance of the control animals as a reference set equal to 100%, the basal diet group had a converting efficiency of 71% compared to the controls, whereas the experimental group had approximately a 40% efficiency for conversion of diet to weight gain (2). Although the starting weights of the dams were similar, the total weight gains of each group were very different. Total weight gain during pregnancy is known to be correlated with birth weight. The litter size was increased among the mothers having the smallest pups, especially the experimental compared to the control diet dams. In reviewing the literature, we found that in many studies of experimental intra-

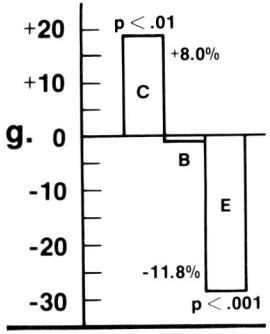

FIG. 2. Net maternal weight change refers to maternal weight minus the weight of the conceptus. The conceptus = fetuses plus placentas plus uterus. Dams on the experimental diet lost approximately 12% of their prepregnant weight at term. (See ref. 2 for details.)

C = CONTROL DIET, n = 4
B = BASAL DIET, n = 17
E = EXPER. DIET, n = 15

uterine growth retardation engendered by diet in rats, litters are selected for comparison which contain a similar number of the fetuses. The different starting weights, total weight gains, and durations of gestation usually are not taken fully into account. A better assessment of the effect of the diet on fetal growth is obtained if one standardizes the values and adjusts for (i.e., statistically controls for) the size of the litter, actual duration of gestation, maternal prepregnant weight, length, and weight gain. The birth weights, brain weights, and placental weights, but not lengths of fetuses from dams on the experimental diet were significantly reduced (Fig. 3).

When the protein concentration of the brains was adjusted for litter size, the maternal prepregnant weight, length, and weight gain during pregnancy, and the duration of pregnancy (20, 21, or 22 days), the protein concentration and content of the brains in the experimental pups was significantly reduced compared to that of the basal and control diet pups. The apparent increase in the protein content of their placentas was not statistically significant (Fig. 4). We interpret the reduction of birth weight and brain weight, and brain protein concentration and content, without significant reduction in length or placental weight, as evidence of fetal malnutrition. In these experiments, the catabolism of maternal tissues did not prevent fetal malnutrition, contrary to the thesis of Naismith (4).

TABLE 2. *Converting efficiency of the diet calculated as intake per gram total weight gain with reference to performance of the control group*

Diet group	Total intake (g)	Wt gain (g)	Intake/g wt gain	Converting efficiency (%)
Basal	301	50.3	5.98	71
Experimental	247	23.3	10.60	40
Control	272	63.8	4.26	100

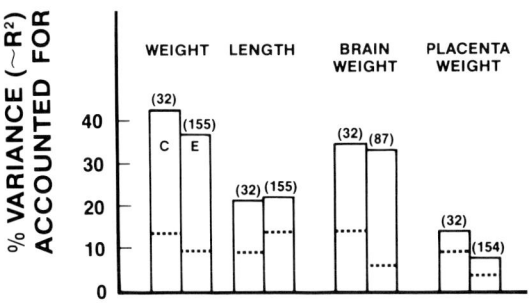

FIG. 3. The proportion of the variance in the fetal measures accounted for by maternal characteristics in the control and experimental group relative to the basal diet group is illustrated. The *dotted line* refers to the proportion of the variance due to the diet effect alone. (See ref. 2 for details.)

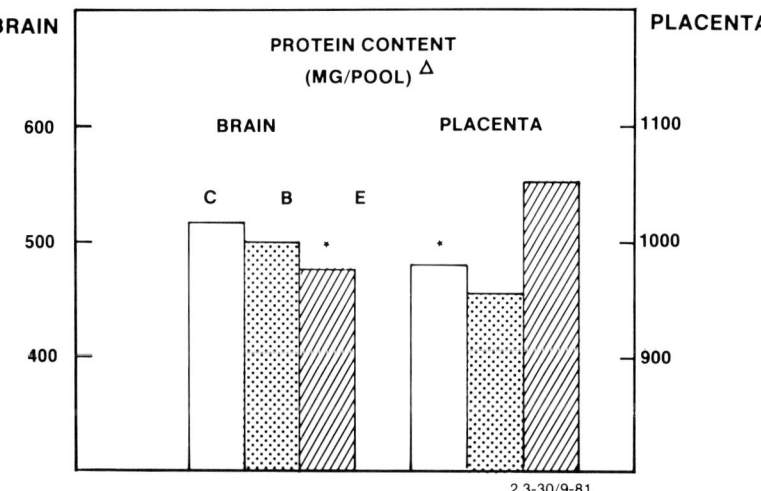

FIG. 4. The protein content of the brain in the experimental group was less than that in the basal group while that of the placenta in controls was more than that observed in the basal diet reference group after adjusting for the variables illustrated by the symbol Δ. "Pool" refers to the pooled tissues from a single litter. Mean values for all litters per group are illustrated.

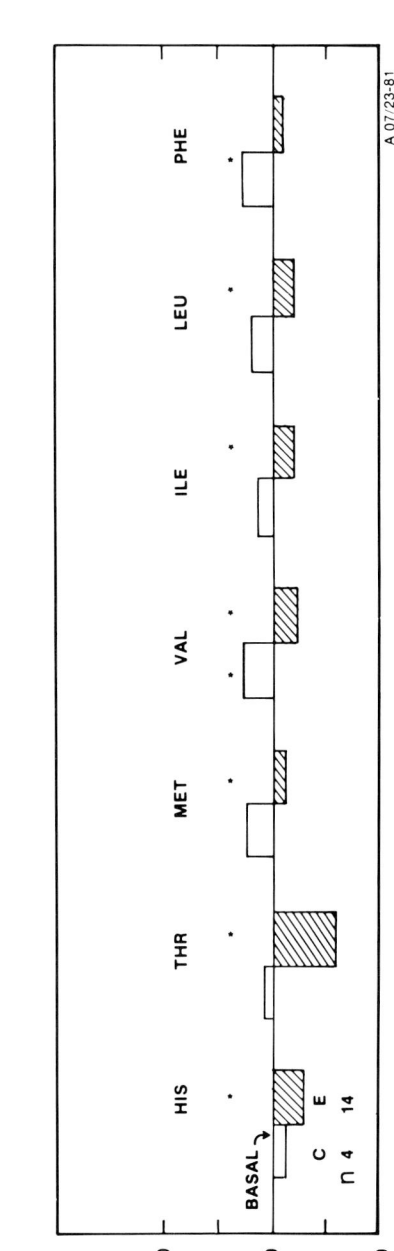

FIG. 5. The level of the maternal plasma essential amino acids in the basal group is set at 1, and values for the control (C) and experimental (E) diet dams are related to the basal. The deviations are negative for the experimental diet animals with the exception of phenylalanine; and positive for the control animals, although the values for histidine, threonine, methionine, isoleucine, and leucine do not differ significantly from values observed in the basal diet group. These measurements were made on plasma obtained at term, immediately after delivery of the fetuses.

At term, the experimental dams had significantly lower mean values for the essential amino acids in plasma, and the control animals had higher values, compared to the basal diet dams (Fig. 5). Using multiple regression analysis, we attempted to identify the best subset of plasma amino acid levels which accounted for the largest proportion of the difference (i.e., the best "predictors") in the plasma threonine level between control diet animals and the basal diet group (Table 3). The contribution of small neutrals was essentially reduced to alanine, which accounted for about 33% of the variance in the threonine level. The large neutrals accounted for about 69% of the variance in the level of threonine. This observation is consistent with those of Tews, and indicates that a dietary imbalance with excess small or large neutral amino acids will affect metabolism of threonine.

Stepwise multiple regression analysis also was used to assess the relative contributions of maternal factors to the birth weight of the pups. Diet was the major contributor to the difference between the control and the basal diet pups; but, duration of pregnancy, prepregnant weight, and maternal plasma levels of methionine, alanine, glutamic acid, arginine, histidine, and phenylalanine also were significant contributors. Although we selected dams with prepregnant weights between 220 and 240 g, the 20 g difference apparently

TABLE 3. *Combinations of amino acids best predicting maternal plasma level of threonine*[a]

Amino Acid Sets (C vs B)	t	% Variance (r^2) accounted for
Small neutrals		
SER	ns	
GLY	ns	
ALA	2.61	33.2
Large neutrals[b]		
ILE	−1.46	
LEU	−2.31	
VAL	5.47	68.8
PHE	1.23	
TYR	−3.47	
HIS	2.25	

[a] Stepwise multiple regression analysis with plasma level of threonine as the dependent variable and comparing the control (C) vs the basal (B) diet groups indicates that alanine, among the small neutral amino acids, accounts for 33.2% of the variance in the plasma level of threonine. The predicting equation for the large neutrals simplifies to the arrangement indicated in footnote b, and accounts for 68.8% of the variance in plasma threonine. The *t*-values are for the partial correlation coefficients.

[b] Simplifies to = VAL + 0.08 (VAL + PHE + HIS) − 95 (ILE + LEU + TYR).

did have a significant influence upon the maternal weight gain and upon birth weight of the pups (Table 4). In the experimental versus the basal group, the diet, duration of pregnancy (21 or 22 days), plasma levels of histidine, phenylalanine, and valine, maternal weight gain, litter size, and prepregnant weight, were significant contributors (Table 4). With respect to the brain, a similar type of analysis indicated that the plasma levels of cystine, isoleucine, methionine, lysine, leucine, and glycine could account for a significant proportion of the variance between the brain weights of the control and basal diet pups (Table 5). The difference between brain weights for the experimental compared

TABLE 4. Stepwise regression of pup birth weight on maternal variables[a]

Control vs basal		Experimental vs basal	
Variable	F	Variable	F
Control diet	30.5	Experimental diet	19.4
Duration pregnancy	76.9	Duration pregnancy	66.3
Methionine	32.5	Histidine	20.9
Alanine	8.9	Weight gain	11.5
Glutamic acid	9.8	Litter size	21.8
Arginine	10.1	Prepregnant weight	11.9
Prepregnant weight	9.0	Phenylalanine	7.7
Histidine	7.0	Valine	12.8
Phenylalanine	12.0		
$df\ (N-2) = 18$		$df\ (N-2) = 28$	

[a] Prepregnant weight, weight gain, length, litter size, and plasma amino acid levels.

TABLE 5. Stepwise regression of pup brain weight on maternal variables[a]

Control vs basal		Experimental vs basal	
Variable	F	Variable	F
Control diet	611.8	Experimental diet	11.3
Cystine	172.1	Valine	87.0
Isoleucine	69.0	Proline	39.0
Methionine	88.6	Tyrosine	13.8
Lysine	43.1	Glycine	11.3
Leucine	24.2	Arginine	7.9
Glycine	14.3	Prepregnant weight	5.9
		Ma Length	15.8
		Weight Gain	6.9
		Aspartic Acid	6.6
$df\ (N-2) = 12$		$df\ (N-2) = 15$	

[a] Prepregnant weight, weight gain, length, litter size, and plasma amino acid levels.

to the basal diet pups was largely accounted for by the differences in the maternal plasma amino acid levels of valine, proline, tyrosine, glycine, arginine, and aspartic acid. Prepregnant weight, maternal length, and weight gain also were important contributing variables. The items which contributed most to the variance in birth weight difference between the control and basal and experimental versus basal diet pups were maternal weight gain, litter size, and plasma levels of methionine, alanine, glutamic acid, and valine. For the pup brain weight, maternal weight gain, length, and the plasma levels of histidine, threonine, glycine, valine, methionine, isoleucine, and leucine (Table 6).

Dietary imbalance of amino acids during pregnancy, such as that resulting from an excess of neutral amino acids when the threonine content of the diet is limited, impairs fetal somatic and brain growth. The mechanism cannot be inferred from these studies, but the observations on fetal growth are consistent with those of Tews for postnatal growth. The amino acid imbalance presumably limits protein synthesis, possibly by interfering with uptake of some essential amino acids by cells.

CONCLUSIONS

We conclude from these preliminary experiments that fetal malnutrition can be produced in pregnant rats by dietary threonine imbalance augmented by an excess of nonessential amino acids. The fetally malnourished pups have smaller brains with reduced protein concentration and content. In the pregnant dams, amino acid imbalanced diets reduced the efficiency for conversion of food intake to tissue stores. The plasma levels of six large neutral amino acids appeared to account for about 69% of the variance in their plasma threonine levels. Stepwise multiple regression analysis selected combinations of some maternal characteristics and a few plasma amino acid levels which could account for a significant proportion of the variance in birth weight of these malnourished pups.

TABLE 6. *Different maternal variables contribute ($p < 0.05$) to regression (C vs B, E vs B)[a]*

Birth weight	Brain weight	
Diet	Diet	Valine
Weight gain	Cystine	Proline
Litter size	Isoleucine	Tyrosine
Methionine	Methionine	Arginine
Alanine	Lysine	Prepregnant weight
Glutamic acid	Leucine	Maternal length
Valine	Aspartic acid	Weight gain

[a] Summary of data presented in Tables 4 and 5. C, control; B, basal.

ACKNOWLEDGMENTS

We wish to express appreciation to Mr. Richard Luff for superior technical assistance, to Mr. Kenneth C. Day for assistance with data processing, and to Dr. Roger Whitehead, Director, Dunn Nutritional Laboratories, MRC, for making it possible to carry out these experiments.

REFERENCES

1. Metcoff, J. (1981): Association between fetal growth and maternal nutrition. In: *Nutrition in Health and Disease and International Development.* Symposia from the XII International Congress on Nutrition, pp. 629–641. Alan R. Liss, N.Y.
2. Metcoff, J., Cole, T. J., and Luff, R. (1981): Fetal growth retardation induced by dietary imbalance of threonine and dispensable amino acids, with adequate energy and protein-equivalent intakes, in pregnant rats. *J. Nutr.,* 111:1411–1424.
3. Metcoff, J., Costiloe, P., Crosby, W. et al. (1981): Maternal nutrition and fetal outcome. *Am. J. Clin. Nutr.,* 34:708–721.
4. Naismith, D. J. (1969): The foetus as a parasite. *Proc. Nutr. Soc.,* 28:25–31.
5. Tews, J. K., Good, S. S., and Harper, A. E. (1978): Transport of threonine and tryptophan by rat brain slices: Relation to other amino acids at concentrations found in plasma. *J. Neuro. Chem.,* 31:581–589.
6. Tews, J. K., Lee-Kim, Y. W., and Harper, A. E. (1979): Induction of threonine imbalance by dispensable amino acids: Relation to competition for amino acid transport into brain. *J. Nutr.,* 109:304–315.

DISCUSSION

Dr. Guesry: Coming back to your slide where you show that weight gain efficiency was reduced when pregnant rat mothers did not get threonine (Fig. 2), we can see that the pregnant rats not given threonine ate much less than the others, and we know that the weight gain efficiency is reduced when the total food intake is also reduced. Did you afterwards pair-feed pregnant rat mothers with and without threonine?

Dr. Metcoff: The total intake in grams was not very different in the control and experimental animals, 272 versus 247 g. The controls gained 64 g on 272 g of total intake, the experimentals only gained 23 g. Threonine was limiting, but only relatively. It was contained in the casein. The threonine supplement was eliminated in the experimental diet. We did not attempt to pair-feed these animals because we were interested in the efficiency of conversion of food to weight gain. The total caloric intakes were almost identical in the three groups, the difference being not significant.

Dr. Räihä: After meals, there is a dramatic change in the postprandial plasma amino acid concentrations in both animals and humans. Did you always take blood samples in your experiments at the same time after meals, or did time of sampling vary?

Dr. Metcoff: The minimum sampling time in the experimental animals was approximately 24 hr after food intake, and the maximum time was about 28 hr. Food was removed from the cages the day before sacrifice. In the humans, the mothers were supposed to be fasting when the blood samples were taken in the morning. We cannot always guarantee that is the case, but we think that, among these more than 1,000 mothers, most of them were fasting. The amino acid observations in the humans and in the rats are not comparable, since the analyses in the former were at midpregnancy, and, in the latter, at term.

Dr. Greenberg: The question that I think is interesting is how the alterations in maternal composition of nutrient supply produce an alteration of fetal growth. I have been really impressed by Halvor Christensen's continued pounding when we are looking at amino acid transport. We are looking at two transport processes, especially in the placenta: one into the syncytiotrophoblast cells and the other out of them, so that changes in supply to the placenta cannot be assumed to reflect themselves in changes in the release of the amino acids into the fetal compartment. Do you have data on the amino acid composition of blood supplying the fetus? Have you looked at fetal amino acid profiles in this situation?

Dr. Metcoff: That, of course, is one of the important questions, and the answer is: no, not yet. The carcass and organs of the pups are analyzed for total amino acid composition. Blood flow was not measured. Of course, more than a single amino acid is required to achieve protein synthesis. I think we are oversimplifying a complex event by using incorporation of a single amino acid to measure protein synthesis or release of a single amino acid to measure protein degradation, and assuming this reflects *in vivo* metabolism. Most of the data suggest that the amino acid mix will modulate the rates and amount of protein synthesized, other factors being equal. My guess is that what we are seeing in our experiments is a reflection of some aberration in the mix. How it imposes on protein synthesis is uncertain. We know that the situation is very much more complicated than suggested by the multiple regression analysis. For example, computer analysis has shown a significant interaction between plasma lysine levels and plasma iron levels which were closely related to protein synthesis in pregnant women (3). Protein synthesis was measured as ^{3}H-Leucine incorporation into leukocytes, using the leukocytes as a replicating cell model. We tested the computer-determined relationship in the laboratory, and we found that we could inhibit protein synthesis significantly by incubation in a medium containing iron at a high normal concentration and lysine at a low normal concentration, as found in the plasma of these mothers. The interactions between nutrients may be a major factor in regulating protein synthesis. Sooner or later, we must confront this complexity. As long as we confine ourselves to testing the effect of changing only a single variable at a time, we are only going to get an oversimplified, single facet of the story explained.

Dr. Rey: You said that in your previous experiences the amino acid values in the mothers were lower when the growth of the babies was high, and you made the hypothesis that the uptake of amino acids was higher when the growth of the babies was faster, whereas, in this model of threonine imbalance, you have shown that controls have higher values and experimental animals lower ones. So, I wonder if your hypothesis is right. Second, you discuss the converting efficiency of the diet, but it seems that the main part of the energy intake is used for maintenance and not for the growth of the fetus. I would like to ask you what the meaning is of converting efficiency of the diet in the presence of amino acid imbalance when the synthesis of protein is depressed.

Dr. Metcoff: The plasma amino acid levels in the rats were measured at term, when the animals were sacrificed. The values which I showed initially in pregnant women were obtained at 20 weeks of gestation. The two situations are not comparable, so we could not test that portion of the hypothesis. The converting efficiency referred to maternal weight gain, not to the relative weight of the fetuses. The net weight gain in the basal and experimental groups was very small or negative relative to the large amount of diet consumed, possibly because the diet calories *were* used for maintenance in these pregnant rats. Presumably, efficient conversion implies sustained protein synthesis. The converting efficiency of the experimental diet dams probably is a manifestation of depressed protein synthesis, as you suggest, and of increased protein degradation of the maternal tissues. Nonetheless, the fetus was not a successful parasite, since it became growth-retarded and malnourished.

The Use of Intravenous Fat Emulsions in Preterm Infants

Philip Sunshine and John A. Kerner, Jr.

Department of Pediatrics, Division of Neonatology and Gastroenterology, Stanford University School of Medicine, Stanford, California 94305

The first intravenous fat (IVF) preparation used to any great extent in the United States was made from cottonseed oil and marketed under the tradename of Lipomul®. A great deal of experience was gained with the use of this emulsion and, in fact, an entire symposium was published reviewing the data regarding this agent (*Metabolism*, 6:591–831, 1957). Lipomul® was withdrawn from the market in 1965 because of numerous reports of toxicity, including "the fat-overloading syndrome", hemorrhagic tendencies, and liver damage. The toxic accumulation of fat observed with Lipomul® was attributed to its large particle size (1 μ in diameter), and possibly the emulsifying agent, pluronic F-68 (46,76).

In 1961 Schuberth and Wretlind described the use of a parenteral fat emulsion made from soybean oil (65), and in 1981 Wretlind reported that in Sweden over 1.6 million units of this emulsion, Intralipid®, were infused with only 8 cases of suspected untoward reaction. In only one case was a causal relationship probable (79).

After Intralipid® had been used extensively in Europe and Canada, it was finally approved by the FDA for use in the United States in 1975. In 1979 Liposyn® became available in the United States, and, more recently, a third fat preparation, Travamulsion®, has also been released for use.

Intralipid® and Travamulsion® contain soybean oil as a base, while Liposyn® is made from safflower oil. Each product uses purified egg phospholipid as an emulsifier, each contains glycerin to make the solutions isotonic, and, when metabolized appropriately, each will yield 1.1 cal./ml.

Table 1 lists the make-up and notes the differences in each of the products. The particle size of Intralipid® is 0.5 μ while those of Liposyn® and Travamulsion® are 0.4 μ. Both Intralipid® and Travamulsion® contain linolenic acid in significant amounts—8% and 6% respectively; less than 0.5% of this fatty acid is found in Liposyn®. Until recently, linolenic acid deficiency had been recognized only in trout (80) and rats (41), but a 6-year-old child who had received a linolenic-free diet for 5 months developed neurological symptomatology including numbness, weakness, leg pain, and blurring of vision (37). Her symptoms disappeared when she was given linolenic acid via an infusion

TABLE 1. *IVF emulsions (10%)*

	Intralipid®	Liposyn®	Travamulsion®
Base	Soybean oil	Safflower oil	Soybean oil
Glycerin content	2.25%	2.5%	2.25%
Osmolarity (mOsmoles/l)	280	300	270
Particle size (micron)	0.5	0.4	0.4
Fatty acid composition			
Linoleic acid	54%	77%	56%
Oleic acid	26%	13%	23%
Palmitic acid	9%	7%	11%
Linolenic acid	8%	0.5%	6%

of Intralipid®. Thus, one must be cautious in using Liposyn® as the only source of fat for patients receiving long-term parenteral nutrition (10).

Both Liposyn® and Intralipid® are available as 10% and 20% solutions, but Travamulsion® is available only as a 10% solution. To date, experience with the 20% emulsions has been limited in the United States (10), and most reports evaluating this solution have emanated from Europe (78). Two additional soybean preparations are available, Intrafat® (Japan) and Lipofundin-S® (Germany), and a cottonseed oil emulsion, Lipiphysan®, is available in France.

METABOLISM OF INTRAVENOUS FAT

The metabolic pathway for the IVF emulsions is similar to that of naturally occurring chylomicrons. The clearance takes place near the capillary endothelial cells, primarily in adipose tissue and muscle, and is dependent upon the activity of lipoprotein lipase to hydrolyze the circulating protein-bound triglyceride (7,30). The free fatty acids thus liberated can enter adipose tissue, where they are reesterified to triglycerides and stored, or they can be utilized as metabolic fuel in the heart, skeletal muscle, or liver. In the liver, free fatty acids can also be converted to very low density lipoproteins (VLDL), which in turn can be secreted into the plasma.

The clearance of lipid can be enhanced with the concurrent use of heparin, dextrose, or insulin. Adequate calories derived from carbohydrates are necessary for free fatty acids to be oxidized through the citric acid cycle. If there is inadequate carbohydrate to fuel the citric acid cycle, oxidation of fatty acids does not progress properly, and ketone body formation is accelerated. Insulin enhances triglyceride clearance and tissue uptake through lipogenesis and decreases the release of free fatty acids from adipose tissue.

USE OF INTRAVENOUS FAT IN PRETERM INFANTS

While a great deal of experience has been accumulated with the use of IVF in laboratory animals and adult humans, it has been only within the last 10 years that any data have been generated regarding the use of these preparations in preterm infants (11,28,29,47). With the use of IVF, it has become possible to provide the infants with a more balanced nutritional regimen, to avoid the problems of essential fatty acid deficiency, and, at the same time, to allow physicians to utilize peripheral rather than large-caliber central veins to infuse nutriments parenterally. The major stimulus for the use of IVF was provided by the work of Cashore and co-workers, who demonstrated that infants given glucose, casein hydrolysate, and IVF regain their birthweights by 8–12 days of age and grow at approximately the same rate they would have, had they remained *in utero* (11).

In addition, physicians recognize that infants receiving parenteral nutrition that is free of fat soon develop signs and symptoms of fatty acid deficiency (26,31,35,36). This is especially true in small prematurely born infants and infants who are small for gestational age, as they often have less than 1% of their body weight as fat. Essential fatty acids are necessary for a large number of important physiological functions, including the maintenance of membrane integrity (26,49), prostaglandin synthesis (44,58), wound healing, immunocompetency (35), and integrity of the central nervous system (36). Often the signs and symptoms of fatty acid deficiency are not recognized readily, and, in some infants, these signs can occur within several days to a week of being on a fat free intake (23). In addition to a reduced rate of growth, these infants demonstrate a characteristic scaly dermatitis, which at times can develop into a weeping erythematous rash, impaired wound healing, decreased resistance to infection, abnormal platelet aggregation, and thrombocytopenia, as well as increased fragility of red cells (22). Laboratory documentation of fatty acid deficiency consists of monitoring the ratio of eicosatrienoic to arachidonic acid (triene/tetraene ratio), and a ratio of 0.4 or greater is indicative of essential fatty acid deficiency (34).

In the past, in order to prevent fatty acid deficiency in infants receiving parenteral nutrition, physicians provided some fat enterally whenever that was possible, or else they infused fresh frozen plasma which had been drawn from a suitable donor who had ingested a high-fat meal prior to the collection. While this technique, at times, could transiently reverse essential fatty acid deficiency, the long-term effectiveness was minimal, and the plasma provided few, if any, calories for the infant. In addition, attempts to prevent the essential fatty acid deficiency with use of medium-chained triglycerides were also unsuccessful (33). One-half to 1.0 g/kg/day of IVF is adequate to prevent essential fatty acid deficiency.

IVF preparations have also been shown to provide protein-sparing effects similar to those demonstrated with intravenous glucose, and have resulted in infants demonstrating a marked improvement in nitrogen retention (59). In fact, an infusion of glucose and amino acids, as well as intravenous fats, would seem to be the preferred way of providing a balanced nutritional intake. With the use of IVF the amount and concentration of glucose needed for infusion can be decreased, the need to use a large-caliber vessel for infusions can be obviated, and the fat emulsion itself seems to offer a protective effect to the blood vessel through which the solution is infused.

Because the fat emulsion breaks down if mixed with hypertonic solutions, the fat must be administered separately, usually through a Y-connector attached as near as possible to the point of entry of the catheter or needle into the vein. The infusion is usually best tolerated if given as a constant infusion over 24 hr.

In most situations the infusion of fat need not exceed 2 g/kg/day. Thus, if IVF is given to infants receiving 12.5% dextrose and 2.0% amino acids, the fat will provide 24% of the calories if the glucose–amino acid solution is infused at the rate of 100 ml/kg/day (75 cal./kg/day); 20% of the total calories if the rate is 120 ml/kg/day (85 cal./kg/day); and 17% of the calories if the rate is 150 ml/kg/day (105 cal./kg/day). This type of caloric distribution may be appropriate for the preterm infant, even though the contribution of fat to total caloric intake is less than that found in most formulas, including breast milk. Data from the studies of Riechman and co-workers show that very-low-birth-weight infants, who are fed enterally an infusion wherein the fat makes up greater than 50% of the total calories, have a much greater fat content in their body composition than they would have had had they remained *in utero* (32% vs. 10%–12%) (57).

In very-low-birth-weight infants or infants who have severe respiratory disease, where fluid restriction is desired, the lipids can be given as a 20% solution rather than as a 10% solution. On occasion an increased amount of IVF may be desired or indicated, especially if a greater caloric intake is necessary; however, it is unusual for more than 3 g/kg/day to be infused into very-low-birth-weight infants.

TOLERANCE OF IVF IN PRETERM INFANTS

Although normal term infants are able to tolerate and metabolize IVF at rates similar to those of adults, preterm infants are unable to tolerate the fats as well (18,60). Studies by Shennan and co-workers (60), as well as by Filler and co-workers (18), suggest that immature infants metabolize IVF slowly, at rates that are approximately one-third those of mature infants. The incidence of hyperlipidemia in infants who are less than 33 weeks gestation and who weigh less than 1,500 g is triple or quadruple that of mature infants (18). Interestingly, these immature infants increase their capabilities to tolerate IVF after the first week or two of extrauterine life (54,55).

Similarly, infants who are small for gestational age (SGA) also have a decreased rate of utilization of IVF compared with infants who are appropriate for gestational age (AGA) (2,29,50). Often the incidence of decreased tolerance in SGA infants is greater than that found in preterm infants who are AGA, and concentrations of triglycerides and free fatty acids in serum following infusions of IVF are two to three times greater than that found in preterm infants who are AGA (1).

In addition, infants who are hypoxic, acidotic, septic, or who have intercurrent illnesses, have intolerances for IVF even at rates of infusion that had been tolerated before these problems became evident (9).

Thus, while infants who are AGA can metabolize 0.15 g/kg/hr (3.6 g/kg/day), very immature infants and infants who are SGA may accumulate plasma lipids at this rate, and slower rates of infusion are necessary for these patients (29).

The reason for this impaired rate of infusion has been thought to be due to decreased activity of lipoprotein lipase as well as decreased amounts of adipose tissue present in these infants. Dhanireddy and co-workers have demonstrated that immature infants of 25 and 26 weeks gestation have about one-third of post-heparin lipolytic activity as compared with infants of more than 27 weeks gestation (15). This is indirect evidence that the activity of tissue lipoprotein lipase is also decreased. Data in humans are lacking, but studies in laboratory animals show that the activity of lipoprotein lipase in lungs follows a developmental pattern that is very low in activity in the immediate newborn period and increases as the animal matures (32).

Although heparin has been shown to release lipoprotein lipase from tissue and enhance the clearance of IVF in the serum of patients receiving Intralipid®, (29) Coran and co-workers have shown that the addition of 150 IU/kg/day of heparin did not significantly alter the rate of clearance of fat from the serum of immature infants (13). Recently, Zaidan and co-workers (81) have shown that continuous intravenous administration of 1 U/ml of heparin to very-low-birth-weight infants receiving Intralipid® enhanced the clearance of triglycerides from serum, but at the same time appreciably increased the concentration of free fatty acids in serum. Thus, the routine addition of heparin to IVF solutions has not been completely evaluated, especially in the very-low-birth-weight infants.

COMPLICATION OR ADVERSE REACTIONS

The incidence of complication or adverse reactions of IVF is low even in the preterm infant if the rate of infusion does not exceed 0.15 g/kg/hr. However, there are numerous complications, actual and theoretical, that should be anticipated if IVF is to be used.

Allergic Manifestations

Allergic manifestations, painful extremities, fever, headaches, and vomiting have been described in older infants, children, and adults; these complications, however, are difficult to recognize and assess in preterm infants (38). Eosinophilia is not an uncommon finding in infants (6), but it may be due to a variety of factors, such as ingestion of cow's milk protein, frequent blood transfusions, cutaneous applications of various dermatological preparations, and oral and parenteral infusions of pharmacological agents. Thus, documentation of allergic reaction to IVF in preterm infants is difficult, if not impossible.

Cholestasis

Cholestasis is a complication frequently encountered in infants receiving total parenteral nutrition (TPN), and the longer the infant receives TPN, the greater likelihood that cholestasis will be encountered (66). It was hoped that the use of IVF would decrease the incidence of cholestasis; unfortunately, this is not the case. Conversely, the use of IVF has not resulted in an increased incidence of cholestasis in these infants. The pathophysiological factors that are responsible for the development of cholestasis in the affected infants are incompletely understood at present.

Fat-Overloading Syndrome

The fat-overloading syndrome, consisting of hyperlipemia, fever, liver damage, and coagulopathy, which was described primarily in adults, has been encountered infrequently, if at all, in infants and children (4,48). This is due primarily to the fact that infants are given relatively small amounts of IVF as compared with adults.

Impaired Utilization of Glucose

Rapid infusions of IVF have caused hyperglycemia in infants receiving glucose and amino acid solutions at rates that they had tolerated prior to the time the IVF was given. In recently reported studies, infusions of IVF at rates of 0.5 g/kg/hr for 2 hr, and even at rates of 0.25 g/kg/hr, have resulted in glucose intolerance in low-birth-weight infants (75). Mechanisms by which hyperglycemia has been produced is not completely understood, but a significant increase in the concentration of plasma insulin occurs during the infusion of IVF, mitigating the hypothesis that insulin activity is depressed. Whether the IVF reduces the rate of glycolysis or enhances gluconeogensis has not been elucidated in these patients.

Impairment of Pulmonary Function

Greene and co-workers were the first to note the relationship between IVF-induced hyperlipemia and decreased pulmonary function (27). They noted a decrease in pulmonary membrane diffusion at rest, and also following exercise, in normal healthy adults. In addition, they demonstrated that rabbits infused with Intralipid® had erythrocytes coated with lipid particles in their lungs. Friedman and co-workers reported two infants of low-birth-weight who received IVF and had fat globules in their alveolar macrophages and capillaries at necropsy (25). Levene and co-workers described fat accumulation in the lungs of eight prematurely born infants who expired in the neonatal period and who had received a 20% solution of IVF (42). The *maximum* rate of infusion of fat in seven of eight of these infants had exceeded 0.15 g/kg/hr, but the *mean rate* of infusion exceeded 0.15 g/kg/hr in only one infant. Andersen and co-workers performed postmortem examinations not only of preterm infants who had received IVF, but also of those who had received only intravenous glucose and human milk enterally (3). They found similar findings to those reported by Levene and co-workers in both groups of infants, and they felt that pulmonary accumulation of fat could occur in infants whether they received fat enterally or parenterally. Dahms and Halpin suggested that lipid deposition in pulmonary walls was probably derived from IVF, but occurred in vessels that had been damaged secondary to pulmonary hypertension, chronic lung disease, or congenital heart disease (14).

Sun and co-workers demonstrated a reduction in PaO_2 in term infants when given 1 g/kg of Intralipid® over a 15-min period (69). Although they could demonstrate no alteration in pulmonary function per se, Pereira and co-workers were able to detect a significant decrease in PaO_2 in preterm infants given 1 g/kg of fat emulsion over a 4-hr period (55). This drop in PaO_2 was more pronounced in infants less than a week of age than in older preterm infants and seemed to be correlated with increased concentrations of both triglycerides and free fatty acids in plasma. We have also noted significant drops in $P_{Tc}O_2$ in patients who receive IVF emulsions, especially in those with severe cardiopulmonary disease.

In classic studies carried out in an anesthetized sheep model, McKeen, Brigham, and others showed that the reduction in arterial PO_2 during and following the infusion of fat emulsions in amounts that were usually given to humans was not due to hyperlipidemia (45). They clearly demonstrated that the IVF was associated with an increase in pulmonary lymphatic flow, an increase in pulmonary arterial pressure, and a decrease in arterial oxygen tension. While treatment with heparin cleared the serum of triglyceride, it did not affect the increased pulmonary lymphatic flow, the increased pulmonary arterial pressure, or the fall in PaO_2. However, pretreatment of the animals with indomethacin, a potent inhibitor of prostaglandin synthesis, prevented these changes.

It appears that infusions of fat emulsions to preterm infants are associated with an increase in the rate of pulmonary lymphatic flow, and this in turn increases pulmonary arterial pressure, which may cause a decrease in PaO_2. In infants with chronic lung disease or heart disease who already have increased lung water and increased pulmonary lymphatic flow, infusions of IVF even at rates of less than 0.15 g/kg/hr may potentiate an already undesirable condition. Not only does the PaO_2 decrease, but, in patients who become relatively hypoxic, fat is poorly metabolized, and plasma triglycerides and free fatty acids may remain elevated for a prolonged period of time and potentiate this vicious cycle of events. This creates a very difficult clinical situation, because as one tries to provide adequate calories for infants with chronic lung or heart disease, the solution used to provide the calories may potentiate the hypoxia and lead to acidosis as well.

Diminished Immune Responsiveness Secondary to IVF

Deposition of fat in the macrophages of the reticuloendothelial system of infants who have received IVF has been noted by a number of investigators (40,52,74). Fischer and co-workers showed that IVF impaired bacterial clearance and enhanced bacterial virulence in mice and inhibited chemotaxis of human neutrophils in an *in vitro* situation (19,20).

Palmblad et al. could not demonstrate that IVF affected the function of neutrophils of adults (51), and English and co-workers showed that chemotaxis inhibition was due to the glycerol in the Intralipid® preparation (17). This inhibition was probably a result of "hypotonic shock." They also noted that lipid emulsions would have had to have been administered at an "inordinately high rate to cause transient inhibition of circulating neutrophil function" (17).

Generation of Free Bilirubin by Metabolites of IVF

Although the IVF emulsions themselves have been shown not to displace bilirubin from albumin circulating in plasma (71,72), there has been some concern that liberation of free fatty acids during hydrolysis of IVF might displace albumin-bound bilirubin. If infants are icteric, the use of IVF emulsions has been considered hazardous, if indeed, unbound or free bilirubin might potentially increase the risk of kernicterus. There have been several studies suggesting that the use of IVF emulsions may not be dangerous unless the amount of fatty acid liberated increases significantly, so that bilirubin-binding sites on the albumin molecule would be compromised (67). Andrew and co-workers recommended that a safe method to monitor and prevent such complications would be to maintain a free fatty acid to serum albumin molar ratio (FA/SA) at six or less (2). Using a simplified method to measure the FA/SA (5), Kerner and co-workers found that in preterm infants receiving 0.5 to 3.3 g/kg/day of *continuous* IVF infusions, the mean ratio was only 1.1 (39). If, on the other hand, bolus infusions are utilized, the FA/SA ratio might be altered, and the patient might be at risk.

In recent studies, Dr. Levine and co-workers have questioned the role of free or unbound bilirubin as a major factor in producing kernicterus (43). They have demonstrated, at least in laboratory animals made icteric, that alteration of the blood–brain barrier by rapid infusion of hypertonic solutions resulted in deposition of bilirubin into tissues of the central nervous system. Thus, we must be more concerned of the hazards of hypoxia, acidosis, and hyperosmolarity in damaging the blood–brain barrier, than of the potential of utilizing medications or nutriments that may displace bilirubin from the albumin molecule. While the IVF emulsions or free fatty acids themselves may not potentiate the risk of the infant developing kernicterus, it is possible that the rate of infusion of IVF might cause the infant to become hypoxic and acidotic and may increase the risk of the infant developing bilirubin encephalopathy.

No matter what the basic cause of kernicterus is, one must use IVF with caution in infants with indirect hyperbilirubinemia. Often the infusion of IVF will not be initiated until the infant's serum bilirubin has decreased to a level that is considered safe, and the infant is no longer at risk of developing bilirubin encephalopathy.

Hypocarnitinemia

In order for fatty acids to be metabolized completely, they must be acetylated and then transported across the mitochondrial membrane, where, through a process of β-oxidation, they are converted to water, CO_2, and energy (70). Carnitine is a naturally occurring trimethylamine which, in the form of one or several acylcarnitines, facilitates the transport of fatty acids into mitochondria (70). Carnitine can be synthesized from both lysine and methionine, but, in the newborn period, the synthetic pathway does not seem to be functioning appropriately. Carnitine is present in human milk and in Similac® (1 mg/dl), but it is absent in soybean formulas and in any of the currently available amino acid preparations (62).

Preterm and term infants receiving TPN with IVF have been found to have decreased concentrations of total carnitine, acylcarnitine, and free carnitine as compared to infants who have received enteral nutrition containing carnitine. In addition, following an infusion of IVF in preterm infants, concentrations of β-hydroxybuturate as well as free fatty acids and triglycerides rose rapidly in plasma (63).

Although there are reports that adding carnitine to the diet of infants potentiates growth and weight gain (8), there have not been any documented abnormalities encountered in preterm infants who have hypocarnitinemia. In addition, infants have a rapid decrease in urinary excretion of cartinine during TPN, indicating that they are capable of preserving whatever carnitine they possess (53).

Whether hypocarnitinemia is a chemical abnormality in search of a clinical syndrome is purely speculative. However, patients with defects of carnitine biosynthesis have been described who have either cardiomyopathy (73) or a form of lipid storage disease in which patients have episodes of lethargy, somnolence, hypoglycemia, hepatomegaly, and hyperammonemia (12). Families with cardiomyopathy have been described who have markedly decreased serum and tissue levels of carnitine, and those patients with this disorder have been shown to have a beneficial response to oral carnitine intake. Not only did the patients with cardiomyopathy have heart failure and what appeared to be endocardial fibroelastosis, but they also developed severe metabolic acidosis (73).

In newborn infants, especially infants who have abnormalities of the cardiopulmonary system, such as chronic lung or heart disease, the finding of hypocarnitinemia might be significant, and might indicate that these infants have poor myocardial function. Detection of abnormalities with X-rays, electrocardiography, and echocardiography may be important, especially if the dysfunction can be reversed with the addition of oral carnitine.

Thus, hypocarnitinemia is an enigma as far as our present understanding of this biochemical finding is concerned, and a great many more studies have to be accomplished before any definite recommendations regarding its routine use in patients receiving TPN and IVF can be made.

Additional Actual and Theoretical Complications

Several other actual or theoretical complications associated with the use of IVF emulsions are described:

1. Altered rates of synthesis of prostaglandins which might lead to abnormalities of platelet function and possibly abnormalities of pulmonary function (24).
2. Increased concentrations of IVF in plasma which might interfere with several biochemical tests. The first is spurious hyperbilirubinemia, which is encountered when certain spectrophotometric methods are utilized to measure bilirubin (61), and the second is spurious hyponatremia, which is caused by the space-occupying effect of fat. This latter inaccuracy can be corrected if the serum is ultracentrifuged prior to the determination.
3. Transient sinus bradycardia (68).
4. Arachidonic acid deficiency occurring in spite of the high linoleic acid content of IVF (21).
5. Malassezia-Furfur-induced pulmonary vasculitis (56).
6. Decreased concentrations of ionized calcium in serum (77).

MONITORING

Although serum turbidity may reflect increased lipid levels in blood associated with IVF infusion, the gross estimation of turbidity by looking at the serum lactesence has been totally ineffective in evaluating the extent of the increased concentration of lipid in plasma. The use of a micronephelometer to measure the plasma light-scattering index (LSI) and, in turn, the IVF concentration, was thought to be a very sensitive method of monitoring fat levels, especially if the IVF levels increased above 100 mg/dl (9). Schreiner and co-workers adapted a simplified modification of the nephelometer using a fluorometric technique (64). They were able to demonstrate that the *in vitro* fluorometric technique correlated well with the nephelometry measurements, but that the correlations of LSI with free fatty acids, cholesterol, and triglycerides *in vivo* were poor. In a study carried out in 23 infants, D'Harlingue and co-workers noted a positive correlation between serum IVF levels as determined by micronephelometry and triglycerides, but also that the IVF level did not reliably detect elevated levels of triglycerides, cholesterol, or free fatty acid–albumin molar ratios (16). Neonates receiving IVF, therefore, cannot be monitored by nephelometry alone, and adequate monitoring requires the measurement of the specific fractions of lipid in serum. The data also indicate that if the serum triglyceride levels exceed 150 mg/dl, the rates of IVF must be decreased in preterm infants. In some infants, especially those with pulmonary insufficiency, the serum triglyceride concentrations in serum should be maintained at about 100 mg/dl.

REFERENCES

1. Andrew, G., Chan G., and Schiff, D. (1976): Lipid metabolism in the neonate. I. The effects of Intralipid® infusion on plasma triglyceride and free fatty acid concentrations in the neonate. *J. Pediatr.*, 88:273.
2. Andrew, G., Chan, G., and Schiff, D. (1976): Lipid metabolism in the neonate. II. The effect of Intralipid® on bilirubin binding *in vitro* and *in vivo*. *J. Pediatr.*, 88:279.
3. Andersen, G. E., Hertel, J., and Tygstrup, I. (1981): Pulmonary fat accumulation in preterm infants. *Lancet,* i:441.
4. Belin, R. P., Bivins, B. A., Jona, J. Z., et al. (1976): Fat overload with a 10% soybean emulsion. *Arch. Surg.,* 111:1391.
5. Berde, C. B., Kerner, J. A., and Johnson, J. D. (1980): Use of the conjugated polyene fatty acid, parinaric acid, in assaying fatty acids in serum or plasma. *Clin. Chem.,* 26:1173.
6. Bhat, A. M., and Scanlon, J. W. (1981): The pattern of eosinophilia in preterm infants. *J. Pediatr.,* 98:612.
7. Boberg, J., and Carlson, L. A. (1964): Determination of heparin-induced lipoprotein lipase activity in human plasma. *Clin. Chem. Acta,* 10:420.
8. Borniche, P., and Canlorbe, P. (1960): Action clinique et humorale de la carnitine dans les syndromes de denutrition post-infectieux de l'enfance. *Clin. Chem. Acta,* 5:171.
9. Bryan, H., Shennan, A., Griffin, E. et al. (1976): Intralipid®—Its rational use in parenteral nutrition of the newborn. *Pediatrics,* 58:787.
10. Byrne, W. J. (1982): Intralipid® or Liposyn®—Comparable products? *J. Pediatr. Gastroenterol. Nutr.,* 1:7.
11. Cashore, W. J., Sedaghatian, M. R., and Usher, R. H. (1975): Nutritional supplements with intravenously administered lipid, protein hydrolysate, and glucose in small premature infants. *Pediatrics,* 56:8.
12. Chapoy, P. R., Angelinei, C., Brown, W. J., et al. (1980): Systemic carnitine deficiency—A treatable inherited lipid-storage disease presenting as Reye's syndrome. *N. Engl. J. Med.,* 303:1389.
13. Coran, A. G., Edward, B., and Zaleska, R. (1974): The value of heparin in the hyperalimentation of infants and children with a fat emulsion. *J. Pediatr. Surg.,* 9:725.
14. Dahms, B., and Halpin, T. C. (1980): Pulmonary arterial lipid deposit in newborn infants receiving intravenous lipid infusion. *J. Pediatr.,* 97:800.
15. Dhanireddy, R., Hamosh, M., Sivasubraimanian, K. N. et al. (1981): Postheparin lipolytic activity and Intralipid® clearance in very low birth weight infants. *J. Pediatr.,* 98:617.
16. D'Harlingue, A., Hopper, A. O., Stevenson, D. K., et al. (1983): Limited value of nephelometry in monitoring the administration of intravenous fat in neonates. *J. Parent Ent. Nutr.,* 7:55.
17. English, D., Roloff, J. S., Lukens, J. N., et al. (1981): Intravenous lipid emulsions and human neutrophil function. *J. Pediatr.,* 99:913.
18. Filler, R. M., Takada, Y., Carreras, T., et al. (1980): Serum Intralipid levels in neonates during parenteral nutrition: The relation to gestational age. *J. Pediatr. Surg.,* 15:405.
19. Fischer, G. W., Hunter, K. W., Wilson, S. R., et al. (1979): Inhibitory effect of Intralipid on reticuloendothelial function and neutrophil bactericidal activity. *Pediatr. Res.,* 13:494.
20. Fischer, G. W., Wilson, S. R., Hunter, K. W., et al. (1980): Diminished bacterial defenses with Intralipid. *Lancet,* ii:819.
21. Friedman, A., and Frolich, J. C. (1979): Essential fatty acids and major urinary metabolites of the E prostaglandins in thriving neonates and infants receiving parenteral fat emulsions. *Pediatr. Res.,* 13:932.
22. Friedman, Z. (1980): Essential fatty acids revisited. *Am. J. Dis. Child.,* 134:397.
23. Friedman, Z., Dunon, A., Stahlman, M. T., et al. (1976): Rapid onset of essential fatty acid deficiency in the newborn. *Pediatrics,* 58:640.

24. Friedman, Z., Lamberth, E. L., Frolich, J. G., et al. (1977): The effect of parenteral fat emulsions (PFE) on tissue fatty acid composition, the major urinary metabolites of E prostaglandins (PGE-M) and lung histology. *Pediatr. Res.,* 11:443.
25. Friedman, Z., Marks, K. H., Maisels, J., et al. (1978): Effect of parenteral fat emulsion on the pulmonary and reticuloendothelial systems in the newborn infant. *Pediatrics,* 61:694.
26. Goodgame, J., Lowry, S., and Brennan, M. (1978): Essential fatty acid deficiency in total parenteral nutrition: Time course of development and suggestions for therapy. *Surgery,* 84:271.
27. Greene, H. L., Hazlett, D., and Demares, R. (1976): Relationship between Intralipid® induced hyperlipemia and pulmonary function. *Am. J. Clin. Nutr.,* 29:127.
28. Gustafson, A., Kjellmer, I., Olegard, R., et al. (1972): Nutrition in low birth weight infants I. Intravenous injection of fat emulsion. *Acta Paediatr. Scand.,* 61:149.
29. Gustafson, A., Kjellmer, I., Olegard, R., et al. (1974): Repeated intravenous injections of fat emulsions *Acta Paediatr. Scand.,* 63:177.
30. Hallberg, D. (1965): Studies on the elimination of exogenous lipids from the bloodstream. *Acta Physiol. Scand.,* 65(Suppl. 254):1.
31. Heird, W. E., and Winters, R. W. (1975): Total parenteral nutrition: The state of the art. *J. Pediatr.,* 86:2.
32. Hietanen, E., and Hartiala, J. (1979): Developmental pattern of pulmonary lipoprotein lipase in growing rats. *Biol. Neonate,* 36:85.
33. Hirono, H., Suzuki, H., Igarashi, Y. et al. (1977): Essential fatty acid deficiency induced by total parenteral nutrition and by medium-chain triglyceride feeding. *Am. J. Clin. Nutr.,* 30:1760.
34. Holman, R. T. (1960): The ratio of trienoic:tetraenoic acids in tissue lipids as a measure of essential fatty acid requirements. *J. Nutr.,* 70:405.
35. Holman, R. T. (1968): Essential fatty acid deficiency. In: *Progress in the Chemistry of Fats and Other Lipids, Vol. 9,* edited by R. T. Holman, pp. 275–348. Pergamon Press, Elmsford, N.Y.
36. Holman, R. T. (1977): Essential fatty acid deficiency in humans. In *Handbook of Nutrition and Foods,* edited by M. Recheigl. CRC Press, Cleveland.
37. Holman, R. T., Johnson, S. B., and Hatch, T. F. (1982): A case of human linolenic acid deficiency involving neurologic abnormalities. *Am. J. Clin. Nutr.,* 35:617.
38. Kamath, K. R., Berry, A., and Cummins, G. (1981): Acute hypersensitivity reaction to Intralipid. *N. Engl. J. Med.,* 304:360.
39. Kerner, J. A., Cassani, C., Hurwitz, R., et al. (1981): Monitoring intravenous fat emulsions in neonates with the fatty acid/serum albumin molar ratio. *J.P.E.N.,* 5:517.
40. Koga, Y., Swanson, V. L., and Hays, D. M. M. (1975): Hepatic "intravenous fat pigment" in infants and children receiving lipid emulsion. *J. Pediatr. Surg.,* 10:641.
41. Lamptey, M. S., and Walker, B. L. (1976): A possible essential role for dietary linolenic acid in the development of the young rat. *J. Nutr.,* 106:86.
42. Levine, M. J., Wigglesworth, J. S., and Desai, R. (1980): Pulmonary fat accumulation after Intralipid® infusion in the preterm infant. *Lancet,* ii:815.
43. Levine, R. L., Fredericks, A. B., and Rapaport, S. I. (1982): Entry of bilirubin into the brain due to the opening of the blood–brain barrier. *Pediatrics,* 69:255.
44. Marcus, A. J. (1978): The role of lipids in platelet function: With particular reference to the arachidonic acid pathway. *J. Lipid Res.,* 19:793.
45. McKeen, C. R., Brigham, K. L., Bowers, R. E., et al. (1978): Pulmonary vascular effects of fat emulsion infusion in unanesthetized sheep. *J. Clin. Invest.,* 61:1291.
46. Meng, H. C. (1972): Use of fat emulsions in parenteral nutrition. *Drug Intell. Clin. Pharm.,* 6:321.
47. Mestyan, J., Rubecz, I., and Soltesz, G. (1976): Changes in blood glucose, free fatty acids and amino acids in low birth weight infants receiving intravenous fat emulsion. *Biol. Neonate,* 30:74.
48. Monnens, L., Smuldero, Y., and Dekker, W. (1976): Lipid overloading due to Intralipid infusion in an infant with intractable diarrhea. *Z. Kinderchir. Grenzgeb.,* 19:1.
49. *Nutr. Rev.* (1977): Essential fatty acids and water permeability of the skin, 35:303.
50. Olegard, R., Gustafson, A., Kjellmer, I., et al. (1975): Nutrition in low-birth-weight infant. III. Lipolysis and free fatty acid elimination after intravenous administration of fat emulsion. *Acta Paediatr. Scand.,* 64:745.
51. Palmblad, J., Bronstrom, O., Uden, A. M., et al. (1980): Letter. *Lancet,* ii:1138.
52. Passwell, J. H., David, R., Katznelson, D., et al. (1976): Pigment deposition in the reticuloendothelial system after fat emulsion infusion. *Arch. Dis. Child.,* 51:366.

53. Penn, D., Schmidt-Sommerfield, E., and Wolf, H. (1980): Carnitine deficiency in premature infants receiving total parenteral nutrition. *Early Hum. Dev.,* 4:23.
54. Pereira, G. R., Fox, W. W., Stanley, C. A., et al. (1980): Decreased oxygenation and hyperlipemia during intravenous fat infusions in premature infants. *Pediatrics,* 66:26.
55. Pereira, G. R., Stanley, C. A., Fox, W. W., et al. (1978): The effect of postnatal age on the metabolism of intravenous fat emulsion. *Pediatr. Res.,* 12:440.
56. Redline, R. W., and Dahms, B. B. (1981): Malassezia pulmonary vasculitis in an infant on long-term Intralipid therapy. *N. Engl. J. Med.,* 305:1395.
57. Reichman, B., Chessex, P., Putet, G., et al. (1981): Diet, fat accretion and growth in premature infants. *N. Engl. J. Med.,* 305:1495.
58. Robertson, R. P. (1979): Prostaglandins as modulators of pancreatic islet function. *Diabetes,* 28:943.
59. Rubecz, I., Mestyan, J., Varga, P., et al. (1981): Energy metabolism, substrate utilization and nitrogen balance in parenterally fed postoperative neonates and infants. *J. Pediatr.,* 98:42.
60. Shennan, A. T., Bryan, M. H., and Angel, A. (1977): The effects of gestational age on Intralipid tolerance in newborn infants. *J. Pediatr.,* 91:134.
61. Shennan, A. T., Cherian, A. G., Angel, A., et al. (1976): The effect of Intralipid on the estimation of serum bilirubin in the newborn infant. *J. Pediatr.,* 88:285.
62. Schiff, D., Chan, G., Seccombe, D. et al. (1979): Plasma carnitine levels during intravenous feeding of the neonate. *J. Pediatr.,* 95:1043.
63. Schmidt-Sommerfield, E., Penn, D., and Wolf, H. (1982): Carnitine blood concentrations and fat utilization in parenterally alimented premature newborn infants. *J. Pediatr.,* 100:260.
64. Schreiner, R. L., Glick, M. R., and Nordschow, C. D. (1979): An evaluation of methods to monitor infants receiving intravenous lipids. *J. Pediatr.,* 94:197.
65. Schuberth, O., and Wretlind, A. (1961): Intravenous infusion of fat emulsions, phosphatides, and emulsifying agents: Clinical and experimental studies. *Acta Chir. Scand. (Suppl.),* 278:1.
66. Sondheimer, J. M., Bryan, H., Andrews, W. et al. (1978): Cholestatic tendencies in preterm infants on and off parenteral nutrition. *Pediatrics,* 62:984.
67. Starinsky, R., and Shafrir, E. (1970): Displacement of albumin-bound bilirubin by free fatty acids: Implications for neonatal hyperbilirubinemia. *Clin. Chim. Acta,* 29:311.
68. Sternberg, A., Gruenevald, T., Deutsch, A. A. et al. (1981): Intralipid-induced transient bradycardia. *N. Engl. J. Med.,* 304:422.
69. Sun, S. C., Ventura, C., and Verasestakul, S. (1978): Effect of Intralipid-induced lipemia on the arterial oxygen tension in preterm infants. *Resuscitation,* 6:265.
70. Tao, R. C., and Yoshimura, N. N. (1980): Carnitine metabolism and its application in parenteral nutrition. *J. Parent Ent. Nutr.,* 4:469.
71. Thaler, M. M., and Pelger, A. (1977): Influence of intravenous nutrients on bilirubin transport. III. Emulsified fat infusion. *Pediatr. Res.,* 11:171.
72. Thaler, M. M., and Wennberg, R. P. (1977): Influence of intravenous nutrients on bilirubin transport. II. Emulsified lipid solutions. *Pediatr. Res.,* 11:167.
73. Tripp, M. E., Katcher, M. L., Peters, H. A. et al. (1981): Systemic carnitine deficiency presenting as familial endocardial fibroelastosis: A treatable cardiomyopathy. *N. Engl. J. Med.,* 305:385.
74. van Haelst, U. J., and Sengers, R. C. (1976): Effects of parenteral nutrition with lipids on the human liver. An electron-microscopic study. *Virchows Arch. [Cell Pathol.],* 22:323.
75. Vileisis, R. A., Cowett, R. M., and Oh, W. (1982): Glycemic response to lipid infusion in the premature neonate. *J. Pediatr.,* 100:108.
76. Waddell, W. R., Geyer, R. P., Olsen, F. R., et al. (1957): Clinical observations on the use of non-phosphatide (pluronic) fat emulsion. *Metabolism,* 6:815.
77. Whitsett, J., and Tsang, R. C. (1977): *In vitro* effects of fatty acids on serum-ionized calcium. *J. Pediatr.,* 91:233.
78. Wretlind, A. (1978): Parenteral nutrition. *Surg. Clin. North. Am.,* 58:1055.
79. Wretlind, A. (1981): Development of fat emulsions. *J.P.E.N.,* 5:230.
80. Yu, T. C., Sinnhuber, R. O., and Hendricks, J. D. (1979): Reproduction and survival of rainbow trout (*Salmo gairdneri*) fed linolenic acid as the only source of essential fatty acids. *Lipids,* 14:572.
81. Zaidan H., Dhanireddy R., Hamosh M., et al. (1982): Effect of continuous heparin administration on Intralipid clearing in very low-birth-weight infants. *J. Pediatr.,* 101:599.

Nutritional Adaptation of the Gastrointestinal Tract of the Newborn, edited by N. Kretchmer and A. Minkowski. Nestlé, Vevey/Raven Press, New York © 1983.

Nutrient Deposit in Low-Birth-Weight Infants

*G. Putet and **J. Senterre

*INSERM U34 et Departement Neonatale (Professeur B. Salle), Hôpital Edouard-Herriot, 69374 Lyon Cedex 08, France; and
**Université de Liège et Hôpital de Bavière, B-4020 Liège, Belgium

The growth curves of a fetus *in utero* (4) and of a preterm infant are shown in Fig. 1. Following birth, weight is lost and there is a delay until growth is resumed. Afterwards, there is usually little difference between the slope of both curves, and it is only when there is a flattening out of the intrauterine (IU) curve that our preterm infant curve catches up with it. This figure raises an important question: Should we try to have a faster "catching up" of the extrauterine growth in low-birth-weight (LBW) infants?

Another important question can be asked from data on the daily increment of each major nutrient during fetal life as calculated by different authors (9,11): does extrauterine growth mimic, or should it mimic, IU growth qualitatively?

These are important questions, and it is the task of today's neonatologist to answer them.

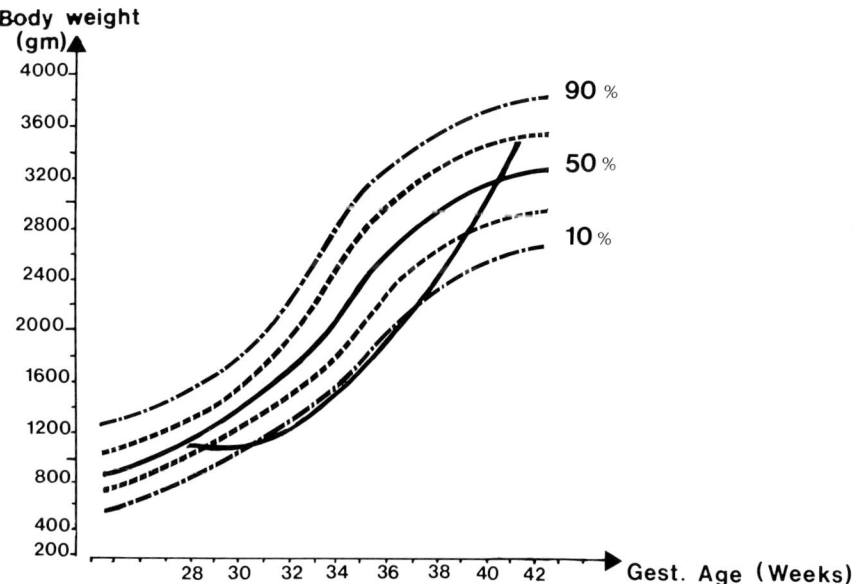

FIG. 1. Intrauterine growth curve from Lubchenko (4) and postnatal growth curve of a preterm infant.

In the following study we have tried to compare growth and quality of growth of preterm infants fed two different regimes. Preliminary results are presented here.

METHODS

The principles of indirect calorimetry (IC) together with urinary nitrogen measurements were used in order to assess energy expenditures and nutrients oxidation (3) of LBW infants. Using an open circuit system (8), 12 to 24 hr continuous IC measurements were performed during a 3-day nutritional balance. Ingesta and excreta were precisely measured according to a carefully designed protocol (7). All biochemical analyses of ingesta and excreta were performed in Senterre's laboratory. By combining these two methodologies (nutrient balances and oxidation measurements by IC), the quantity of each nutrient absorbed and oxidized was calculated (3). The difference between the amount absorbed and the amount oxidized being assumed to be retained in the body as new tissue, we expected to achieve a reflection of growth composition (1,5).

Twelve healthy, orally fed preterm infants were studied. Six were fed human milk (pooled pasteurized human milk) (HM group); six others were fed a specially adapted preterm formula (PF group). Two complete studies (IC measurement and nutrients balance) were done successively on each infant: study 1 and study 2. (Study 2 was performed on all but one infant in each group.) Table 1 gives the infants' gestational age, birth weight, postnatal weight, and age at the time of studies 1 and 2. Milk composition and infants' intakes are summarized in Table 2.

RESULTS AND DISCUSSION

Anthropometry

During study 1 the weight gain (expressed as g/kg/day of weight gain) during the week in which the balance took place was 22.7 ± 4 g/kg/day for the PF group and 13.1 ± 4.6 g/kg/day for the HM group, and during study 2, 19.9 ± 2.5 g/kg/day and 16.9 ± 2 g/kg/day, respectively. If we now consider the mean weight gain achieved in the period between the two studies, PF-fed infants gained 22.5 ± 2.8 g/kg/day versus 13.8 ± 2.3 g/kg/day for HM-fed infants. However, there were no statistically significant differences between the two groups in length gain (expressed in centimeters per week): 1.35 ± 0.3 cm (PF group) versus 0.95 ± 0.3 (HM group); and, in head-circumference growth (expressed in centimeters per week): 1.12 ± 0.06 cm versus 0.96 ± 0.26 cm.

TABLE 1. Clinical data

	PF group	HM group
Gestational age (weeks)	30 ± 1.6	30.3 ± 1.5
Birth weight (g)	1,353 ± 255	1,318 ± 155
Postnatal age (days)		
Study 1	29.5 ± 1 (34 weeks)[a]	20.6 ± 5.8 (33.2 weeks)[a]
Study 2	45.2 ± 1.4 (36.5 weeks)[a]	38.5 ± 7.7 (35.8 weeks)[a]
Postnatal weight (g)		
Study 1	1,641 ± 98	1,453 ± 118.6
Study 2	2,160 ± 111	1,907 ± 95.3

[a] Gestational age at the time of the study.

TABLE 2. Milk composition and milk intakes

	PF Group	HM Group
Composition of milk (per 100 ml)		
Carbohydrates (g)	9.7	6.6 ± 0.2
Lactose	7.3	5.5
Maltodextrins	2.4	
Lipids (g)	3.4	3.03 ± 0.3
MCT	1.36	
Protein (g)	2	1.4 ± 0.14
Casein	40%	
Whey	60%	
Energy (kcal)	77	61
Volume intake (ml/kg/day)		
Study 1	159 ± 6	177 ± 12
Study 2	161 ± 6	173 ± 14

Utilization of Nutrients

Energy, protein, and fat intakes, losses, and oxidations are shown in Tables 3 (study 1) and 4 (study 2). (These are only preliminary data calculated from results of four balances in the HM group and of six in the PF group.)

During study 1 PF infants received a higher energy intake than HM infants (121 kcal/kg/day versus 97 kcal/kg/day) despite a lower volume intake (Table 2). This discrepancy was increased by higher energy losses in stools in the HM group, almost totally owing to the fact that HM fat was not as well absorbed as the PF milk fat (67% and 89% absorption rate, respectively). As a conse-

TABLE 3. Energy, protein, and fat balance during Study 1[a]

	Energy (kcal/kg/day)		Protein (g/kg/day)		Fat (g/kg/day)	
	HM	PF	HM	PF	HM	PF
Intake	97	121	2.4	3.16	4.68	5.56
Losses	16.5	8.2	0.4	0.32	1.53	0.6
Oxidation	39.3	56.5	0.4	0.44	1.83	1.83
Accretion	41.2	56.3	1.5	2.4	1.32	3.13

[a] Preliminary results of four nutritional balances in the HM group and of six in the PF group.

quence, the amount of fat absorbed at that age was twice as much with PF (3.13 g/kg/day) as compared with HM (1.32 g/kg/day). The same amount of protein was oxidized in both groups (around 0.4 g/kg/day), but, as PF contained more proteins, the retention of protein was higher with PF (2.4 g/kg/day) than with HM (1.5 g/kg/day).

During study 2 the difference in energy intake between both groups lessened (123 kcal/kg/day for PF versus 114 kcal/kg/day for HM group). Energy losses in stools were similar (6.05 kcal/kg/day versus 5.6 kcal/kg/day, respectively) and almost entirely due to fat losses; however, at that postnatal age, the HM group achieved the same fat-absorption rate as the PF group (93% versus 91%). Protein retention was again higher with PF than with HM because of a higher intake.

In Fig. 2, these preliminary results on nutrient retention are expressed as daily increment (in grams per day) of weight, proteins, and lipids and compared with IU daily accretion of each nutrient calculated from Ziegler (11).

HM-fed preterm infants grew at the rate of 19.3 g/day and 29.3 g/day, respectively during studies 1 and 2. This is less than could be expected from the IU curve. However, the slope of the curve drawn between the two points is similar to that of the IU curve.

TABLE 4. Energy, protein, and fat balance during Study 2[a]

	Energy (kcal/kg/day)		Protein (g/kg/day)		Fat (g/kg/day)	
	HM	PF	HM	PF	HM	PF
Intake	114	123	2.41	3.17	5.9	5.45
Losses	5.6	6.05	0.38	0.55	0.4	0.5
Oxidation	50.7	60.53	0.53	0.57	2.8	1.87
Accretion	57.7	56.4	1.5	2.05	2.6	3.08

[a] Preliminary results of four nutritional balances in the HM group and of six in the PF group.

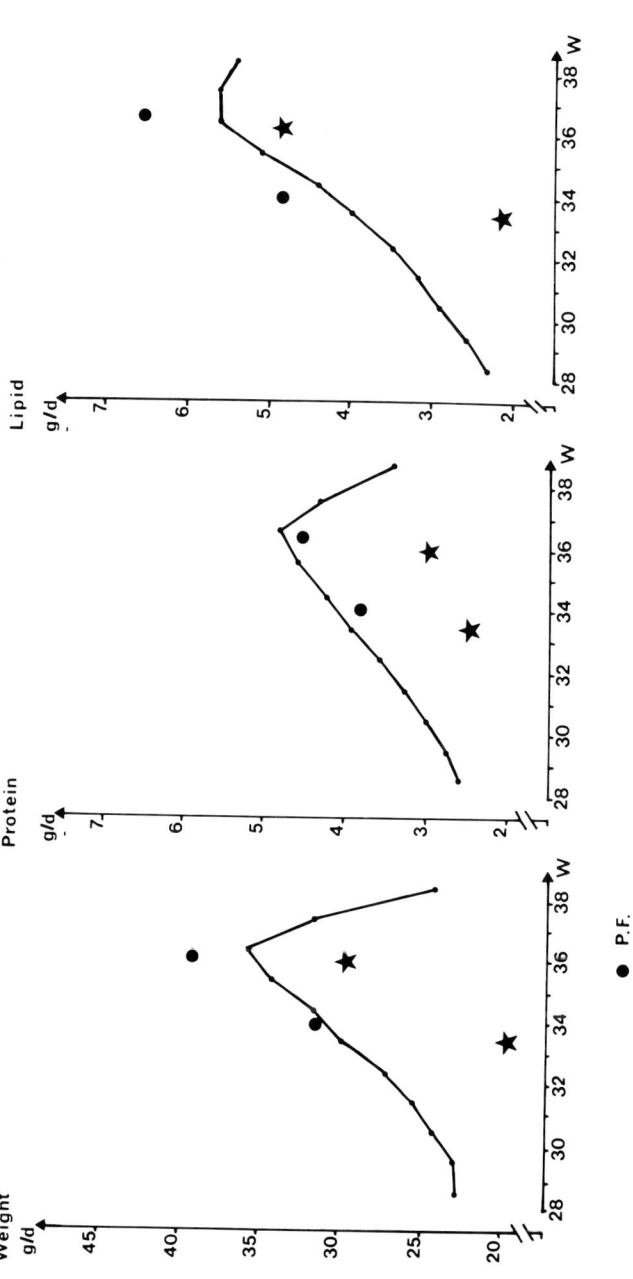

FIG. 2. Daily increment of weight, protein, and lipid during studies 1 and 2. The curve represents IU increment as calculated from Ziegler (11).

Protein retention was 2.34 g/day and 2.82 g/day, respectively during studies 1 and 2. It represented 12% and 9.6% of the weight gain, whereas a fetus of similar gestational age would have retained 13% and 14%, respectively, of his weight gain as protein. These data indicate that net protein retention was lower in the HM group when compared with the fetus. Fat accretion was calculated to be 2.06 g/day and 4.88 g/day during studies 1 and 2, respectively, and was much lower than the net amount which would have been deposited in the fetus, particularly at the time of the first study. However, the accretion rate which represented 10.6% (study 1) and 16% (study 2) of the weight gain correlated well with the IU fat deposition rate of 12% of the weight gain between weeks 28 and 32, and 19.8% between weeks 36 and 40.

As seen in Fig. 2, the results of the PF group are quite different; in this group, weight gain was 31.8 g/day and 39 g/day, protein retention 3.79 g/day and 4.5 g/day, and fat deposition 4.96 g/day during studies 1 and 2.

The net amount of protein retained was almost identical to the IU amount and represented 12% of the weight gain during both studies (vs. 12.2% and 13.9% for the fetus at the same gestational age). Fat accretion was higher than during fetal life, especially during the second study. It accounted for 15.5% and 17% of the weight gain for studies 1 and 2, respectively, as compared with 12% and 19.8% during fetal life at the same gestational age.

CONCLUSIONS

If we take the fetus growth as a model of growth (11), these preliminary data suggest that pooled, pasteurized human milk does not fulfill the criteria for an adequate growth with the volume intakes used in this study, its inadequacy being particularly marked when considering protein retention. However, Fig. 2 does not show a significant difference between the slopes of the two curves (IU growth curve and curve indicated by the two points obtained in our studies): there is no catching up in the interval between the two studies. PF gave a protein deposition similar to that obtained *in utero* (Fig. 2), but weight and fat retention were higher than for the fetus of the same gestational age. Therefore, at a postconceptional age of 42 weeks, these prematures would have a different body composition from the normal fullterm newborn.

A few recent studies have dealt with nutrient accretion and growth of the LBW infant, trying to evaluate the impact of nutrient intake on growth and body composition (1,5,6). They are difficult to compare since protein, energy intake, and protein/energy (P/E) ratio, as well as gestational age of the infants studied are different. For instance, by giving prematures (with a postconceptional age of 32.3 weeks) 148 kcal/kg/day of a formula, Reichman et al. (5) found a daily weight increment of 16.8 g/kg/day with a fat deposition of 5.4 g/kg/day, which is almost three times greater than in our HM group and two times greater than our PF group during study 1 (with corresponding gestational age). The same caloric intake would have needed 210 to 230 ml/kg/day of

HM (if we calculate an energy density of 65–70 kcal/100 ml of milk), an amount seldom given. In Reichman's study, protein deposition accounted for 1.9 g/kg/day versus 1.5 g for our HM group and 2.05 g for our PF group. The P/E ratio (10) was 2.1 g/100 kcal, both in Reichman's study and in our HM group, versus 2.6 in our PF group. This suggests that, at this particular time, too low a P/E ratio would require a high energy intake in order to fulfill "adequate" protein deposition (i.e., equal to that of the fetus) and would promote a higher amount of energy to be deposited as fat. Obviously, numerous factors need to be taken into account when comparing nutrient quality, and many more studies are necessary to give precise data on weight gain composition during extrauterine life and its long-term consequences.

REFERENCES

1. Brooke, O. G., Alvear, J., and Arnold, M. (1979): Energy expenditure and growth in healthy immature infants. *Pediatr. Res.*, 13:215–220.
2. Brooke, O., and Barley, J. (1978): Loss of energy during continuous infusions of breast milk. *Arch. Dis. Child.*, 53:344–348.
3. Jequier, E. (1980): Métabolisme énergétique. *Encycl. Méd. Chir. Paris Nutr.*, 10371, A 10.
4. Lubchenco, L. O., Hansman, C., Dressler, M., and Boyd, E. (1963): Intrauterine growth as estimated from liveborn birthweight data at 24 to 42 weeks of gestation. *Pediatrics*, 32:793–800.
5. Reichman, B., Chessex, P., Putet, G., Verellen, G., Smith, J. S., Heim, T., and Swyer, P. R. (1981): Diet, fat accretion and growth in premature infants. *N. Engl. J. Med.*, 305:1495–1500.
6. Sauer, P. J. J., Dance, H. J., Pearse, R. G., and Visser, H. K. A. (1981): Energy requirements for growth in the neonate. In: *Metabolic Adaptation to Extrauterine Life*, edited by R. de Meyer, pp. 191–207. Martinus Nijhoff, The Hague.
7. Senterre, J. (1976): *Alimentation optimale du prématuré*. Vaillant Carmanne S.A., Liège.
8. Swyer, P. R., Putet, G., Smith, J. M., and Heim, T. (1978): Energy metabolism and substrate utilisation during total parenterale nutrition in the newborn. In: *Intensive Care of the Newborn, II*, edited by L. Stern, W. Oh, and B. Friis-Hansen, pp. 307–316. Masson, N.Y.
9. Widdowson, E. M. (1968): *Biology of Gestation, Vol. 2*, edited by N. S. Assalied, pp. 1–49. Academic Press, N.Y.
10. Young, Y. R. (1981): Protein–energy interrelationships in the newborn: A brief consideration of some basic aspects. In: *Textbook of Gastroenterology and Nutrition in Infancy*, edited by E. Lebenthal. Raven Press, New York.
11. Ziegler, E. E., O'Donnell, A., Nelson, S. E., and Fomon, S. J. (1976): Body composition of the reference fetus. *Growth*, 40:329.

DISCUSSION

Dr. Räihä: I would first of all like to congratulate Guy Putet for this very nice study and the elegant way he has set up the balance studies, because this is not easy to do. My first question concerns the human milk group. It seems that the volume intake of human milk was very low, and as I will show in my paper, if you give preterm infants 170 ml of pooled human milk, you will probably not achieve optimal weight gain, which you can achieve only by giving over 185 ml, usually up to 200 ml. The second thing is that the value of 61 calories per deciliter of human milk is also very low—I think it has been reported in our studies to be about 68, and in some other studies over 70, calories per deciliter. Finally, I would like to ask if those length and head-circumference differences you found between the formula-fed and human-milk-fed infants were statistically significant. My final question is as follows: what did you do with the mother's own breast milk, or didn't any of these mothers give any of their own breast milk? We found that it is very difficult to define a study for preterm infants where we give only pooled human milk, because, at least in our country, most of the mothers of preterm infants bring their own milk, and we then feel obliged to give this milk to the infants.

Dr. Putet: The first question concerns the quantity of milk given. In our unit, we give around 180 ml/kg/day of HM, because we consider it an amount below which we usually have no abdominal problems (distensions, regurgitations, etc.). We recognize now that our pooled pasteurized milk does not suit all the nutritional needs, and, since then, we have modified quantitatively our HM. On the other hand, giving more than 180 ml/kg/day of PF leads to a growth rate which we judge to be unreasonably high. So we think that the intake should be adapted to the energy density of the milk.

The second question concerns the energy density of our HM. The latter has been calculated: knowing the amount of fat, carbohydrates, and protein by biochemical analyses, we apply the caloric value of each nutrient to obtain the total energetic value of the milk. Our low results can be explained by the fact that it is pooled pasteurized human milk which is transferred several times to different recipients (2).

The third question concerns length and head-circumference increments. There were no statistically significant differences between the two groups (preliminary data).

Finally, we agree that there could be a change in results if the infants received their own mothers' milk, especially if given fresh and untreated. However, and because of some contamination problems, we never give a premature baby his own mother's milk directly.

Dr. Rey: I would like to congratulate you for this very sophisticated study. I believe also that the limiting factor in your study with human milk is energy (available energy); you could probably obtain a better growth with a higher energy density human milk than the pooled human milk (61 kcal/100 ml) you have been using. It seems to me that the most striking finding is the increase in fat deposition in these premature babies after birth. My question is: What is the significance of this increase in fat? Probably, it is an adaptation to the extrauterine life, as other investigators have shown that subcutaneous fat increases dramatically when you remove the premature baby from the incubator. I think that one of the best questions is also: Why do humans deposit fat during gestation?

Dr. Putet: Apparently, during extrauterine life the premature infant behaves in the same way as a full-term newborn.

We all know that after birth and during the following 4 months, fat accounts for around 40% of the weight gain. In a study (7) on premature infants fed a formula at an energy intake level of 148 kcal/kg/day, fat was found to account for 32% of the weight gain from 30 to 35 weeks after conception; here, in the PF group fed 121 kcal/kg/day, by the same sort of calculation, we find that fat accounts for 18% of the weight gain, and, in both studies, the net amount of fat deposited is higher than during fetal life. So the postnatal changes in body composition found in both studies resemble the changes that normally take place in the full-term infant. The consequences of this change in body composition in relation to subsequent growth and development are not known.

Dr. Eeckels: It's beautiful to see what can be done with two groups of 6 babies. I was very impressed by the very high fat absorption of your formula-fed infants; what kind of fat did you have in the formula, and in what proportions?

Dr. Putet: The specially adapted formula utilized contains 3.4 g of fat/100 ml with 40% medium-chain triglycerides, 40% butter fat, and 20% vegetable oil.

Nutrition of the Low-Birth-Weight Infant

Niels C. R. Räihä

Department of Pediatrics, University of Lund, 214 01 Malmö, Sweden

There are three major considerations affecting the quantity and quality of protein to be given to a low-birth-weight baby. These are (a) requirements for normal growth and body composition, (b) development of protein and amino acid metabolism, and (c) renal function.

A number of different techniques have been used to estimate the requirements in adults, for example, nitrogen balance, body composition, amino acid turnover, fractional nitrogen excretion, and calorimetry. The application of these methods to the problem of determining the protein requirement of the small preterm infant is very difficult, because the optimal rate at which preterm infants *ex utero* should accumulate protein has yet to be determined.

The classical factorial method has been used to estimate protein requirements. The results suggest that the amount of protein in human milk and in many formulas designed for normal babies is inadequate (33). The calculations assume that the *in utero* growth rate remains optimal *ex utero* and that the body composition of the developing fetus is adequately known. Also, many empirical studies have shown that babies fed expressed human milk gain weight at a slower rate than those receiving a cow's milk-based formula (5,8,20,32). But the question remains, does this difference in weight gain have any advantage? Is the difference in weight gain due to a difference in protein intake or to other factors, for example, a lower energy content or a lower sodium content in human milk compared with cow's milk-based formulas.

In any case, it is not sufficient merely to estimate protein requirements on the basis of theoretical calculations from *in utero* accumulation rates or to administer large quantities of protein in order to attain intrauterine growth rates in the immediate extrauterine environment. The biochemical immaturity of the human preterm infant makes him nutritionally very vulnerable, and the margin between an adequate protein intake and protein undernutrition or overnutrition with possible adverse effects is small. There is an incomplete development of several amino acid metabolic pathways in the newborn infant, especially in the small preterm infant (22). Thus, many of the amino acids previously thought to be nonessential, for example, cysteine, taurine, may be essential, at least for the immature organism, and must be supplied in the diet. Also, amino acid catabolism is incomplete, and an administration of protein in quantities which exceed the needs for synthesis stress the infants metabolic machinery for disposing of excess nitrogen and results in hyperaminoacidemia, metabolic acidosis, and hyperammonemia. Recent reviews have been published (19–22). Few of the classic studies (5,8,17,20,32) which showed that preterm infants gained weight better with high-protein formulas than with human milk measured metabolic effects.

The proteins of human milk have been reviewed recently (4,7,12,16). The protein content of human milk is about 1.2 g/dl (1.8 g/100 kcal) when expressed as total nitrogen × 6.38 and 0.9 g/dl (1.3 g/100 kcal) when expressed as amino acid nitrogen × 6.38. Transitional human milk (6 to 10 days postpartum) contains 1.6 g/dl and colostrum (first 5 days postpartum) 2.3 g/dl. The milk of women delivering prematurely contains approximately 20% more nitrogen for the first 14 days of lactation than milk of mothers delivering at term (3,10,28), but not all studies show this (2,27). The whey proteins represent more than 70% of the total proteins in human milk, but less than 20% in cow's milk (12,16). β-Lactoglobulin is the main whey protein in cow's milk but is absent from human milk, which is rich in α-lactalbumin, lactoferrin, and immunoglobulins. The whey proteins used in some formulas are thus very different in composition from the whey proteins in human milk. Human milk from milk banks can be enriched with components of human milk such as fat or protein, etc. (human milk engineering), but further careful clinical evaluation is needed (11,18).

Most commercial formulas used for feeding healthy term infants have a caloric density of 67 kcal/dl and a protein content of 1.5 to 2.0 g/dl, thus containing 2.2 to 3.0 g protein/100 kcal. The major part of the protein is whey (whey/casein 60:40), but there are a number of "unadapted" cow's milk-based formulas available with a whey/casein ratio of 18:82.

Formulas specifically designed for low-birth-weight infants have a higher caloric density, usually from 75 to 81 kcal/dl, but also a somewhat higher protein content, from 1.8 to 2.4 g/dl, than the formulas generally used for term infants. These formulas thus contain about 2.2 to 3.2 g protein/100 kcal.

Despite its limitations, the factorial method of assessment provides a means to estimate these protein requirements. As discussed above, it provides no information on whether the amount provided by the diet can be absorbed or utilized after absorption. Intakes of 4.0 g/kg (3.1/100 kcal) for growth from 800 to 1200 g and 3.5 g/kg (2.7/100 kcal) for growth from 1200 to 1800 g have been suggested (33), but experimental evidence that they can be utilized is lacking.

Even if the protein content of breast milk is accepted as 1.2 g/dl (i.e., total nitrogen × 6.38), these advisable protein intakes could be achieved only with intakes of mature human milk around 300 ml/kg/day. Although such high intakes have been recorded (30), they are not common. The minimum intake of 2.25 g/kg/day recommended by the American Academy of Pediatrics' Committee on Nutrition (1) could, however, be achieved by feeding about 185 ml/kg/day. Intakes of 185 to 200 ml/kg/day are common practice, and there is new evidence showing that moderately-low-birth-weight babies (>1.5 kg) thrive and achieve an intrauterine rate of weight gain without signs of metabolic stress (6,14) on 185 ml of human milk/kg.

Two reports suggest that very-low-birth-weight babies (<1.5 kg) may benefit in terms of weight gain from preterm milk—presumably because of its somewhat higher protein content (9,21). This interesting finding requires confirmation and further evaluation. In the meantime, during the early weeks of life, when survival may be in doubt and when the "protective factors" in human milk may be of great value, clinical experience in some centers suggests that it is reasonable to accept the theoretically suboptimal protein content of breast milk. For this reason, it is acceptable to provide mature milk or, better, the mothers own preterm milk fed at 185 ml/kg/day or more when full volume intake can be accepted clinically. Perhaps any deficiencies of growth or body composition might be repaired after this critical period for survival is over (23,29). Recent studies have also shown better fat absorption and higher intraluminal bile acid concentration in preterm infants fed human milk as compared with formula-fed infants (13,15,31).

Formulas specially designed for low-birth-weight babies require thorough study and evaluation before routine use is justified, but the following guidelines may be helpful. There is today documented experience of feeding low-birth-weight babies (<1500 g) with formulas containing 1.5 g protein/dl (1.8 g/100 kcal) (30), and thus there is at present little justification for designing a formula for low-birth-weight babies which contains less protein than this. Since many low-birth-weight babies thrive on such formulas, it is suggested that the lower limit for protein content be set at 1.5 g/dl or 1.8 g/100 kcal; when fed at the level of 130 kcal/kg/day, it will provide 2.3 g/kg/day. If the upper estimate reached by the factorial method (33) of 4 g/kg/day is accepted, then at the level of 130 kcal/kg/day it implies a protein:energy ratio of 3.1 g/100 kcal. A number of formulas are available with such a protein:energy ratio, but detailed documented experience, particularly data on metabolic tolerance (e.g., plasma concentration of ammonia, amino acids, urea, hydrogen ion, urinary concentration) is very limited. One study found that an intake of 3.0 g/100 kcal compared with an intake of 2.3 g/100 kcal, (fed at 117 kcal/kg, i.e., 2.5–3.2 g/kg) did not lead to faster growth, but a quarter of the babies developed late metabolic acidosis (29). Formulas containing 3.0 g of protein/100 kcal (>2 g/dl) should be used with caution, particularly during the first week or so of life, until additional systematically recorded experience becomes available.

Formulas with protein content greater than this, for example, 3.8 g/100 kcal (3 g/dl/78 kcal, fed at 150 ml/kg, i.e., 117 kcal and 4.5 g protein/kg/day) are associated with high plasma concentrations of aromatic amino acid, ammonia and hydrogen ion, particularly if the protein is mainly casein (24,25). Although it is not established conclusively that such metabolic abnormalities are harmful, neither can it be said that they are safe. Formulas with a higher whey/casein ratio are associated with lower plasma aromatic amino acid concentration (26).

Formulas for low-birth-weight babies should contain predominantly whey protein. This will ensure an intake of cysteine at least equal to that of the breastfed baby. Babies who receive dietary taurine, for example, in breast milk or added to a formula, excrete taurine in the urine (25) and have a higher taurine to glycine ratio in their bile acids (14). Until there is evidence of definite clinical benefits, however, we have at present no justification for urging that formulas for low-birth-weight babies contain taurine. This is an area of active investigation which needs close observation.

REFERENCES

1. American Academy of Pediatrics' Committee on Nutrition. (1977): Nutritional needs of low-birth-weight infants. *Pediatrics,* 60:519-30.
2. Anderson, D., Pittard, W., Shulman, P., Mitman, F., Merkatz, R., and Kerr, D. (1981): Comparative nutrient composition of human milk. *Pediatr. Res.,* 15:525.
3. Atkinson, B. A., Bryan, M. H., and Andersson, G. H. (1978): Human milk: Difference in nitrogen concentration in milk from mothers of term and premature infants. *J. Pediatr.,* 93:67-69.
4. Bezkorovairy, A. (1977): Human milk and cholostrum proteins: A review. *J. Dairy Sci.,* 60:1023-1037.
5. Crosse, V. M., Hickmans, E. M., Haworth, B. E., and Aubrey, J. (1954): The value of human milk compared with other feeds for premature infants. *Arch. Dis. Child.,* 29:178.
6. Davies, D. P. (1977): Adequacy of expressed breast milk for early growth of preterm infants. *Arch. Dis. Child.,* 52:296.
7. George, E. D., and Lebenthal, E. (1981): Human breast milk in comparison to cow's milk. In: *Textbook of Gastroenterology and Nutrition in Infancy,* edited by E. Lebenthal, pp. 295-320. Raven Press, N.Y.
8. Gordon, H. H., Levine, S. Z., and McNamara, H. (1947): Feeding of premature infants: A comparison of human and cow's milk. *Am. J. Dis. Child.,* 73:442-452.
9. Gross, S. J. (1981): Growth and metabolic response of preterm infants fed preterm and mature breast milk. *Pediatr. Res.,* 15:533.
10. Gross, S. J., David, R. J., Bauman, L., and Tomarelli, R. M. (1980): Nutritional composition of milk produced by mothers delivering preterm. *J. Pediatr.,* 96:641-644.
11. Hagelberg, S., Lindblad, B. S., Lundsjö, A., Carlsson, B., Fonden, R., Fujita, H., Lassfolk, G., and Lindqvist, B. (1982): The protein tolerance of very low weight infants fed human milk protein enriched mother's milk. *Acta Paediatr. Scand.,* 71:597.
12. Hambraeus, L. (1977): Proprietary milk versus human breast milk in infant feeding. *Pediatr. Clin. North Am.,* 24:17-36.
13. Järvenpää, A.-L.: Feeding the low-birth-weight infant: IV. Fat absorption as a function of diet and duodenal bile acids. *Pediatrics (in press).*
14. Järvenpää, A.-L., Räihä, N. C. R., Rassin, D. K., and Gaull, G. E. (1983): Preterm infants fed human milk attain intrauterine weight gain. *Acta Paediatr. Scand.,* 72:239-243.
15. Järvenpää, A.-L., Rassin, D. K., Kuitunen, P., Gaull, G. E., and Räihä, N. C. R.: Feeding the low-birth-weight infant: III. Diet influences bile acid metabolism. *Pediatrics, (in press).*
16. Jenness, R. (1979): The composition of human milk. *Semin. Perinatol.,* 3:225-239.
17. Levin, B., Mackay, H. M. M., Neil, C. A., Oberholzer, V. G., and Whitehead, T. P. (1959): Weight gains, serum protein levels, and health of breast fed and artificially fed infants. *Spec. Rep. Ser. Med. Res. Coun.,* No. 296, p. 115. HMSO, London.
18. Lucas, A., Lucas, P. J., Chavin, S. I., Lyter, R. L. J., and Baum, J. D. (1980): A human milk formula. *Early Hum. Dev.,* 4(1):15-18.
19. Malloy, M. H., and Gaull, G. E. (1979): Enteral protein and amino acid nutrition in preterm infants. *Semin. Perinatol.,* 3:315-320.
20. Omans, W. B., Barness, L. A., Rose, C. S., and György, P. (1961): Prolonged feeding studies in premature infants. *J. Pediatr.,* 59:951-957.

21. Pearce, J. L., and Buchanan, L. F. (1979): Breast milk and breast feeding in very low-birth-weight infants. *Arch. Dis. Child.,* 54:897–899.
22. Räihä, N. C. R. (1980): Protein in the nutrition of the preterm infant. Biochemical and nutritional considerations. *Adv. Nutr. Res.,* 3:173–206.
23. Räihä, N. C. R. (1981): Handicaps of amino acid metabolism and optimal protein nutrition of preterm infants. In: *Physiological and Biochemical Basis of Perinatal Medicine,* edited by M. Monset-Couchard and A. Minkowski, pp. 79–89. S. Karger, Basel.
24. Räihä, N. C. R., Heinonen, K., Rassin, D. K., and Gaull, G. E. (1976): Milk protein quality and quantity in low-birth-weight infants: I. Metabolic responses and effects on growth. *Pediatrics,* 57:659–674.
25. Rassin, D. K., Gaull, G. E., Järvenpää, A.-L., and Räihä, N. C. R. (1983): Feeding the low birth weight infant: II. Effects of taurine and cholesterol supplementation on amino acids and cholesterol. *Pediatrics,* 71:179–186.
26. Rassin, D. K., Gaull, G. E., Räihä, N. C. R., and Heinonen, K. (1977): Milk protein quantity and quality in low-birth-weight infants. IV. Effects on tyrosine and phenylalanine in plasma and urine. *J. Pediatr.,* 90:356–360.
27. Sann, L., Bienven, J., Bienven, F., Lahet, C., and Bethenod, M. (1981): Comparison of the composition of breast milk from mothers of term and preterm infants. *Acta Paediatr. Scand.,* 70:115–116.
28. Schander, R. J., and Oh, W. (1980): Composition of breast milk obtained from mothers of premature infants as compared to milk obtained from donors. *J. Pediatr.,* 96:679–681.
29. Svenningsen, N. W., Lindroth, M., and Lindquist, B. (1982): Growth in relation to protein intake of low birth weight infants. *Early Hum. Dev.,* 6:47–58.
30. Valman, H. B., Brown, R. J. K., Palmer, T., Oberholzer, V. G., and Levin, B. (1971): Protein intake and plasma amino acids of infants of low birth weight. *Br. Med. J.,* 4:789–791.
31. Watkins, J. B., Järvenpää, A.-L., Szczepanik Van-Leeuven, P., Klein, P. D., Rassin, D. K., Gaull, G., and Räihä, N. C. R. Feeding the low-birth-weight infant: V. Effects of human milk, taurine and cholesterol on bile acid kinetics. *Gastroenterology (in press).*
32. Young, W. F., Poynet-Wale, P., Hymphreys, H., Finch, E., and Broadbent, I. (1950): Protein requirements in infants. 3. The nutrition of premature infants. *Arch. Dis. Child.,* 25:31–51.
33. Ziegler, E. E., Biga, R. L., and Fomon, S. J. (1981): Nutritional requirements of premature infants. In: *Pediatric Nutrition,* edited by R. M. Suskind, pp. 29–39. Raven Press, N.Y.

DISCUSSION

Dr. Koldovský: When you increase the volume from 170 ml to 185 ml, which is about 10%, the weight gain increases from 12.8 g to 15.1 g, so that by giving 10% more you actually get a 20% better weight gain. What could be the explanation?

Dr. Räihä: We are increasing the intake of electrolytes, the caloric intake, and the protein intake, so I cannot really answer your question. There is, however, a definite difference in the rate of weight gain, and with the high volumes, the weight gain is close to, if not identical with, the IU weight gain.

Dr. Rey: The maintenance energy requirement of a human or of an animal is the energy expenditure without growth. If you increase the energy intake above the maintenance requirement, you increase the weight proportionately to the energy available for growth, so there is nothing surprising at all in finding that a 10% increase in energy intake results in 20% or 30% or more weight increase.

Dr. Hagelberg: As you pointed out at the beginning, the preterm milk contains more protein than term milk, and that seems good because the preterm infants need more protein. However, it might be interesting to know what kind of protein is increased in the preterm milk, because if it is secretory IgA, for example, it is not very interesting from a nutritional point of view, since it is not absorbed in the gut.

Dr. Räihä: There is good evidence that it is partly secretory IgA. In fact, the difference in the protein concentration lasts a very short time—only 2 to 3 weeks—and I don't think it has much nutritional importance on a long-term basis.

Dr. Hagelberg: It has been postulated that the preterm milk is a sort of prolonged colostrum, and it seems, therefore, logical to assume that IgA is increased. Did you see any adverse effects of increasing the volume up to 200 ml/kg?

Dr. Räihä: Yes, I am aware of the work by Oh and others who experienced clinical problems with high volumes. The volume of 200 ml/kg/day is, of course, high, but we did not see any adverse effects in our infants.

Dr. Gamarra: What do you recommend to give to very-low-birth-weight premature infants, less than 32 weeks old, for whom the intake of water must be limited because of respiratory distress?

Dr. Räihä: All the cases that we have studied were preterm infants that we were able to feed enterally. On the basis of our results, I cannot answer your question. I would think, however, that in a case of severe respiratory distress when the baby weighs, say, 1,200 g and is on a respirator, we would keep the baby on a very-low-volume intake during the first few days. We give the baby fresh breast milk in very small volumes— 1 to 5 ml/hr—and then supplement it with intravenous feeding: glucose, sometimes amino acids if the intravenous feeding has to be prolonged for more than 5 or 6 days. We hardly ever use Intralipid®, and we don't worry too much about the caloric intake during those first days when the infant is very sick. We try to increase the volume of breast milk, and in our experience, it is not impossible to maintain some breast milk intake even in babies who are on the respirator. This may be due to the fact that the emptying of the stomach is much faster with human milk than with formula, for instance. I don't think we should push those babies, nor should we try to give them optimal caloric and amino acid amounts, because this is also a source of metabolic stress. The albumin always goes down in preterm infants on human milk. We let it go down, and it will eventually rise within some weeks. This is the usual trend. Of course, there is a possibility that lower serum albumin levels may even be beneficial for the kidney function and glomerular filtration rate.

Dr. Eeckels: I just wanted to ask you how low the lowest safe figure is for albumin in the premature infant?

Dr. Räihä: We have seen some preterm infants at around the 4th to 6th week, with serum albumin as low as 30 g/liter. Very few of those infants show edema or any clinical signs of being ill. We just follow them, and then they begin to improve. This was shown by Crosse many years ago and may be of physiological significance. I think we are getting back to the fact that the preterm infant is a special biological entity. We don't really know what is normal and what is abnormal, and I don't think we should try to bring them up to IU standards of weight gain or even of amino acid levels.

Nutritional Adaptation of the Gastrointestinal Tract of the Newborn, edited by N. Kretchmer and A. Minkowski. Nestlé, Vevey/Raven Press, New York © 1983.

Parenteral Nutrition in the Very-Low-Birth-Weight Infant

J. Rigo and J. Senterre

Department of Paediatrics, State University of Liege, Bavière Hospital, B-4020 Liège, Belgium

In preterm infants an optimal nutritional supply must be provided early during the neonatal period. Indeed, undernutrition leads to growth retardation which may be hazardous for brain development (18). Growth rate is maximum during the last trimester of gestation and corresponds to about 60 cm/year (19). Therefore, contrary to young children, preterm infants after an arrest of growth, whatever the cause, cannot achieve a complete return to normal growth. This fact is clearly illustrated by the follow-up of very-small-for-gestational age infants in spite of a high protein, mineral, and energy intake. Oral nutrition alone cannot maintain adequate growth in very-low-birth-weight (VLBW) infants because of their poor clinical condition and the immaturity of their gastrointestinal tract. Total or supplemental parenteral nutrition has been shown to improve the neonatal growth of VLBW infants by enhancing their caloric and nitrogen supply (4,24). In this chapter, we shall present some guidelines about nitrogen, amino acid, energy, and mineral intakes for infants on total parenteral nutrition (TPN).

NITROGEN REQUIREMENT AND AMINO ACID METABOLISM

Nitrogen requirement of VLBW infants on TPN may be estimated by nitrogen balance studies. Nitrogen retention depends upon nitrogen intake and energy available for growth (25,29). A nitrogen retention of about 300 mg/kg/day, similar to that *in utero* (Fig. 1), can be obtained with a supply of 450 mg nitrogen or 3.1 g amino acids/kg/day provided that the energy supply is adequate.

However, such a high intake may impose a metabolic stress because of the immaturity of several enzymatic pathways and the amino acid imbalance in the parenteral solution. In a previous study, we analyzed the factors influencing the serum amino acid concentration in 163 LBW infants fed either parenterally ($N = 54$) or orally with human milk or adapted formulas ($N = 109$). We reported that threonine metabolism is reduced in preterm infants (Fig. 2) probably because of the low activity of the serine threonine dehydratase, the principal enzyme involved in the threonine metabolism (23).

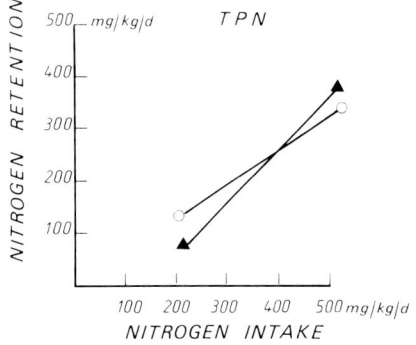

FIG. 1. Relationship between nitrogen retention and nitrogen intake in VLBW infants. Circles, Zlotkin et al. (29) ($r = 0.91$, $N = 18$); triangles, this study ($r = 0.92$, $N = 20$). $y = 1.03x - 152$; $r = 0.92$, $p < 0.001$.

The metabolism of aromatic amino acids is also impaired in preterm infants (22). In our study, for a similar intake, serum phenylalanine concentration was higher in infants fed parenterally than in those fed orally (Fig. 3). This might be due to the bypass of the portal circulation during parenteral nutrition and possibly also to a decrease of enzymatic activities in the liver. In parenteral nutrition, tyrosine intake is very low because of its poor solubility. Neverthe-

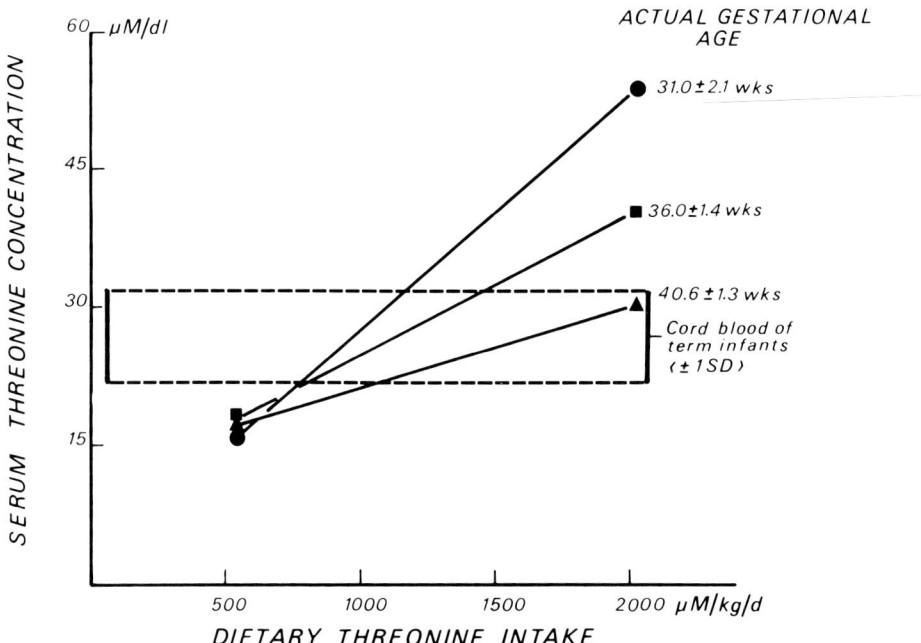

FIG. 2. Influence of the actual gestational age on the relationship between the serum threonine concentration and the intake in LBW infants fed orally or on TPN. $z = 0.017x$ (intake) $- 0.66y$ (AGA) $+ 29.67$, $r = 0.66$, $p_x < 0.001$, $p_y < 0.001$.

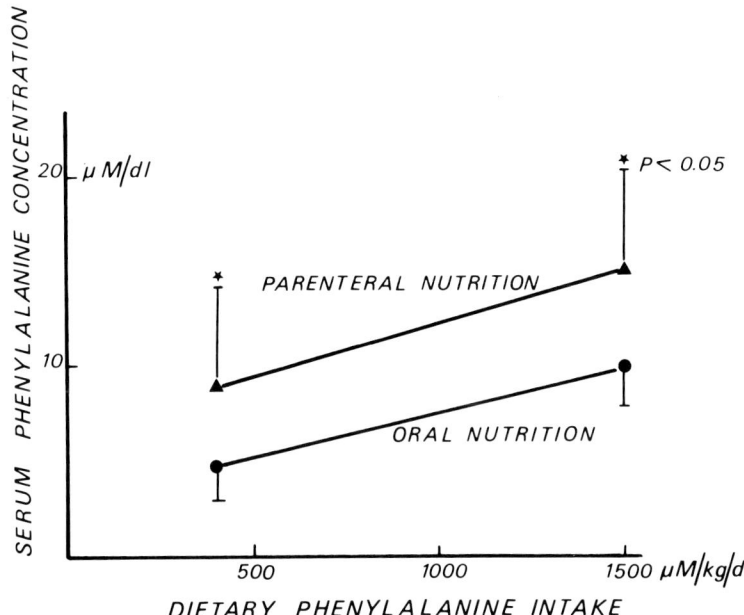

FIG. 3. Influence of the mode of administration on the relationship between serum phenylalanine concentration and phenylalanine intake in LBW infants fed orally (*circles*) or parenterally (*triangles*). Orally: $y = 0.0046x + 2.93$, $r = 0.31$, $p < 0.01$, $N = 109$. Parenterally: $y = 0.0056x + 6.78$, $r = 0.26$, $p = 0.07$, $N = 54$. Difference between levels: $p < 0.05$.

less, the serum levels of tyrosine are similar in preterm infants fed parenterally and in those fed orally (Fig. 4). Therefore, the phenylalanine hydroxylase activity seems to be satisfactory, and tyrosine must be considered as a semiessential rather than as an essential amino acid even in preterm infants. Similar conclusions have been drawn by others (10,16).

By contrast, Zlotkin and coworkers (27) and Anderson and coworkers (1) observed normal phenylalanine and low tyrosine serum concentrations in preterm infants with similar aromatic amino acid intakes (Table 1). The high branched-chain amino acids, in particular, the high leucine concentration in their parenteral solution, might be responsible for the low serum aromatic amino acid concentration. Indeed, experiences with parenteral nutrition in patients with hepatic failure have shown that high branched-chain amino acid intakes can decrease the serum level of aromatic amino acids (6). However, further studies are necessary to confirm this hypothesis.

In preterm infants, sulfur amino acid metabolism is impaired because of the low cystathionase and cystein sulfinic acid decarboxylase activities (9). In parenteral nutrition, cystine supply is low because of its poor solubility. In our study the increase in serum methionine concentration was less marked in parenteral than in oral nutrition (Fig. 5). Serum cystine concentration was

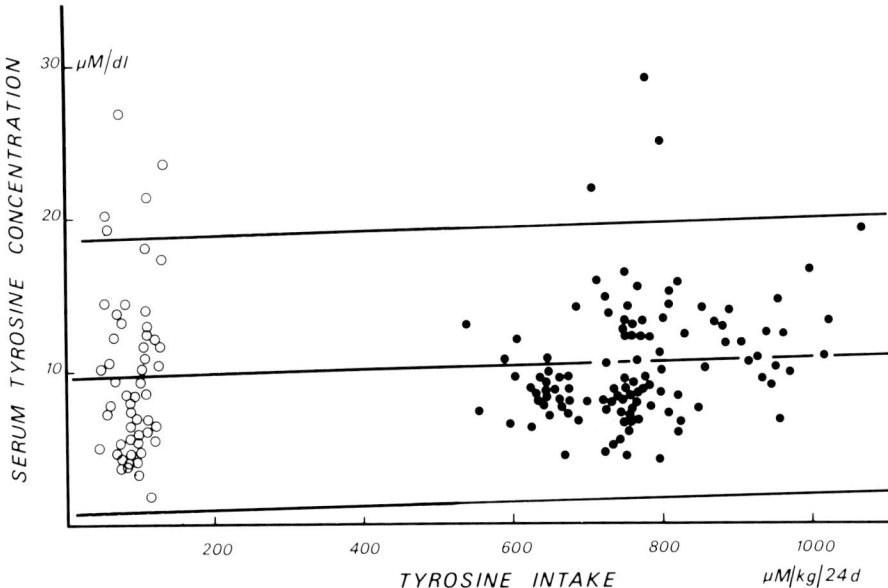

FIG. 4. Absence of relationship between serum tyrosine concentration and tyrosine intake in LBW infants fed orally (*closed circles*) or parenterally (*open circles*). $y = 0.0012x + 9.68$, $r = 0.09$, $p > 0.05$, $N = 163$.

related to the serum methionine concentration (Fig. 6). However, at low serum methionine concentration (2 μmoles/dl), cystine level was lower in parenteral than in oral nutrition. By contrast, when serum methionine level was high (6 μmoles/dl), serum concentration of cystine was similar in both groups. In addition, serum cystine concentration also increased according to actual gestational age (Fig. 7). These observations were confirmed by recent studies of Zlotkin and collaborators (27,28). In LBW infants on TPN supplemented with cystein, they observed an increase of the plasma cystine concentration without

TABLE 1. *Aromatic amino acid intake (μmoles/kg/day) and serum amino acid concentration (μmoles/kg/dl) in LBW infants on TPN*

	Ghadimi (10) Jones (16)	Zlotkin et al. (29) Anderson et al. (1)
Phenylalanine		
Intake	423–910	500–1100
Serum concentration	8–15	5–7
Tyrosine		
Intake	25–60	70–140
Serum concentration	7–12	2–4

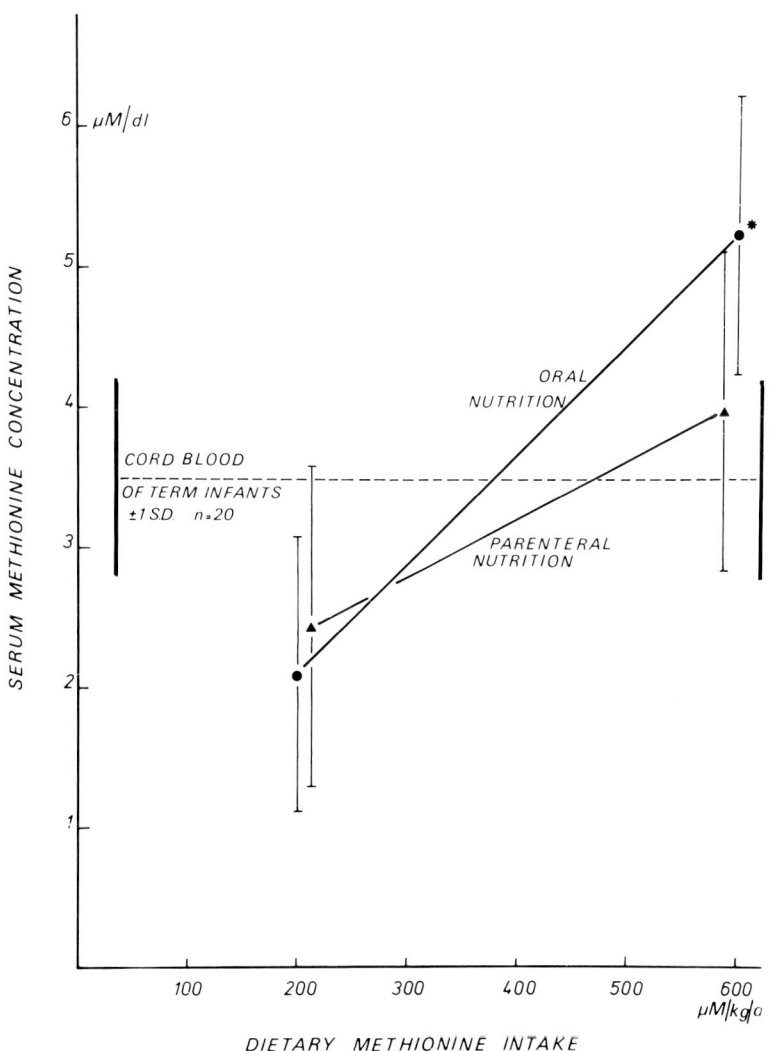

FIG. 5. Relationship between serum methionine concentration and intake in LBW infants fed orally (*circles*) or parenterally (*triangles*). Orally: $y = 0.0078x + 0.54$, $r = 0.69$, $p < 0.001$, $N = 109$. Parenterally: $y = 0.0041x + 1.56$, $r = 0.36$, $p < 0.05$, $N = 54$. Slope difference $p < 0.05$.

any change in nitrogen retention or in growth. They also reported a significant activity of cystathionase in the liver, the adrenal glands, and the kidney of preterm infants. These studies and our observations suggest that the cystathionase activity is sufficient to maintain an adequate level of cystine even in the most premature infants, provided the methionine supply is sufficient.

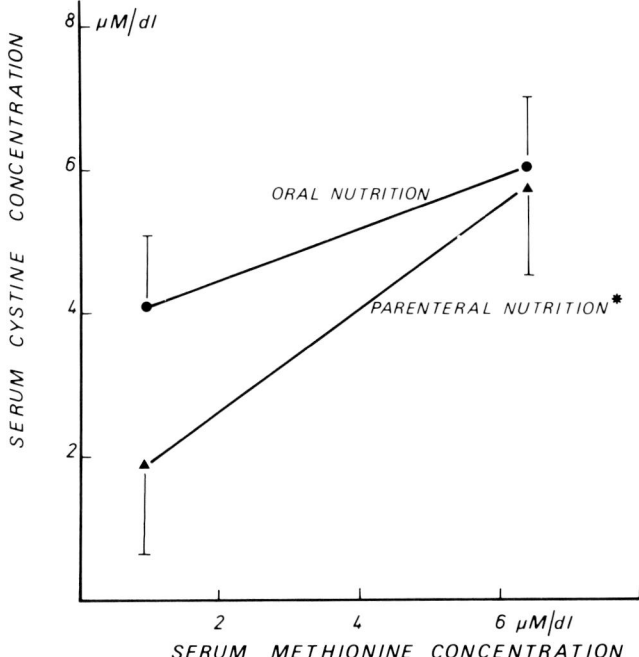

FIG. 6. Relationship between serum cystine concentration and serum methionine concentration in LBW infants fed orally (*circles*) or parenterally (*triangles*). Orally: $y = 0.36x + 3.77$, $r = 0.45$, $p < 0.001$, $N = 109$. Parenterally: $y = 0.712x + 1.22$, $r = 0.57$, $p < 0.001$, $N = 54$. Slope difference $p < 0.05$.

Therefore, cystine must be considered as a semiessential amino acid rather than an essential one.

The serum branched-chain amino acid levels increased with the intake in LBW infants fed orally and parenterally. However, branched-chain amino acid metabolism was higher in preterm than in full-term infants. Indeed, as shown in Fig. 8 for valine, for a similar intake, the serum concentration was lower in the preterm than in the full-term infants.

INNOCUOUS SERUM AMINO ACID CONCENTRATION IN PRETERM INFANTS

Serum amino acid concentration in the cord blood is stable during the last trimester of gestation (12). It is not influenced by conditions of delivery (vaginal or cesarean section) (21); it is similar to the values determined by umbilical venous puncture by MacIntoch and collaborators in 10 fetuses (20) and reflects the fetal amino acid level. During gestation, serum amino acid concentration in the fetus is elevated. They provide nutrients for growth and are regulated

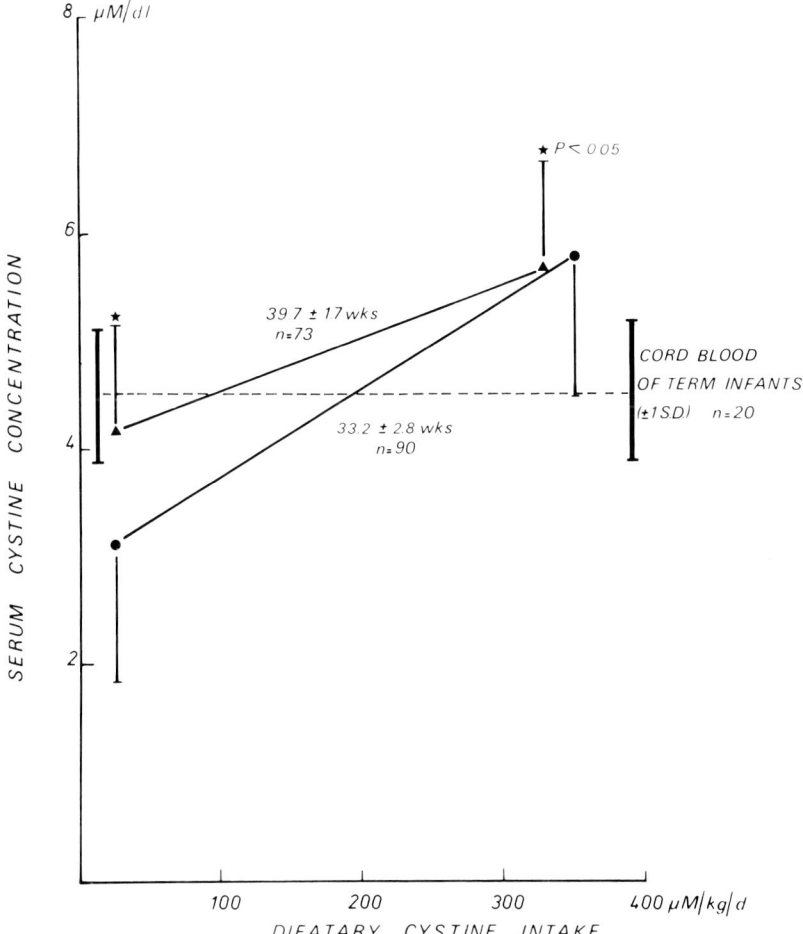

FIG. 7. Influence of gestational age on the relationship between serum cystine concentration and intake in LBW infants. $z = 0.0064x$ (intake) $+ 0.084y$ (AGA) $+ 0.40$; $r = 0.58$; $N = 163$; $p_x < 0.001$; $p_y < 0.01$.

by the transplacental exchanges. The normal serum level of aromatic amino acids at birth in phenylketonuric infants of healthy mothers clearly demonstrates this fact (15).

The high serum amino acid concentrations in the fetus may be related to its high rate of growth. Indeed, in tissue culture, there is a relationship between the nitrogen uptake and the amino acid concentration in the culture medium. Consequently, it can reasonably be assumed that a blood amino acid concentration similar to that *in utero* is innocuous for the preterm infant and is, perhaps, a good condition to promote growth and brain development.

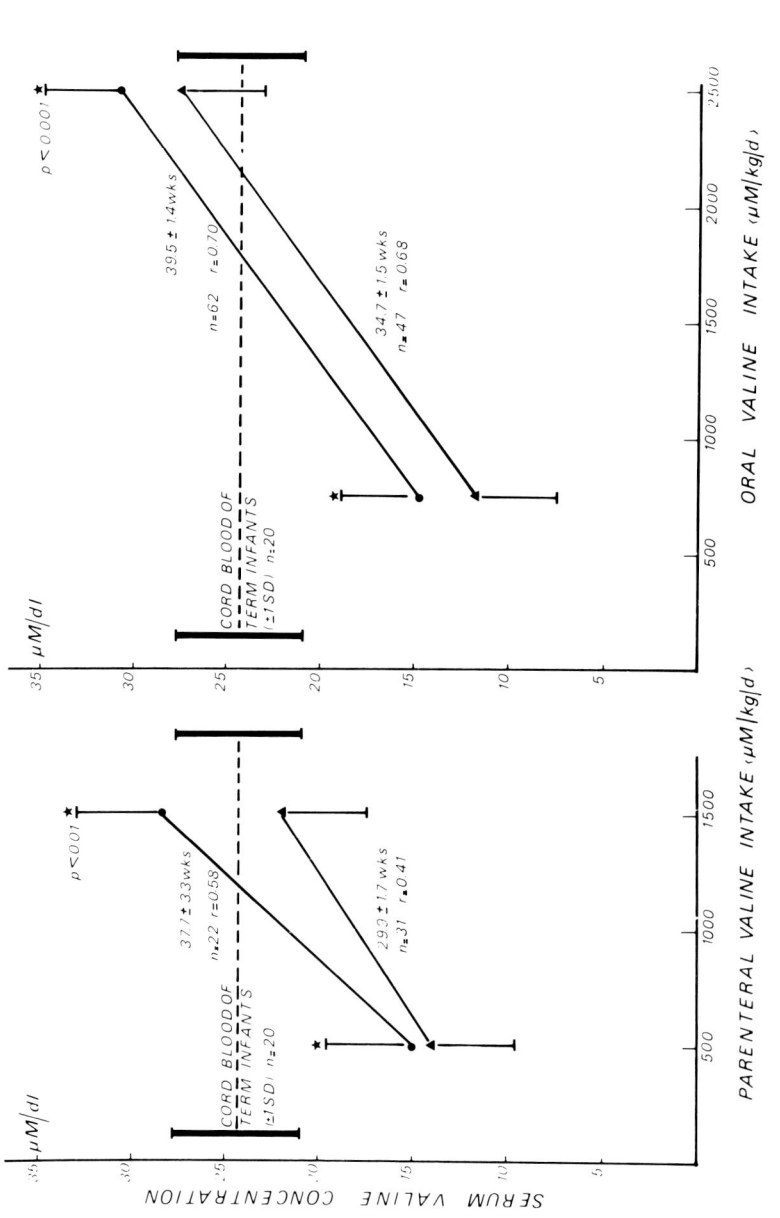

FIG. 8. Influence of gestational age on the relationship between serum valine concentration and intake in LBW infants fed orally **(right)** or parenterally **(left)**. *Orally:* $z = 0.0088x$ (intake) $+ 0.43y$ (AGA) $- 8.88$, $r = 0.67$, $N = 109$, $p_x < 0.001$, $p_y < 0.01$. *Parenterally:* $z = 0.0098x$ (intake) $+ 0.42y$ (AGA) $- 3.93$, $r = 0.56$, $N = 54$, $p_x < 0.001$, $p_y < 0.01$.

OPTIMAL AMINO ACID INTAKE IN PRETERM INFANTS ON PARENTERAL NUTRITION

In preterm infants, the amino acid intake must be sufficient to fulfill nitrogen requirements and to assure growth without overload in amino acids and nitrogen metabolites. By multivariate analysis of our data, we have calculated the amount of each amino acid necessary to obtain a serum concentration similar to that of the fetus *in utero* (Table 2). These amounts are similar in oral and in parenteral nutrition except for phenylalanine.

The total intake corresponds to 3.1 g of amino acids or 480 mg of nitrogen per kilogram body weight per day with one-half as essential amino acids. These values are in agreement with the results of nitrogen balance studies carried out in preterm infants on oral or parenteral nutrition (25,29). However, it appears that the amino acid composition of parenteral solutions is not fully adapted for preterm infants. In particular, these solutions are generally too rich in threonine and aromatic amino acids, and deficient in branched-chain amino acids, lysine, and taurine. Therefore we believe that solutions with better balanced amino acid composition must be developed to promote growth and brain development without overloading the enzymatic systems of the immature infant.

ENERGY REQUIREMENTS IN PRETERM INFANTS ON TPN

VLBW infants need a high caloric intake (13). The energy necessary for basal metabolism, thermoregulation, and muscular activity corresponds to

TABLE 2. *Optimal amino acid intake in preterm infants*

Amino acids	µmoles/kg/day	mg/kg/day
Threonine	970	115
Leucine	2375	311
Isoleucine	1235	162
Valine	2315	271
Methionine	377	56
Phenylalanine orally	750	124
TPN	400	66
Lysine	2925	427
Histidine	750	116
Tryptophane	245	50
Tyrosine orally	400	72
TPN	150	27
Cystine	244	59
Taurine	140	19
TEAA	11942	1632
TAA	24879	3100
TEAA/TAA	0.48	0.53

about 70 kcal/kilo body weight/day, whereas the total energy requirement for growth, synthesis, and storage represents about 45 kcal/kg or 3 kcal/g of body weight gain. In parenteral nutrition, fecal and urinary losses of energy are generally low. Therefore, the total energy requirement can be estimated at about 100 to 120 kcal/kg/day. This requirement can be met by fats and carbohydrates.

Fat solutions provide the essential fatty acids necessary for growth. Intralipid®, the most widely used parenteral fat solution, contains 54% of linoleic acid and it must be utilized with caution.

VLBW infants do not seem able to clear more than 2 g of lipids/kg/day. Indeed, it has been reported that lipid serum concentration increases with the intake and that hyperlipemia may be induced by an intake of less than 3 g/kg/day (5).

Griffin and co-workers (11) have reported an increase in the plasma concentration of free cholesterol, phospholipid, and lipoprotein X during continuous Intralipid® infusion. According to these authors, 50% of the increase of plasma free cholesterol derives from endogenous sources, whereas the hyperphospholipemia is attributed to the lipid concentration. The exact process responsible for the lipoprotein X formation is not clearly established. Calorimetric studies (13) have shown that endogenous fat oxydation decreases with the caloric intake. In preterm infants at 70 kcal/kg/day, endogenous fat oxydation is null on parenteral nutrition with amino acids, glucose, and fat. With a caloric intake over 80 kcal, the percentage of energy derived from fat oxydation does not reach more than 30% regardless of the fat intake. It has been calculated that preterm infants do not metabolize more than 2 to 3 g of Intralipid®/kg/day and that too much intake leads to tissue deposition.

Studies of body fat composition (2,8) have shown an increase in the relative linoleate content and a decrease in the relative arachidonate content. These modifications may lead to prostaglandin deficiency (2), to pulmonary and reticuloendothelial dysfunctions (7), and to potential changes in myelin configuration and function (3). We therefore prefer to limit the lipid intake to 2 g or 20 kcal/kg/day until additional information is available.

Most of the calories therefore must be provided by carbohydrates. However, particularly during the first weeks of life, high glucose infusion leads to hyperglycemia. Fructose, which is present in some parenteral amino acid solutions, may have theoretical advantages because of its rapid utilization and its lack of dependence on insulin for its metabolism. However, acute infusion may lead to acidosis, depletion of ATP, hyperuricemia, and hyperuricosuria. Therefore, fructose utilization in parenteral nutrition for LBW infants is still controversial (26).

We have analyzed the effect of carbohydrate tolerance in VLBW infants under 1,500 g (body weight: 1,186 ± 196 g; length: 37.8 ± 2.7 cm; gestational age: 30.2 ± 2.4 weeks). The infants parenterally received amino acids, fats, and carbohydrates (either glucose alone, or $2/3$ glucose and $1/3$ fructose). In

infants fed on TPN with glucose alone, the serum glucose concentration increased with the intake (Fig. 9). However the slope of the regression line was significantly higher during the first 10 days of life than thereafter. The relationship between serum insulin concentration and serum glucose level was similar during both periods. Thus hyperglycemia during the first days of life seems to be due more to a peripheral resistance to insulin than to a relative lack of insulin secretion.

During the first 10 days of life (Fig. 10), the slope of the regression line was significantly lower in infants receiving a glucose–fructose solution than in those fed on glucose alone. Nevertheless, the relationship between serum insulin concentration and glucose level was similar in the two groups. After 10 days of life, glucose tolerance was higher and no further difference was observed between the two groups. No adverse effects such as acidosis or an increase of uric acid excretion were observed during fructose infusion. The serum fructose concentration averaged 15 mg/dl and was always below 30 mg/dl.

Therefore, during the first days of life, a supply of 25% of carbohydrate such as fructose could be used for increasing the caloric intake.

MINERAL REQUIREMENTS

Rickets has been reported in preterm infants on TPN. Adequate mineral supply is sometimes difficult to provide because of the precipitation of calcium phosphate (14,17). In our parenteral solution prepared at the pharmacy of the hospital, calcium gluconate was added to the amino acid solution. The calcium seems to be chelated to the amino acids. This solution was then diluted with glucose and electrolyte solutions. Finally, phosphorus was added as Sörensen buffer. The parenteral solution contains 33 mg of calcium, 30 mg of phosphorus, and 3.3 mg of magnesium per 100 ml. Under these conditions, a positive retention can be obtained (Table 3) and rickets may be prevented, provided vitamin D is given.

CONCLUSION

Adequate nutrition in VLBW infants is frequently difficult to achieve because of their clinical condition and the immaturity of the gastrointestinal tract. Total or supplemental parenteral nutrition is necessary to avoid undernutrition and to promote growth of VLBW infants. Satisfactory growth and nitrogen retention can be obtained on an energy intake of 100 to 120 kcal/kg body weight/day and a nitrogen intake of 400 to 450 mg or about 3 g of amino acid/kilo body weight/day. However VLBW infants are particularly vulnerable to high amino acid intakes because of the immaturity of some enzymatic pathways; new solutions with a better amino acid balance should therefore be developed. Fat intake must be limited to 2 g/kg body weight/day in order to avoid hyperlipemia and its possible toxic effects. Most of the energy intake

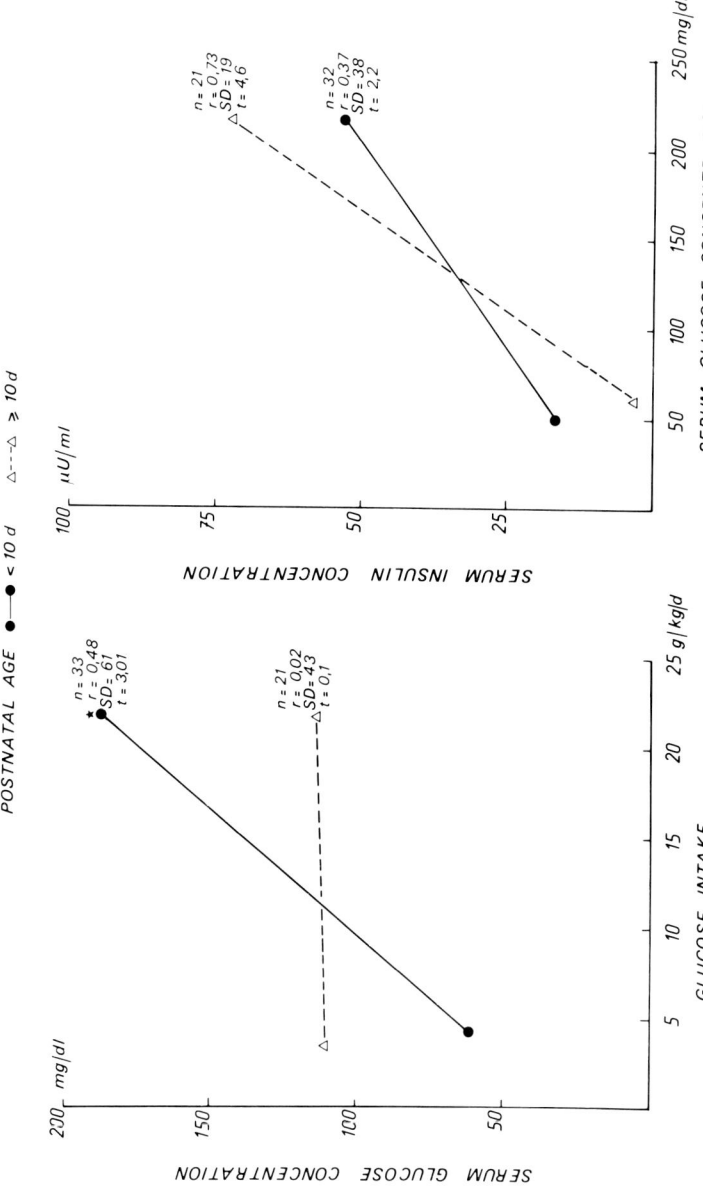

FIG. 9. Influence of postnatal age on the relationship between serum glucose concentration and glucose intake (**left**) and serum insulin concentration and serum glucose concentration (**right**) in VLBW infants fed parenterally (BW < 1,500 g). z (glycemia) = 0.0043x (intake) − 3.61y (postnatal age) + 97.24, r = 0.46, t = 2.68, N = 55, p_x < 0.01, p_y < 0.01. z (insulinemia) = 0.33x (glycemia) − 0.16y (postnatal age) − 5.69, r = 0.45, t = 2.54, N = 53, p_x < 0.01, p_y < 0.05.

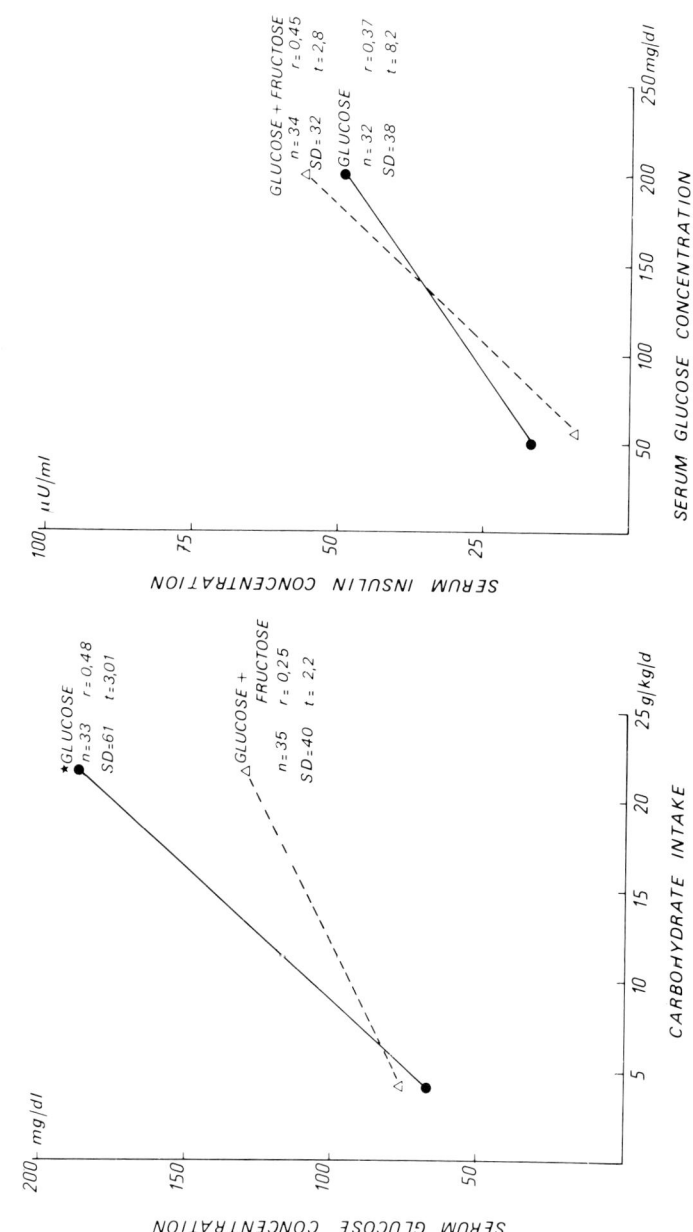

FIG. 10. Relationship between serum glucose concentration and carbohydrate intake (**left**) and between serum insulin concentration and serum glucose concentration (**right**) in VLBW infants (BW < 1,500 g) on parenteral nutrition with glucose (*circles*) or glucose and fructose (*triangles*) during the first 10 days of life. **Left:** *Glucose:* $y = 0.0068x + 39.16$, $r = 0.48$, $p < 0.01$, $N = 33$. *Glucose + fructose:* $y = 0.0031x + 63.17$, $r = 0.35$, $p < 0.05$, $N = 35$. Difference of level $p < 0.05$. **Right:** *Glucose:* $y = 0.22x + 5.71$, $r = 0.37$, $p < 0.05$, $N = 32$. *Glucose + fructose:* $y = 0.37x - 12.08$, $r = 0.45$, $p < 0.01$; $N = 34$.

TABLE 3. *Calcium, magnesium, and phosphorus retention in LBW infants on TPN (mg/kg/day)*

	Calcium (N = 18)	Magnesium (N = 19)	Phosphorus (N = 18)
Intake	48 ± 17	3.6 ± 1.4	30 ± 11
Urinary excretion	5 ± 5	1.1 ± 0.9	10 ± 9
Retention	42 ± 16	2.6 ± 1.6	20 ± 15

should be derived from carbohydrates, essentially glucose. During the first week of life, glucose tolerance is limited and some fructose might be helpful as a substitute. It is also necessary to provide sufficient calcium, phosphorus, and magnesium in order to achieve a positive mineral retention.

Nevertheless, several problems remain to be resolved. Among these, we shall mention the need to achieve an optimal intake of trace elements and vitamins in long-term parenteral nutrition. The factors responsible for liver cholestasis must be studied. Last but not least, follow-up studies are needed to show if better neurological development can be achieved by improving nutrition during the neonatal period.

REFERENCES

1. Anderson, T. L., Muttart, C. R., Bieber, M. A., Nicholson, J. F., and Heird, W. C. (1979): A controlled trial of glucose versus glucose and amino acids in premature infants. *Pediatrics,* 94:947.
2. Ballabriga, A. (1979): Parenteral nutrition of the newborn and infant. In: *Nutrition and Metabolism of the Foetus and Infants,* edited by H. K. A. Visser, p. 402. M. Nijhoff, The Hague, Boston, London.
3. Bryan, H., Shennan, A., Griffin, E., and Angel, A. (1978): Intralipid®: Its rational use in parenteral nutrition of the newborn. *Pediatrics,* 58:787.
4. Driscoll, J. M., Jr., Heird, W. C., Schullinger, J. N., Gongaware, R. D., and Winters, R. W. (1972): Total intravenous alimentation in low-birth-weight infants: A preliminary report. *J. Pediatr.,* 81:145.
5. Filler, R. M., Takada, Y., Carreras, T. H., and Heim, T. (1980): Serum intralipid levels in neonates during parenteral nutrition: The relation to gestational age. *J. Pediatr. Surg.,* 15:405.
6. Fischer, J. E., Rosen, H. M., Ebeid, A. M., et al. (1976): The effect or normalization of plasma amino acids on hepatic encephalopathy in man. *Surgery,* 80:77.
7. Friedman, Z., Marks, K. H., Maisels, M. J., Thorson, B. S., and Waeye, R. (1978): Effect of parenteral fat emulsion on the pulmonary and reticuloendothelial systems in the newborn infant. *Pediatrics,* 61:694.
8. Friedman, Z., and Frolich, J. C. (1979): Essential fatty acids and the major urinary metabolites of the E prostaglandins in thriving neonates and in infants receiving parenteral fat emulsions. *Pediatr. Res.,* 13:932.
9. Gaull, G. E., Rassin, D. K., Räihä, N. C. R., and Heinonen, K. (1977): Milk protein quantity and quality in low-birth-weight infants. III. Effects on sulfur amino acids in plasma and urine. *J. Pediatr.,* 90:348.
10. Ghadimi, H. (1975): Newly devised amino acid solutions of intravenous administration. In: *Total Parenteral Nutrition: Premises and promises,* edited by H. Ghadimi, p. 393. Wiley, New York, London, Sydney, Toronto.
11. Griffin, E., Breckenridge, W. C., Kuksis, A., Bryan, M. H., and Angel, A. (1979): Appearance and characterization of lipoprotein X during continuous intralipid infusions in the neonate. *J. Clin. Invest.,* 64:1703.

12. Hayashi, S., Sanada, K., Sagawa, N., Yamada, N., and Kido, K. (1978): Umbilical vein–artery differences of plasma amino acids in the last trimester of human pregnancy. *Biol. Neonate,* 34:11.
13. Heim, T., Putet, G., Verellen, G., Chessex, P., Swyer, P. R., Smith, J. M., and Filler, R. M. (1981): Energy cost of intravenous alimentation in the newborn infant. In: *Intensive Care in the Newborn. III,* edited by L. Stern, B. Salle, and B. Friis-Hansen, p. 219. Masson, New York, Paris.
14. Heird, W. C. (1975): Disorders of calcium and phosphorus metabolism. In: *Intravenous Nutrition in the High Risk Infant,* edited by R. W. Winters, and E. G. Hasselmeyer, p. 249. Wiley, New York, London, Sydney, Toronto.
15. Hsia, D. Y. Y., Berman, J. L., and Slatis, H. M. (1964): Screening newborn for phenylketonuria. *J.A.M.A.,* 188:203.
16. Jones, A. B. (1978): Study of the use of total parenteral nutrition in neonates suffering from necrotizing enterocolitis. In: *Advance in Parenteral Nutrition,* edited by I. D. Johnston, p. 281. MTP, Lancaster, England.
17. Knight, P. J., Buchanan, S., and Clatworthy, H. W., Jr. (1980): Calcium and phosphate requirements of preterm infants who require prolonged hyperalimentation. *J.A.M.A.,* 243:1244.
18. Lloyd-Still, J. D., Hurwitz, I., Wolff, P. H., and Shwachman, H. (1974): Intellectual development after severe malnutrition in infancy. *Pediatrics,* 54:306.
19. Lubchenco, L. L., Hansman, C., Dressler, M., and Boyd, E. (1963): Intrauterine growth as estimated from liveborn birth-weight data at 24 to 42 weeks of gestation. *Pediatrics,* 32:793.
20. McIntosh, N., Rodeck, C. H., and Heath, R. (1981): Plasma amino acids of the mid trimester foetus. *Pediatr. Res.,* 15:1189.
21. Pohlandt, P. F. (1978): Plasma amino acid concentrations in umbilical cord vein and artery of newborn infants after elective cesarean section or spontaneous delivery. *J. Pediatr.,* 92:617.
22. Raiha, N. C. R. (1974): Biochemical basis for nutritional management of preterm infants. *Pediatrics,* 53:147.
23. Rigo, J., and Senterre, J. (1980): Optimal threonine intake for preterm infants fed on oral or parenteral nutrition. *J. Parenter. Enter. Nutr.,* 4:15.
24. Rigo, J., Senterre, J., and Oger, J. (1979): Improvement of neonatal growth by parenteral nutrition in low-birth-weight infants. *Acta Paediatr. Belg.,* 32:35.
25. Senterre, J., and Rigo, J. (1980): Protein requirements of low-birth-weight infants. In *The Samuel Z. Levine Conference: The Physiological and Biochemical Basis for Perinatal Medicine,* edited by A. Minkowski, p. 125. Karger, Basel.
26. van den Berghe, G., and Hers, H. C. (1978): Dangers of intravenous fructose and sorbitol. *Acta Paediatr. Belg.,* 31:115.
27. Zlotkin, S. H., and Anderson, G. H. (1982): The development of cystathionase activity during the first year of life. *Pediatr. Res.,* 16:65.
28. Zlotkin, S. H., Bryan, M. H., and Anderson, G. H. (1981): Cystein supplementation to cysteinfree intravenous feeding regimes in newborn infants. *Am. J. Clin. Nutr.,* 34:914.
29. Zlotkin, S. H., Bryan, M. H., and Anderson, G. H. (1981): Intravenous nitrogen and energy intake required to duplicate *In utero* nitrogen accretion in prematurely born human infants. *J. Pediatr.,* 99:115.

DISCUSSION

Dr. Perman: I am interested in your recommendation regarding the administration of fructose in total parenteral nutrition solutions in the low-birth-weight infants. As you pointed out, low-birth-weight infants are relatively fructose-intolerant, and I am curious as to whether you see in these infants a response which you might see in an infant with hereditary fructose intolerance. You mentioned that you measured the phosphorus balance, and I am wondering whether these infants had decreased phosphorus levels and perhaps increased uric acids.

Dr. Rigo: In low-birth-weight infants, kinetic studies of fructose and glucose infusions have shown that renal fructose threshold level is lower than renal glucose threshold level. In addition, acute fructose infusion may lead to metabolic acidosis, hypophosphatemia, and high urinary excretion of uric acid. In our study, fructose infusion corresponded to about 30% of the carbohydrate intake. Under these conditions, fructose tolerance was good: serum fructose level was below 30 mg/dl and urinary excretion of fructose represented less than 3% of the fructose intake. Serum phosphorus level and urinary excretion of uric acid were similar in the infants receiving glucose and in those infused with a mixture of glucose and fructose.

Dr. Räihä: You said that you feel that the fetal plasma amino acid level is optimal. I wonder why you come to that conclusion, because we don't use the fetal PO_2 as optimal in the newborn glucose level either. I think you can call them a reference point, but we may not want to strive at those levels.

Dr. Rigo: Regarding PO_2, I think that we can agree that oxygen consumption is not the same before and after birth. About amino acids, plasma amino acid level of the fetus *in utero* is high during the whole period of gestation and is similar to cord blood values. This level is probably necessary for his development and nontoxic for his brain. It is quite difficult to define an optimal reference for preterm infants. Indeed, prematurity is not a physiological status. Amino acid levels are dependent not upon only the protein intake but also upon the nitrogen retention. If we want to have a postnatal growth and a nitrogen retention similar to that existing *in utero,* we shall have a higher amino acid level than the one observed in term infants fed human milk. Human milk is not exactly a physiological diet for a preterm infant. So we may not consider the plasma amino acid level of low-birth-weight infants fed on human milk as a reference level. What I would conclude is that, if not a reference level, cord blood amino acid levels may be considered at least as a safe level for preterm infants.

Dr. Metcoff: Do you think that constant enteral infusion would be better than constant parenteral infusion with respect to amino acids?

Dr. Rigo: When feeding the low-birth-weight infant, we frequently carry out continuous enteral feeding or very frequent meals every 1 or 2 hrs. Except for phenylalanine, we did not observe any difference between enteral and parenteral nutrition when we consider the relationship between serum amino acids level and dietary amino acid intake.

In our unit, we tend to reduce total parenteral nutrition for very-low-birth-weight infants—we use supplemental parenteral nutrition, and the data that I gave earlier were related to the growth of infants on supplemental parenteral nutrition. However, the data presented on amino acid metabolism in preterm infants were collected in infants on total parenteral nutrition, because some years ago we used more parenteral nutrition over a longer period for infants of very low birth-weight and for those with surgical problems. I think that for the study of the metabolism of amino acids, we need to have total parenteral nutrition. Now, we have decreased the frequency of total parenteral nutrition and increased the supplemental parenteral nutrition for the low-birth-weight infant. The duration of parenteral nutrition has also decreased, and after 10 days we stop parenteral nutrition and replace it by oral nutrition. We use human milk, supplemented with protein, phosphorus, and calories, or we use a mixture of human milk and specially adapted formula for low-birth-weight infants.

Dr. Räihä: I have a question for Dr. Putet. When comparing growth in your two groups, do you think it is really an advantage for the infant to gain weight at 21.4 g instead of 15 g/kg/day? We are not so much concerned about weight gain in our infants on breast milk—they usually pick up later anyway.

Dr. Putet: I am glad that you have asked this question, because it was one of our first questions: Should we try to reach the IU growth rate? I am not sure at all, but I believe that there is no answer at the moment. In babies gaining weight at the rate of 20 g/kg/day, we don't know what is the total body water. We need this type of information to evaluate the quality of the weight of these babies.

Dr. Metcoff: Our own data in rats as well as a myriad of other data indicate that plasma levels of amino acids correlate very poorly with levels of amino acids in almost any other tissue—muscle and liver as well. I am becoming increasingly cautious about interpreting plasma amino acid levels for any meaningful purpose.

Dr. Räihä: I think we all agree about that, but can you suggest how we could analyze amino acids from anything else? I know that Bill Hurd at Columbia has studied newborn pups on total parenteral nutrition and he has been able to show that a 10% increase or decrease in certain plasma amino acids may indicate a 100% increase in the tissue level. So I would be very worried by a change in the plasma level, because that level may indicate that the tissue level is many, many times higher or lower.

Dr. Metcoff: In response to your question, we have found a fair correlation between leucocytes and muscle. Leucocytes are fairly easy to obtain, and they can be analyzed using very small quantities of blood.

Dr. Räihä: I think that is very important and I know Bo Lindbladt in Stockholm is looking at red cell amino acids. We may have to get into that, but the reason why we are still measuring plasma amino acids is that we now have a big pool of data on plasma amino acids with various diets. If we now suddenly turn to looking at leucocyte amino acids or red cell amino acids, then we would have to do all the clinical trials and studies again, because we cannot compare the red cells to the plasma values.

Modifications of Human Milk Composition During the Early Stages of Lactation

B. Ribadeau Dumas

*Institut National de la Recherche Agronomique,
C.N.R.Z., 78350 Jouy-en-Josas, France*

This chapter deals with the modifications of human milk composition during the early stages of lactation and the possible implications of these modifications as far as the needs of the newborn are concerned.

Figure 1 illustrates how difficult human milk is to work on, especially that from the first part of lactation (Fig. 1). This figure, based on results of a study carried out recently in Australia (3), shows the tremendous modifications that occur in milk composition during the prepartum period. The composition of prepartum colostrum remains quite constant, as far as lactose and total proteins are concerned (Fig. 1, *top*). Within a few hours after delivery, however, the composition of milk changes dramatically. Therefore, when one has to study the composition of milk during this period, it is very hard to present data representative of an average human milk composition.

Figure 2 compares the protein composition of human milk and of colostrum with that of cow's milk. This figure shows that there are major differences between human and bovine milks, and also important differences between human milk and human colostrum. Figure 2 *top* shows the differences in the proportion of casein and whey protein, and the fairly high proportion of low-molecular products containing nitrogen in human milk and colostrum. Among them is taurine, which might be important for the newborn.

Figure 2 *bottom* shows the differences in composition between human milk and cow's milk, human colostrum, and mature human milk as far as the individual whey proteins are concerned. It is well known that a given protein exists only in a single species; that is to say, when comparing two species, one generally finds similar sets of proteins with similar functions, but in most cases, the homologous proteins are different. The more different the species, the more different the proteins. In Figure 2 *bottom,* for example, both human and cow's milks contain lactoferrin, but this does not mean that these proteins are identical. Indeed they are *different.* The proportions of the individual proteins are very different in the two milks. Furthermore, β-lactoglobulin, the main whey protein in cow's milk, is absent in human milk. Figure 2 *bottom* also shows the relative importance of lactoferrin and lysozyme in human milk. In any

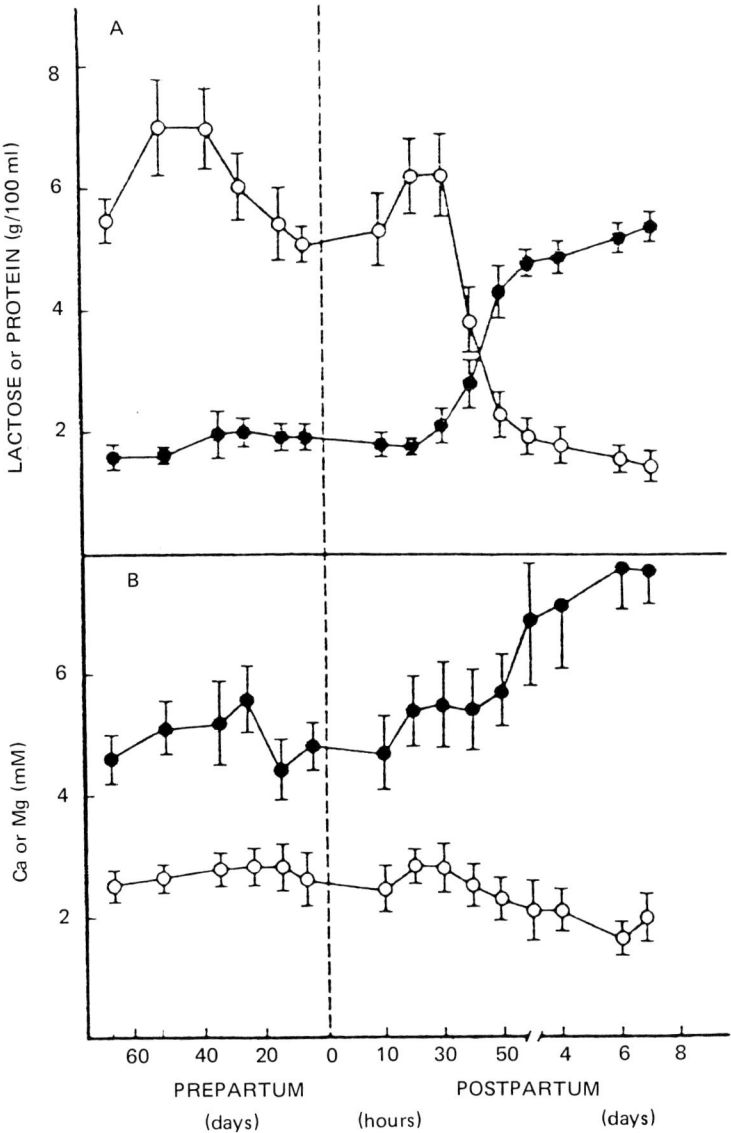

FIG. 1. Modifications in milk composition during the prepartum period. Based on data from ref. 3. See text for details.

case, the concentration of proteins is higher in colostrum than in mature milk, and this is true for all animal species.

Following is a review of data that have been obtained in collaboration with Dr. Gamarra. The study, which was carried out a few years ago, was concerned with the changes in the composition of human milk during the early days after

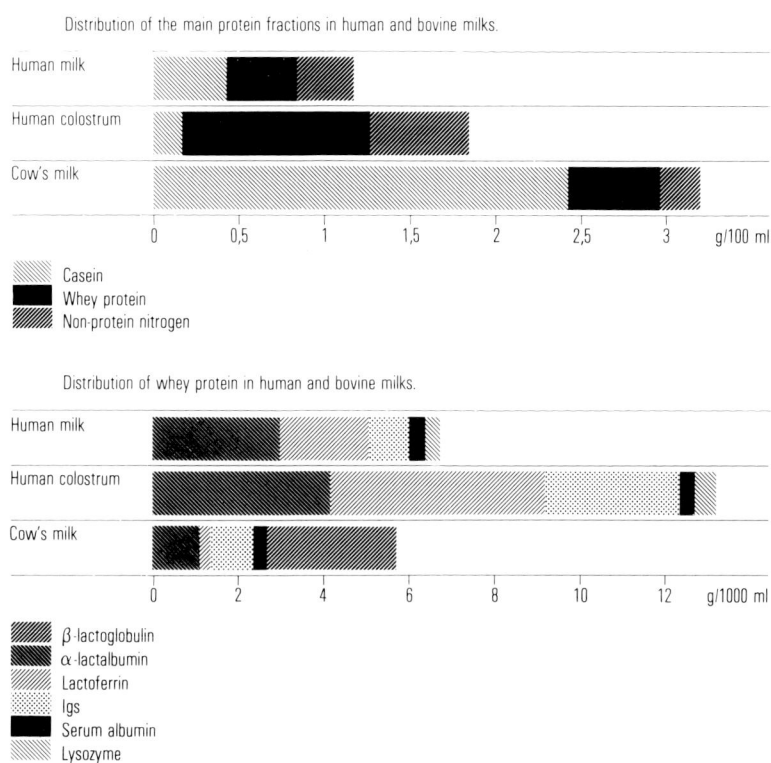

FIG. 2. Distribution of main protein fractions **(top)** and whey protein **(bottom)** in human and bovine milk.

delivery. Two sets of data have been included in Fig. 3. Closed circles and triangles represent data obtained in collaboration with Dr. Gamarra, while open circles and triangles correspond to data obtained in another study by Atkinson et al. (2). The figure represents the variations in nitrogen content of samples of human milk collected from 76 women (49 women from our study and 27 from Atkinson's study). The scattering of points at any time after delivery is striking, thus clarifying the difficulties in deciding what a newborn needs in terms of protein during the early days. Only a range of concentrations, perhaps an average concentration, can be deduced from such a study. In fact, the purpose of our study was to compare milk from preterm and full-term mothers. Our results are quite similar to those of Atkinson et al. A statistical analysis was carried out on both sets of data. It indicates that there is no significant difference between the two types of milk as far as the nitrogen content is concerned, which is at variance with the conclusions drawn by Atkinson et al. (2) in 1978 and more recently by the same authors (1).

I would like to add that milk proteins have several functions. The first one

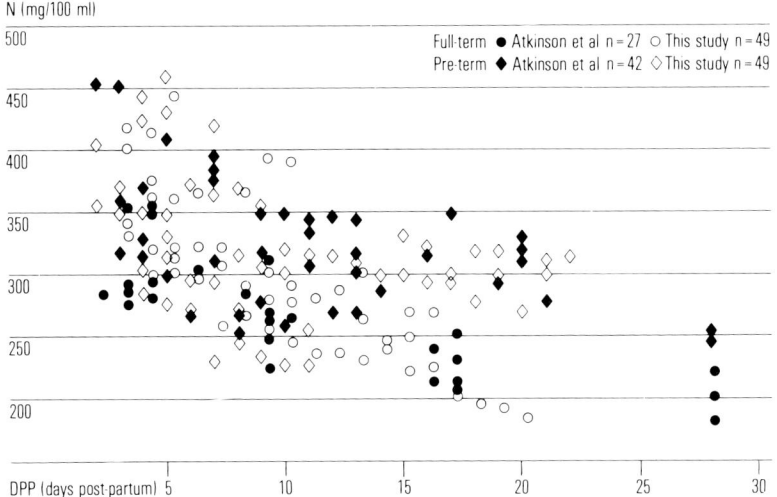

FIG. 3. Changes in nitrogen content in milk during the early days after delivery. *Closed circles and triangles,* data from Ribadeau Dumas and Gamarra. *Open circles and triangles,* data from Atkinson et al. (2). See text for details.

is obviously to provide the young child with nitrogen, essential amino acids, and calories. This may not be the only role of these proteins. Specific milk proteins such as IgA, lactoferrin, and lysozyme are supposed to have a physiological role; whether they play it or not is difficult to know. We have carried out several studies to discover if lactoferrin has any bacteriostatic activity in the gut of newborns, and for the moment we have not been able to show any such action, but this does not mean that it does not exist! There is an increasing number of components that are believed to play a role in the newborn gut, but apart from IgAs, in no case has this action been proved *in vivo*. For example, lysozyme has never been shown to interact *in vivo* with the bacterial flora of the gut. I believe that the only good data that have been obtained so far are those dealing with IgAs. The proportions and concentrations of IgAs of different classes in colostrum are quite different from one species to another. In human colostrum there is a fairly high amount of IgA and a low proportion of IgG. It is the opposite in ruminants. It now seems well established that IgAs directed against the microorganisms of the mother's environment are present in her milk and protect the baby's gut against them. The role, if any, of IgMs and IgGs in human milk is still unknown.

Human milk is certainly the best food for the human baby. But, apart from the hygienic aspect, this assertion is based mainly on the fact that human milk has been the only food for the human infant for more than 1 million years. More research is needed to establish its value on a sound scientific basis.

REFERENCES

1. Anderson, G. H., Atkinson, S. A., and Bryan, M. H. (1981): Energy and macronutrient content of human milk during early lactation from mothers giving birth prematurely and at term. *Am. J. Clin. Nutr.,* 34:258–265.
2. Atkinson, S. A., Bryan, M. H., and Anderson, G. H. (1978): Human milk: Difference in nitrogen concentration in milk from mothers of term and premature infants. *J. Pediatr.,* 93:67–69.
3. Kulski, J. K., and Hartmann, P. E. (1981): Changes in human milk composition during the initiation of lactation. *Austr. J. Exp. Biol. Med. Sci.,* 59:101–114.

DISCUSSION

Dr. Semenza: Milk, of course, contains a lot of hormones, and I imagine that they may well be of great importance for premature infants. I wonder if there are any data as to how much of a given hormone is present in milk at the beginning of lactation and how much it changes during lactation.

Dr. Ribadeau Dumas: Several investigators have studied the level of hormones in milk and especially of prolactin. It has been shown that prolactin is indeed present, but nobody knows whether it plays a real role in the gastrointestinal tract of the newborn.

Dr. Shwachman: Would you please comment on the accuracy or inaccuracy of the measurement of electrolytes in milk? I am specifically referring to the milk of women with cystic fibrosis. There was one report years ago that it is dangerous for a baby born from a mother with cystic fibrosis to be fed her milk. We have not been able to verify this information and the reason for this is the inaccuracy of the measurement of electrolytes in milk.

Dr. Ribadeau Dumas: I would like to say first that I am not a specialist of electrolytes, but I know something about the determination of electrolytes in milk. When one looks at results dealing with electrolytes one should verify *when* the figures were obtained. *Nowadays,* with appropriate techniques, the measurements usually give good-quality data. Atomic absorption and emission spectrometry are very accurate techniques.

Dr. Ferguson: You mentioned that the importance of IgAs in milk is well established. Your talk made me realize that I don't know of any study on the composition of milk in women who are IgA-deficient. Approximately one in 700 individuals is IgA-deficient, and most of these individuals have normal gastrointestinal function and no evidence of a predisposition to gastrointestinal infection. You may know of some work on the nature of the milk in IgA-deficient women. For example, is there a great deal more IgM under these circumstances?

Dr. Ribadeau Dumas: It is true that IgAs may play a role, but something which has not been much emphasized in this meeting is important and this is the bacterial population of the intestine of the newborn. It is not only the population by itself that is important but also the pattern of establishment of this flora. Dominant bacterial species in the gut change with time after birth, and this occurs following a rather strict pattern. It may well be possible that in the children of IgA-deficient women, as it is the case in many normal children, the "good" flora establishes itself rapidly and remains in the gut, preventing the occurrence of pathogenic bacteria.

Introduction of Weaning Foods into the Infant's Diet

Olikoye Ransome-Kuti

Department of Paediatrics and Primary Care, Institute of Child Health and Primary Care, College of Medicine, University of Lagos, P.M.B., 12003 Lagos, Nigeria

Weaning has been recognized as a dangerous process in many developing countries since Ceciley Williams described kwashiorkor in 1935. The term weaning has been described as ambiguous by David Morley and should be avoided because "the following two meanings are possible: (a) It is equivalent to the French 'sevrage' i.e. cessation of breast feeding; (b) the time or period in which solid foods or food other than milk are introduced into the baby's diet."

To avoid the confusion, he adopted the definition proposed by Scrimshaw for the "weaning period" which "commences when solids are introduced and continued until 3 months after suckling has been discontinued."

Jelliffe describes the weaning period as the prolonged phase from complete breast feeding until the infant is entirely on an adult diet (12). Others define weaning as the period from the first consistent addition of a food supplement until breast or bottle feeding ends.

Weaning could begin either when any food other than breast milk is introduced into the baby's diet, which includes cow's or goat's milk, or when any diet other than a milk diet (breast or animal) is given to a baby.

At the time when cow's milk was regarded as a suitable substitute for breast milk, it was reasonable to propose the commencement of the weaning period when solids were introduced into the baby's diet. Recent studies have indicated that the ingestion of cow's milk by the baby, particularly during the first 3 months of its life could have adverse immunological, psychological, and nutritive consequences. For this reason weaning should be defined as commencing when any food other than breast milk is introduced into the child's diet. Such a definition will alert the health worker to the dangers of early artificial feeding.

Two phases of weaning now become clear. The first is the early introduction of bottle or formula feeding, the second the feeding of solids or semisolids to the infant.

FORMULA FEEDING IN EARLY INFANCY

The decline in the percentage of women who are breast feeding leading to early formula feeding of the infant has been well documented in many parts of the world (21) (Table 1).

Dietary histories of cases of malnutrition in Lagos in 1968 indicated that bottle feeding during the first month of life was universal. The situation is the same today. From the records of infants attending village child welfare clinics in Kampala, Welbourn described the decline in breast feeding between 1950 and 1955. He further demonstrated that the children fed supplements were 1 to 2 lbs. lighter than the average for Buganda children at ages from 4 to 14 months. Even when cow's milk is sterile, it interferes with the development of the baby's immune system and protective mechanisms against infection (2).

In Mulago Hospital (Kampala), the enteral infection rate in the special care baby unit among low birth weight babies and birth weight above 2,500 g fed formula milk was 13.2% and 1.9%, respectively, in 1977. Of all possible sources of infection, milk is the only source of infection which could be excluded with certainty since sterilized milk preparations were regularly sent for bacteriologic culture and were always found to be negative (13).

Gastroenteritis was rampant in the neonatal wards of the Lagos University Teaching Hospital prior to 1980 in spite of all aseptic measures. It reduced

TABLE 1. *Percentage of breastfeeding mothers giving regular supplements by 2 to 3 months*

Country	% of mothers
Nigeria	
Urban elite	98
Rural	35
Ethiopia	
Urban elite	57
Rural	31
Zaire	
Urban elite	28
Rural	35
Chile	
Urban elite	60
Rural	56
Guatamala	
Urban elite	91
Rural	12
Sweden	4

Data from WHO, ref. 21.

considerably when feeding with only pooled freshly expressed breast milk was instituted in 1981 (Ahmed, *personal communication*). Both instances demonstrate the increased susceptibility of newborns to enteral infection when they are formula fed.

In newborn units, particularly in developing countries, pooled expressed breast milk should be fed to babies. Because of the lack of infrastructure and technology to establish and maintain milk banks, mothers who are constantly present in the unit can be taught to provide clean breast milk daily. Sustained encouragement by the nurses and intensive health education are however needed to maintain supplies.

Before the feeding of expressed breast milk to babies in the Neonatal Unit of the Lagos University Teaching Hospital was instituted, the parents were interviewed regarding their attitude toward feeding their breast milk to other babies. Ninety-five percent of fathers were both willing to permit their wives to donate for other babies and for their babies to receive donated milk. On the other hand, 72% of mothers were willing to donate for other babies, and only 28% were willing for their babies to receive milk from other mothers. The most common fear, expressed by 40% of the women, was that disease or personality characteristics may be transmitted by the donor, and 26% just disliked the idea (see Table 2). Following a series of health education programs, feeding with pooled expressed breast milk was readily accepted.

In the community, two factors may operate in causing diarrhea. These are (a) the difficulties in preparing sterile formula feeds and (b) the increased danger from infection. Early bottle feeding may lead to a failure to empty the breast resulting in a dampening of the "let-down" reflex and reduced breast milk output. The need for bottle feeding is thereby increased and ultimately predominates. When, because of poverty or ignorance, dilute formula feeds are thereafter given to the baby, marasmus occurs.

As early as 1911, Woodbury studied the records of groups of babies from eight American cities, that is, exclusively artificially fed and partially breast

TABLE 2. *Willingness to donate or receive breast milk, by sex of the parent*

	Donate				Receive			
	Fathers		Mothers		Fathers		Mothers	
	No.	%	No.	%	No.	%	No.	%
Willing	19	95	43	72	19	95	17	28
Unwilling	1	5	17	28	1	5	43	72
Total	20	100	60	100	20	100	60	100

Data from Luth (1979) and M.T.C. Egri-Okwaji and A. Bamisaiye (*unpublished data*).

fed. In relative terms, the disadvantage of bottle feeding was greatest during the first 6 months; the greatest relative risk occurred at 4.7 months of age, a pattern that was consistent for all disease categories except deaths due to congenital malformations. This situation is analogous to that in many developing countries at this time.

In the rural areas of India, Chandra (4) found a higher rate of infection among formula-fed babies than those breast-fed. Diarrhea was the most frequently observed illness in both groups. Compared with similar studies in Canada, the same relationship was found regarding rates of infection in both groups but in Canada, respiratory infections had the highest rates (Table 3).

In Chile, at 4 weeks, 3 months, and 6 months, mortality rates in bottle-fed babies were twice those in babies receiving breast milk only. Breast-fed babies who were also given cow's milk fared no better than those given cow's milk alone, indicating that if a baby is to benefit from breast feeding, he must be given breast milk alone (7).

In Guatemalan children, Mata and co-workers (14) state that concomitant with increasing amounts of supplemental foods provided to the breast-fed child, a shift of fecal flora from almost exclusive bifidobacteria to that more typical of the adult was observed. The subtle shift in fecal flora observed with progressive weaning correlated with the intestinal invasion by enteric pathogenic bacteria, parasites and viruses. These fecal microorganisms have been found in very large numbers in the upper small intestine of malnourished children in the Gambia (8).

Jackson & Golden (11) have proposed that cow's milk, evolved to promote bacterial growth in the calf's upper small bowel, may, when fed to an infant, predispose to the multiplication of fermentation bacteria in the infant's upper gastrointestinal tract. Deprived of the immediate effect of passive immunity and possessing limited or impaired capacity to develop active immunity, a process may be set in motion ultimately leading to diarrhea, lactose or cow's milk protein intolerance, and eventually malnutrition.

TABLE 3. *Infection-related morbidity in breast-fed and formula-fed infants in India and Canada*

	No. of episodes of illness over a 24-month period			
	India		Canada	
Disorder	Breast-fed ($N = 35$)	Formula-fed ($N = 35$)	Breast-fed ($N = 30$)	Formula-fed ($N = 30$)
Respiratory infection	57	109	42	98
Otitis	21	52	9	86
Diarrhea	70	211	5	16
Dehydration	3	14	0	3
Pneumonia	2	8	—	—

From Chandra, ref. 4, with permission.

The most common reason given by a large number of mothers for early bottle feeding is "insufficient breast milk" (21). In Egypt, 17% of the urban elite, 10% of the urban poor, and 5.8% of traditional rural mothers gave this reason for early supplementation with bottle feeding. Among the urban elite the use of contraceptive pills (another novel danger) was found to be the second common reason (19%) and the fourth among the urban poor (7.7%) (6).

In Brazil (16,17) and the Far East (15), inadequate production of breast milk was the reason for early bottle feeding, and in the case of Brazil, as early as the first month of life.

In England, studies have shown that breast-fed babies tend to be supplemented later (13.8 weeks) than bottle- (7.8 weeks) or mixed-fed (9.6 weeks) babies. The most common reason for weaning is hunger. The data suggest that babies are more satisfied with breast milk than cow's milk or formula for a longer period (22).

Monthly weights of babies recorded on a weight chart should indicate when breast milk becomes inadequate to maintain the baby's growth. This usually occurs between the 4th and 6th months of life.

The controversy regarding the time of commencement of weaning was reopened following a report from the Gambia that African women were unable to produce enough milk to sustain their baby's growth after 3 months of age (20). To many who have supervised breast feeding and found it to be adequate for the first 4 to 6 months of life, the finding came as a complete surprise. Waterlow et al. (20) calculated the rates of growth of babies from longitudinal studies of weights and heights from different countries and came to the conclusion that "the rate of growth falls off substantially, compared with the U.K., between three and four months and in many cases earlier." They noted that in the WHO Collaborative Study on Breast Feeding (21), it was shown that in less developed countries, by 2 to 3 months, from 10% to 50% of mothers in the rural areas, although continuing to breast feed, were giving supplementary foods: the commonest reason given was not enough milk. In Ibadan, however, the reason given by mothers for early supplementation of breast feeding was to give the baby "health and strength," concepts popular in Nigerian culture and used frequently in food advertising (15). In Lagos, it was because the mothers "took a fancy" to bottle feeding. These examples indicate that answers purporting "hunger in the baby" as a cause for early supplementary feeding may mask other reasons for doing so. F. C. Steady (18) suggests that the availability of another option—bottle feeding—may create a conflict, leading to anxiety and stress in the mother.

In view of the need to ensure the full development of the babies protective and immune mechanisms, a prescription to begin bottle feeding before the age of 2 to 4 months must be considered with great caution, particularly in developing countries where the environment is so highly contaminated.

At the same time, the increase in the percentage of mothers breast feeding in developed countries must be noted. Biering-Sorenson et al. (3) and Bacon and Wylie (1) observed signs of increasing breast feeding in 1974–1975, especially among the higher social classes and commented: "Perhaps the higher social classes will lead a swing back to breast-feeding, just as they led the fashion to the bottle 40 years ago." Similarly, we hope that the richer countries, which have led the poorer countries to the bottle with such disastrous results, will, in time, lead them back to breastfeeding. However, in developing countries, the better educated continue to lead the march toward bottle feeding.

FEEDING WITH SOLIDS AND SEMISOLIDS

The British DHSS report of 1977 recommended that the early introduction of cereals and other foods into the diet of babies before 4 months of age should be strongly discouraged (5). Nevertheless culture plays a major role in many communities regarding food to be given and also when they are to be given. There are foods to be avoided because of taboos and superstitions, others are an integral part of the culture. For example, in Malaysia, there is great faith in the strength-giving qualities of rice, the major staple food. For this reason, it is given to the infant a few days after birth. The Yorubas of Nigeria wean their infants on a maize gruel. This practice is a major cause of malnutrition. The high prevalence of diarrhea and malnutrition in many parts of the world is due to inappropriate feeding practices at the weaning period whereby culture or ignorance dictates that predominantly carbohydrate diets are fed to the infant. This is in spite of the fact that there must be few communities without suitable staple food items for weaning infants successfully.

Attempts by international and charitable organizations to introduce special foods into various developing countries have had limited success because these foods confront their culture, food taboos, and superstitions. Again, "although their production is directed primarily towards the lower income groups, their cost, unavailability from most slum neighbourhood retailers or lack of status in comparison to commercially advertised products often stand in the way of their widespread use. Distribution seems to be most successful when carried out free of charge through an institutional system."

Fortification of staple weaning foods, adopted by many countries, offers an alternative with a greater chance of success.

There is no doubt that commercially advertised weaning foods are gaining ground in many developing countries. These are mainly imported at a high cost of foreign exchange and sold at a price above that which can be afforded by the poor. They are however persuaded to buy them through advertisements and the example of the upper classes. Like formula feeding, the infants are fed inadequate amounts of the cereals and malnutrition is the result.

The aim must be the use of suitable staple foods for weaning the infant. Where fortification of these foods is necessary, means should be found to do so locally. The most important and difficult achievement must be a change in attitude and practice of the members of the community, breaking down barriers of culture, superstition, and taboos towards their staple foods which will result in better infant feeding during the weaning period.

Hibbert and Golden (9) studied samples of bottle feeds brought to the clinic by mothers of 90 well-nourished and 11 undernourished children and found them to be heavily contaminated. They make the point that when the child has been breast fed and is healthy with an intact immune system, gastric acidity, intestinal motility, and a normal resident flora, the contaminated feed can be ingested with relative impunity. However, when this situation does not exist, there is the likelihood of enteral infection and the organisms establishing themselves in the gastrointestinal tract. This likelihood is increased by an attack of measles. Should the weaning period be protracted, the inflammation of the intestinal mucosa and diminished motility of the intestine caused by malnutrition permit bacterial overgrowth. These features may be the cause of the malabsorption observed in malnutrition. Malabsorption associated with a high incidence of weaning diarrhea, growth retardation, and impaired xylose absorption has been demonstrated in children in East Pakistan.

Weaning in many developing countries ends between the 18th and 24th months. In these countries, a quarter of the children born at the beginning of the period would have died. Many of the survivors have suffered illnesses because of interference with their normal biological development based on the mother's ignorance and professional medical misdirection, misguided cultural practices, and a lack of national political will to correct them. Hovering over this dismal scene are the commercial forces, hitherto, of formula, now of weaning foods, continually undermining the ability of mothers to be self-reliant and her confidence to feed her infant effectively during this critical period of the baby's life. Until her confidence in breast feeding is restored and relevant and effective weaning practices practiced by her, our present knowledge about infant feeding would have been acquired in vain.

REFERENCES

1. Bacon, C. J., and Wylie, J. M. (1976): *Br. Med. J.*, 1:308.
2. Ballabriga, A., Hilbert, H., and Isliker, H. (1974/75): Immunity of the infantile gastrointestinal tract and implication on modern infant feeding. In: *Nestlé Research News*, Nestlé, Vevey.
3. Biering-Sorenson, F., Hilden, J., and Biering-Sorenson, K. (1980): Breastfeeding on the increase: Editorial: *J. Trop. Pediatr.*, 26:ii, iii.
4. Chandra, R. K. (1979): Prospective study of the effect of breast feeding on incidence of infection and allergy. *Acta Pediatr. Scand.*, 68:692.
5. Department of Health and Social Security (1977): Present-Day Practice in Infant Feeding. Department of Health and Social Studies, HMSO, London.
6. El-Mougi, M., Mostafa, S., Osman, N. H., and Ahmed, K. A. (1971): Social and medical factors affecting the duration of breast feeding in Egypt: *J. Trop. Pediatr.*, 27:5–11.
7. Gerrard, J. W. (1974): Breast-feeding: Second thoughts. *Paediatrics*, 54:757–763.
8. Heyworth, B., and Brown, J. (1975): Jejunal microflora in malnourished Gambian children. *Arch. Dis. Child.*, 50:27–33.
9. Hibbert, J. M., and Golden, M. H. N. (1981): What is the weanings dilemma? Dietary faecal bacterial ingestion of normal children in Jamaica: *J. Trop. Pediatr.*, 27:255–258.
10. Iwtengan, C. U. (1976): Nutritional evaluation of breast feeding practices in some countries in the Far East. *J. Trop. Pediatr. Environ. Child Health*, 22:63–67.

11. Jackson, A. A., and Golden, M. H. N. (1978): The human rumen: *Lancet,* ii:764–767.
12. Jelliffe, D. B. (1968): *Infant Nutrition in the Tropics and Subtropics,* 2nd Ed. WHO Monograph Series No. 29. WHO, Geneva.
13. Masembe, R. N. (1977): The pattern of bacterial diarrhoea of the newborn in Mulago hospital (Kampala). *J. Trop. Paediatr. Environ. Child Health,* 23:61–65.
14. Mata, L. J., Hejicanos, M. L., and Jimenez, F. (1972): Studies on the indigenous gastrointestinal flora of Guatemalan children. *Am. J. Clin. Nutr.,* 25:1380.
15. Orwell, S., and Murray, J. (1974): Infant feeding and health in Ibadan: *J. Trop. Pediatr. Environ. Child Health,* 20:206–219.
16. Roberto, V. (1975): The decline of breast feeding in Brazil: *J. Trop. Paediatr. Environ. Child Health,* 21:212–213.
17. Sousa, P. L., Barros, F. C., Pinkeiro, G. N. M. and Gonzalle, R. V. (1975): The decline of breast feeding in Brazil. *J. Trop. Paediatr. Environ. Child Health,* 22:12–17.
18. Steady, F. C. (1981): Infant feeding in developing countries: Combating the multinational imperative. *J. Trop. Pediatr.,* 27:215–220.
19. Waterlow, J. C., Ashworth, A., and Griffiths, M. (1980): Faltering in infant growth in less developed countries. *Lancet,* ii:1176–1177.
20. Whitehead, R. G., Rowland, M. G. M., Hutton, M., Prentice, A. M., Miller, E. E., and Paul, A. (1978): Factors influencing lactation performance in rural Gambian mothers. *Lancet,* ii:178–181.
21. W.H.O. (1981): *Contemporary Patterns of Breastfeeding: Report on the WHO Collaborative Study on Breast Feeding.* WHO, Geneva.
22. Wilkinson, P. W., and Davies, D. P. (1978): When and why are babies weaned. *Br. Med. J.,* 1:1682–1683.

DISCUSSION

Dr. Zetterström: One of the main issues in infant feeding is when to introduce supplementary food if the infants are thriving on just breast milk. In Sweden we have now come to the conclusion that it shouldn't be introduced before the age of 6 months, and one reason is that since 20% of children have a disposition to develop allergic diseases, we don't want to introduce too much foreign foodstuff until the age of 6 months. I should like also to mention that the prevalence of breast feeding now in Sweden at the age of 2 months is 85%, so it is now as high in Sweden as it used to be in the 1940s. May I just make a third comment: an ancestor of my mother 250 years ago noticed that freshly expressed human milk stayed fresh for 3 to 4 days whereas cow's milk products were destroyed within a very short period of time.

Dr. Ransome-Kuti: I can only say that those who have promoted breast feeding were a bit alarmed by the findings in Gambia that African mothers could not sustain the growth of their children for more than 2 to 3 months without supplementation. The charts in our clinics indicate that the majority of mothers can maintain their baby's growth on breast milk for at least 6 months. I think we do need to collect more information in this area before the confidence of the mothers in their ability to breast feed their children erodes. When we started collecting pooled expressed breast milk in the teaching hospital, we got the mothers to express the milk in as clean a condition as possible, and we cultured the pooled expressed breast milk and found that the specimens were virtually sterile. We then kept the milk refrigerated for 24 hr and cultured it again and found that there was hardly any growth at all in the milk.

SUBJECT INDEX

Subject Index

Absorption, protein, *see* Protein absorption
Alkaline phosphatase, 53
Allergies
  and intravenous fat emulsions, 167
  and weaning foods, 222
Allograft rejection, and small intestinal mucosa, 61–62
Amino acid(s)
  absorption, 85–88, 103; *see also* Protein absorption
  concentration, in preterm infants, 196–198
  dietary imbalance, and fetal malnutrition, 151–159, 160–161
    amino acid combination and threonine level, 157
    diet efficiency and, 154
    and maternal variables, 158–159
    nutrient variables at midpregnancy, 152
    protein content, 154, 155
    weight loss, 153, 154
  intake, in preterm infants, 199
  and intestinal peptide uptake, 81
  metabolism, in low-birth-weight infants, 191–196
Aminoglycosides, in necrotizing enterocolitis, 112
Amniotic fluid, and intestinal development, 28
Ampicillin, in necrotizing enterocolitis, 112
Antibiotics, and necrotizing enterocolitis, 121
Antigens, intestinal, and cell-mediated immunity, 67–69
Arachidonic acid deficiency, 172
Atresia, intestinal, 28

Bacteria, and necrotizing enterocolitis, 116–118, 126–127
Bilirubin generation, and intravenous fat emulsions, 170–171
Birth weight, 177–188, 191–207

Blood flow, and intrauterine malnutrition, 134
Bradycardia, sinus, 172
Brain involvement, and intrauterine malnutrition, 134
Breast milk, *see* Human milk
Brown fat, and intrauterine malnutrition, 136, 148
Brunner's gland cells, and intestinal development, 12–13
Brush border
  enzymes, fetal, 53–56, 57
  hydrolysis, and peptide uptake, 82
  and protein digestion, 79
  and SI complex anchoring, 30–34, 42

^{13}C-lipid breath tests, 97–98
Calcium
  and intravenous fat emulsions, 172
  and low-birth-weight infants, 201
Calorie intake, and very-low-birth-weight infants, 199–200
Carbohydrate(s)
  digestion assessment, 98
  intake
    and lactase activity, 45–48
    and sucrase activity, 44–45
    and very-low-birth-weight infants, 201, 203
  testing, in feces, 100
  tolerance, in very-low-birth-weight infants, 200–201
Carnosine absorption, 84
Carotene measurements, 96
Cell-mediated immunity, intestinal, 60–69
  animal models, 60–67
  allograft rejection and small intestinal mucosa, 61–62
  intestinal mucosal changes and graft-versus-host reaction, 62–64
  phases of mucosal reactions, 64–65

225

SUBJECT INDEX

Cell mediated immunity, intestinal (contd.)
  animal models (contd.)
    T-cell mediated damage to intestine, 65–67
    induction to fed antigen, 67–69
Cellular differentiation, and intestinal development, 8–22
  crypt cells, 11–13
  endocrine cells, 11
  villous cells, specialized, 13–22
Cellular maturation, and intestinal development, 22–23
Cephalexin absorption, 84
Cholestasis, 168
Commercial formulas, see Formula feeding
Crypt cell differentiation, and intestinal development, 11–13
  Brunner's gland cells, 12–13
  Paneth cells, 11–12
  undifferentiated crypt cells, 11–12
Crypt hyperplasia, 64, 72
Crypt morphogenesis, and intestinal development, 6–7
Crypt-villus columns, and enzyme activity, 46–48
Cystic fibrosis, 106
Cystine intake, and very-low-birth-weight infants, 194, 197
Cytosol, and sucrose-isomaltose malabsorption, 38

Diarrhea, and weaning foods, 217
Digestion, protein, see Protein, digestion
Disaccharidase activity, and carbohydrate intake, 43–48
Disaccharide(s)
  absorption tests, 100
  hydrolysis, 100–103
Dopamine levels, and intrauterine malnutrition, 139, 145

Electrolytes, and human milk, 213
Endocrine cell differentiation, and intestinal development, 11
Energy loss, and low-birth-weight-infants, 179, 180–182
Energy requirements, in preterm infants, 199–201
Enteric feedings, and necrotizing enterocolitis, 114–116

Enterocolitis, necrotizing, see Necrotizing enterocolitis
Epithelial morphogenesis, and intestinal development, 4–11
Epithelial proliferation, and intestinal development, 4–11

Fat(s)
  balance, and low-birth-weight-infants, 180–182
  determination, fecal, 99
  digestion assessment, 95–98
  emulsions, intravenous, in preterm infants, 163–173
    and allergic manifestations, 167
    and cholestasis, 168
    and free-bilirubin generation, 170–171
    and glucose utilization impairment, 168
    and hypocarnitinemia, 171–172
    and immune responsiveness, 170
    list of emulsions, 164
    monitoring, 172–173
    and pulmonary function impairment, 168–169
    tolerance of, 166–167
    usage of, 164–166
  metabolism, intravenous, 164
  overloading syndrome, 168
Fatty acid deficiency, in preterm infants, 165
Fetal intestinal development, see Intestinal development
Formula feeding
  in early infancy, 216–220
  and low-birth-weight infants, 186–188
Free fatty acids, and intrauterine malnutrition, 135

Gastroenteritis, and weaning foods, 216–217
Gastrointestinal evaluation, noninvasive, see Noninvasive gastrointestinal evaluation
Gentamicin, in necrotizing enterocolitis, 121
Glucose
  intake, and very-low-birth-weight infants, 200–201, 202

metabolism, and intrauterine
malnutrition, 134–135
utilization, and intravenous fat
emulsions, 168
γ-Glutamyltranspeptidase, 54
Glycerol, and intrauterine
malnutrition, 136
^{13}C-Glycocholate breath tests, 99
Glycoprotein digestion, 90
Graft-versus-host reaction, and
intestinal mucosal changes, 62–64

H$_2$ breath tests, 101, 103
Hartnup disease, 87
Hormones, and human milk, 213
Human milk
compared to formula feeding, 216–220
insufficient production, 219
and low-birth-weight infants, 186–187
nutrient deposit, 183–184
modifications during early lactation, 209–212, 213
electrolytes and, 213
hormones and, 213
immunoglobulins and, 212, 213
nitrogen and, 211
prepartum period, 209, 210
protein and, 211–212
and necrotizing enterocolitis, 119–120, 127–128
5-Hydroxyindoleacetic acid, and
intrauterine malnutrition, 140–142
Hyperbilirubinemia, 172
Hypocarnitinemia, 171–172
Hyponatremia
and intravenous fat emulsions, 172
and necrotizing enterocolitis, 110
Hypoxia, 120–121

Immune responsiveness, and
intravenous fat emulsions, 170
Immunity, and necrotizing
enterocolitis, 119
Immunoglobulins, and human milk, 212, 213
Infections
and formula feeding, 218
and necrotizing enterocolitis, 116–118

Insulin absorption, 84
Intestinal development, fetal, 3–25, 28;
see also Intestine
cellular differentiation, 11–22
crypt cells, 11–13
endocrine cells, 11
villous cells, specialized, 13–22
maturation, 22–23
proliferation and morphogenesis, 4–11
cellular differentiation and, 8–11
intestinal tract formation, 4–6
villi and crypt morphogenesis, 6–7
Intestine, 86
atresia and, 28
cell-mediated immunity, 60–69
animal models of, 60–67
induction of, to fed antigen, 67–69
development, see Intestinal
development
T-lymphocytes in, 59–60
mucosal T-cells, 60
Peyer's patch lymphocytes, 59–60
Intracellular junctions, and intestinal
development, 28
Intraepithelial lymphocytes, 60
and lymphokine secretion, 71
Intrafat®, 164
Intralipid®, 163–164
Intrauterine malnutrition, 131–145, 148–149
dopamine levels and, 139
5-hydroxyindoleacetic acid levels
and, 140–142
norepinephrine levels and, 139
organ reduction, 132–136
blood flow and, 134
brain involvement and, 134
brown fat and, 136
free fatty acids and, 135
glucose metabolism and, 134–135
glycerol and, 136
lipids and, 135
neurotransmitter metabolism and, 136
serotonin levels and, 138–139
tryptophan levels and, 141–143
tyrosine levels and, 142–143
weight gain and, 138
Intravenous fat emulsions, see Fat(s),
emulsions, intravenous, in
preterm infants

Ischemia, and necrotizing enterocolitis, 121

Kanamycin, in necrotizing enterocolitis, 121

Lactase activity, 43–48, 49–52
  and carbohydrate intake, 45–48
Lactation, and human milk composition, 209–212, 213
Lactose breath H_2 tests, 101, 103
Lamina propria lymphocytes, 60
Laparotomy, in necrotizing enterocolitis, 113
Leukopenia, and necrotizing enterocolitis, 110
Lipids, and intrauterine malnutrition, 135
Lipiphysan®, 164
Lipolysis measurement, 95–96
Lipomul®, 163
Low-birth-weight infants, 191–207
  nutrient deposit in, 177–184
  nutrition of, 185–188
Lymphokine secretion, and intraepithelial lymphocytes, 60
Lyposyn®, 163–164
Lysine absorption, 91
Lysyl-lysine absorption, 82

M cells, and intestinal development, 14–18
Magnesium intake, and low-birth-weight infants, 201, 204
Malnutrition
  fetal, and amino acid imbalance, 151–159, 160–161
  intrauterine, 131–145, 148–149
Methionine intake, and very-low-birth-weight infants, 194, 196
Micellar solubilization assessment, 99
Mineral requirements, in very-low-birth-weight infants, 201
Monosaccharide absorption tests, 100
Monosaccharide uptake assessment, 100–103
Mucosal changes, intestinal, and graft-versus-host reaction, 62–64
Mucosal function, assessment, 99–103
  nonspecific, 99–100
  specific, 100
Mucosal reactions, intestinal, 64–65

Necrotizing enterocolitis, 107–122, 126–128
  laboratory evaluation, 109–110
  management, 112–114
  pathogenesis, 114–121
    enteric feedings and, 114–116
    hypoxic/ischemic considerations, 120–121
    immunologic considerations, 118–120
    infections and, 116–118
  pathology, 111–112
  prevention, 121–122
  radiographic evaluation, 110–111
  signs and symptoms, 108–109
Neurotransmitter metabolism, and intrauterine malnutrition, 136
Nitrogen content, in human milk, 211
Nitrogen requirement, in very-low-birth-weight infants, 191
Noninvasive gastrointestinal evaluation, 95–104, 106
  intraluminal phase, 95–99
    micellar solubilization, 99
    pancreatic function, 95–98
  mucosal phase, 99–103
    hydrolysis of disaccharides, 100–103
    monosaccharide uptake, 100–103
    nonspecific mucosal function, 99–100
    specific functions, 100
Norepinephrine levels, and intrauterine malnutrition, 139, 145
Nutrient deposit, in low-birth-weight infants, 177–184
  anthropometry, 178
  nutrient utilization, 179–182
Nutrition, and low-birth-weight infants, 177–184, 185–188, 189–190
  commercial formulas, 186–188
  human milk, 186–187
  protein requirements, 185

Oligoaminopeptidase development, 54–56
Oxygen, and peptide transport, 91

Pancreatic function assessment, 95–98
  carbohydrate digestion, 98
  fat digestion, 95–98
  protein digestion, 98

SUBJECT INDEX

Paneth cells, and intestinal development, 11–12
Papain solubilization, and sucrase-isomaltase complex, 31
Paracentesis, and necrotizing enterocolitis, 113
Peptide(s)
  absorption
    assessment, 103
    molecular weight and, 91
    protein absorption of, 80–85; see also Protein absorption
  transport, 91
Peyer's patch lymphocytes, in intestines, 59–60
Phenylalanine intake, and very-low-birth-weight infants, 192–193, 194
Phosphorous intake, and low-birth-weight infants, 204
Pneumatosis, and necrotizing enterocolitis, 110–111
Preterm infants; see also Low-birth-weight infants; Very-low-birth-weight infants
  and intravenous fat emulsions, 163–173
Prostaglandin synthesis, and intravenous fat emulsions, 172
Pro-sucrase-isomaltase (ProSI), 34–35, 42
Proteases, and disaccharidase regulation, 50
Protein(s)
  absorption, see Protein absorption
  balance, in low-birth-weight infants, 180–182
  digestion, 78–79, 90–91
    assessment, 98
    historical perspective, 73
    scheme, 78
  functions, and human milk, 211–212
  requirements, and low-birth-weight babies, 185–188, 189–190
Protein absorption, 73–78, 80–89, 90–91
  amino acids, 85–88
    active uptake, 86
    competition for uptake, 87
    factors affecting, 88
    kinetics of, 87–88
    site of maximal absorption, 88
    structural requirements, 86–87
  small peptides, 80–85
    active uptake of, 80–81
    biologically active peptides, 84
    factors affecting, 83–84
    independence of, 81
    kinetics of, 82
    into portal blood, 84–85
    site of maximal absorption, 82–83
    structural requirements, 81
  whole proteins, 88–89
Proteolytic enzymes, pancreatic, 79
Pulmonary function, and intravenous fat emulsions, 168–169

Rickets, and very-low-birth-weight infants, 201

Semisolids, and weaning foods, 220–221
Serotonin levels, and intrauterine malnutrition, 138–139, 144–145
SI complex, 29–38, 42
Side chains, and amino acid absorption, 87
Small intestine; see also Intestine
  allograft rejection and, 61–62
  amino acid transport and, 86
  grading of pathology in, 62
  sucrase-isomaltase complex, 29–38, 42
Sodium, and peptide transport, 91
Solids, and weaning foods, 220–221
Starch
  balance measurement, 98
  intake, 43–48
Stomach, and protein digestion, 79
Sucrase; see also Sucrase-isomaltase complex
  activity, 43–48, 49–52
  molecular weight, 57
  structural developmental differences, 54–56
Sucrase-isomaltase (SI) complex, 29–38, 42
  anchoring of, in brush border membrane, 30–34, 42
  biological control mechanisms, 30
  biosynthesis, 34–35
  malabsorption, 37–38
  membrane insertion, 34–35
  molecular weights of units, 29

Sucrase-isomaltase (SI) complex (*contd.*)
  phylogenetic considerations, 35–37
  positioning, 32
  properties of subunits, 29–30
Sucrose breath H_2 tests, 101, 103
Sucrose intake, and sucrase and lactase activity, 43–48
Sugars, and peptide absorption, 83
Synchronization, in intestinal development, 28

T-cells
  defect and gut permeability, 71
  and intestinal damage, 65–67
  mucosal, in intestines, 60
T-lymphocytes, in intestines, 59–60
  mucosal T-cells, 60
  Peyer's patch lymphocytes, 59–60
Threonine, 151–159, 160–161
Thrombocytopenia, and necrotizing enterocolitis, 109–110
Thyroliberin absorption, 84
Travamulsion®, 163–164
Triolein breath test, 99
Triton solubilization, and sucrase-isomaltase complex, 31
Tryptophan levels, and intrauterine malnutrition, 141–143, 144–145
Tuft cells, and intestinal development, 13–14
Tyrosine
  intake, in very-low-birth-weight infants, 193, 194
  levels, and intrauterine malnutrition, 142–143, 144

Valine, and very-low-birth-weight infants, 196, 198
Vasculitis, pulmonary, 172
Very-low-birth-weight infants, and parenteral nutrition, 191–204, 205–207
  amino acid concentration, 196–198
  amino acid intake, optimal, 199
  amino acid metabolism, 191–196
  energy requirements, 199–201
  mineral requirements, 201
  nitrogen requirement, 191
Villi morphogenesis, and intestinal development, 6–7
Villous absorptive cells, and intestinal development, 18–22
Villous atrophy, and crypt hyperplasia, 72
Villous cell differentiation, and intestinal development, 13–22
  M cells, 14–18
  Tuft cells, 13–14
  villous absorptive cells, 18–22

Weaning foods, introduction of, 215–221, 222
  formula feeding in early infancy, 216–220
  solids and semisolids, 220–221
Weight gain, and intrauterine malnutrition, 138

X-rays, and necrotizing enterocolitis, 110–111
Xylose tests, 99–100